Advanced Practice Nursing

D1317115

Kathryn A. Blair, PhD, FNP-BC, FAANP, is nurse practitioner option coordinator and professor at Beth El College of Nursing and Health Sciences, University of Colorado at Colorado Springs. Her academic experience spans more than three decades. Dr. Blair has more than 25 years of experience in family medicine and most recently began practicing in allergy and immunology. Dr. Blair remains active in various state and national professional organizations.

Michaelene P. Jansen, PhD, RN-C, FNP-C, GNP-BC, FAANP, is a family and gerontological nurse practitioner at Essentia Health Ashland Clinic in Ashland, Wisconsin. She is also professor emeritus of nursing, College of Nursing and Health Sciences, University of Wisconsin–Eau Claire. Her professional nursing experiences include critical care and trauma. She has coedited four editions of *Advanced Practice Nursing, Core Concepts for Professional Role Development* and edited *Pain Management of the Older Adult* (Springer Publishing).

Advanced Practice Nursing

Core Concepts for Professional Role Development

Fifth Edition

Kathryn A. Blair, PhD, FNP-BC, FAANP
Michaelene P. Jansen, PhD, RN-C, FNP-C, GNP-BC, FAANP

Editors

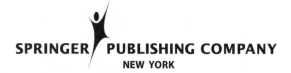

SPRINGER PUBLISHING COMPANY
NEW YORK

Springer Publishing Company, LLC
11 West 42nd Street
New York, NY 10036
www.springerpub.com

Acquisitions Editor: Margaret Zuccarini
Production Editor: Kris Parrish
Composition: GW Tech. Pvt. Ltd.

ISBN: 978-0-8261-7251-8
e-book ISBN: 978-0-8261-7252-5
Instructor's Manual ISBN: 978-0-8261-9434-3
PowerPoint Slides ISBN: 978-0-8261-9433-6

Instructor's Materials: Instructors may request supplements by emailing textbook@springerpub.com

16 17 18/ 5 4

The author and the publisher of this Work have made every effort to use sources believed to be reliable to provide information that is accurate and compatible with the standards generally accepted at the time of publication. The author and publisher shall not be liable for any special, consequential, or exemplary damages resulting, in whole or in part, from the readers' use of, or reliance on, the information contained in this book. The publisher has no responsibility for the persistence or accuracy of URLs for external or third-party Internet websites referred to in this publication and does not guarantee that any content on such websites is, or will remain, accurate or appropriate.

Library of Congress Cataloging-in-Publication Data
Advanced practice nursing (Jansen)
   Advanced practice nursing : core concepts for professional role development / Kathryn A. Blair, Michaelene P. Jansen, editors.—Fifth edition.
      p. ; cm.
   Includes bibliographical references and index.
   ISBN 978-0-8261-7251-8—ISBN 978-0-8261-7252-5 (e-book)
   I. Blair, Kathryn A., editor. II. Jansen, Michaelene P., editor. III. Title.
   [DNLM: 1. Advanced Practice Nursing. 2. Nurse's Role. WY 128]
   RT82.8
   610.7306'92--dc23
                            2014048132

Special discounts on bulk quantities of our books are available to corporations, professional associations, pharmaceutical companies, health care organizations, and other qualifying groups. If you are interested in a custom book, including chapters from more than one of our titles, we can provide that service as well.

For details, please contact:
Special Sales Department, Springer Publishing Company, LLC
11 West 42nd Street, 15th Floor, New York, NY 10036-8002
Phone: 877-687-7476 or 212-431-4370; Fax: 212-941-7842
E-mail: sales@springerpub.com

Printed in the United States of America by Bradford & Bigelow.

CONTENTS

PART III: TRANSITIONS TO THE ADVANCED PRACTICE ROLE

CONTRIBUTORS

Melissa Avery, PhD, RN, CNM, FACNM, FAAN
Professor and Chair
School of Nursing
University of Minnesota
Minneapolis, Minnesota

Beverley Bird, MPH, MSN, B.AppSci, RN, MCHN, FACN
Lecturer (Adjunct)
Faculty of Medicine, Nursing, and Health Sciences
Monash University, Clayton Campus
Clayton, Victoria, Australia

Kathryn A. Blair, PhD, FNP-BC, FAANP
Professor, Family Nurse Practitioner Program Coordinator
Beth El College of Nursing and Health Sciences
University of Colorado–Colorado Springs
Colorado Springs, Colorado

Vicki J. Brownrigg, PhD, FNP
Assistant Professor
Beth El College of Nursing and Health Sciences
University of Colorado–Colorado Springs
Colorado Springs, Colorado

Evelyn G. Duffy, DNP, AGPCNP-BC, FAANP
Associate Professor in the School of Nursing
Associate Director of the University Center on Aging and Health
Francis Payne Bolton School of Nursing
Case Western Reserve University
Cleveland, Ohio

Karen S. Feldt, PhD, GNP-BC
Clinical Educator
Matrix Medical Network
Pownal, Vermont

Cheri Friedrich, DNP, RN, CNP
Clinical Assistant Professor
School of Nursing
University of Minnesota
Minneapolis, Minnesota

Gene Harkless, DNSc, APRN, FAANP, CNL
Associate Professor of Nursing, Chair of Department of Nursing
College of Health and Human Services
University of New Hampshire
Durham, New Hampshire

Michaelene P. Jansen, PhD, RN-C, FNP-C, GNP-BC, FAANP
Family and Gerontological Nurse Practitioner
Essentia Health Ashland Clinic
Professor Emeritus
University of Wisconsin
Eau Claire, Wisconsin

Gail B. Katz, DNP, RN, CNS
Assistant Professor
Beth El College of Nursing and Health Sciences
University of Colorado
Colorado Springs, Colorado

Janet Wessel Krejci, PhD, RN, NEA-BC
Interim Vice President for Academic Affairs and Provost
Illinois State University
Normal, Illinois

Linda L. Lindeke, PhD, RN, CNP, FAAN
Associate Professor
School of Nursing
University of Minnesota
Minneapolis, Minnesota

Catherine G. Ling, PhD, FNP-BC, FAANP
Daniel K. Inouye Graduate School of Nursing
Uniformed Services University
Bethesda, Maryland

Shelly Malin, PhD, RN
Advocate BroMenn Endowed Professor
Illinois State University, Mennonite College of Nursing
Normal, Illinois

Patricia Maybee, EdD, FNP-BC, NP-C, FAANP
Family Nurse Practitioner
Primary Care Department
Gila River Health Care
Sacaton, Arizona

Lorna L. Schumann, PhD, NP-C, ACNP-BC, ACHS-BC, CCRN-R, FAANP
American Academy of Nurse Practitioner Certification Program
Austin, Texas

Rhonda D. Squires, PhD, APRN-BC, FNP
Assistant Professor, Master's/DNP FNP Programs Coordinator
School of Nursing
University of Northern Colorado
Greeley, Colorado

Carole G. Traylor, DNP, RN, CPNP, AE-C
Assistant Professor
Beth El College of Nursing and Health Sciences
University of Colorado
Colorado Springs, Colorado

Shirley E. Van Zandt, MS, MPH, CRNP
Clinical Assistant Professor
School of Nursing
Boise State University
Boise, Idaho

Kathy J. Wheeler, PhD, APRN-FNP, NP-C, FAANP
Assistant Professor
School of Nursing
University of Kentucky
Lexington, Kentucky

Kathryn W. White, DNP, RN, CRNA
Clinical Associate Professor, Program Director and Coordinator
Nurse Anesthesia Specialty
School of Nursing
University of Minnesota
Minneapolis, Minnesota

Patricia A. White, PhD, ANP-BC
Professor of Practice
Director of the DNP Program
Simmons School of Nursing and Health Sciences
Boston, Massachusetts

Jana Gail Zwilling, MSN, FNP-C
Clinical Instructor
College of Nursing and Professional Disciplines
University of North Dakota
Grand Forks, North Dakota

PREFACE

The fifth edition of *Advanced Practice Nursing: Core Concepts for Professional Role Development* carries on the tradition of the previous four editions: updating current trends in practice; reviewing the origins, standards, and competencies of the advanced practice registered nurses (APRNs) in the United States; discussing APRN roles within a nursing context; identifying organizational roles for APRNs; and examining ethics in guiding APRN clinical decision making. Previous editions have focused primarily on nurse practitioners, whereas this edition examines and addresses all four APRN roles. As with similar texts, this edition offers a synopsis of translating research into practice with emphasis on implementing evidence-based practice and how to stay up to date with current research. Useful tools in advanced clinical decision making, practice issues (regulation, certification prescriptive authority, credentialing, and liability), and the exploration of employment opportunities and strategies are reviewed. Content assisting the novice APRN in developing entrepreneur models of care and in transitioning from a professional nursing role to an advanced practice role is included. As advanced practice nursing continues to evolve and expand, new material addressing the upcoming challenges for APRNs has been incorporated into this edition.

For decades the mantra in health care has been the need for collaborative interprofessional teams (IPTs). Chapter 5 explores the role of the APRN in the team's formation and leadership. This chapter discusses the composition of IPTs that will include a variety of health care providers, but in some cases, community leaders, corporate chief executive officers (CEOs), technology experts, and others as well. The author challenges APRNs to assume more prominent leadership roles in health care delivery systems.

With the movement toward expanding the APRN role in collaborative IPT, new skills and understanding of leadership competencies are needed. These concepts are explored in Chapter 7. This revised chapter emphasizes the importance of leadership competencies necessary for the delivery of quality care, evidence-based practice, and patient safety. Different leadership development models and curricula related to leadership in master's and doctorate of nursing practice (DNP) programs are considered.

Health issues have become global, as evidenced by recent infectious disease outbreaks and by the prominence of organizations such as the World Health Organization, Doctors Without Borders, Sigma Theta Tau International Nursing Society, and International Council of Nursing. The demand for APRNs is extending beyond the borders of the United States. A new chapter, Chapter 6, describes the multifaceted roles of APRNs internationally. As the advanced practice role emerges and evolves internationally, new opportunities for APRNs have surfaced. Roles such as (a) developing programs of study for U.S. students, (b) instituting cross-cultural exchange programs, (c) providing direct patient care in the form of mission trips, (d) assisting in the design and evaluation of educational programs for the advanced nursing practice role in developing countries, (e) identifying research partnerships and conducting research, and (f) influencing policies that improve health are presented.

The recent change in health care, the Patient Protection and Affordable Care Act (ACA), has placed APRNs on the front lines of health care reform. This legislation has resulted in an increased demand for APRNs to meet the health care needs of those previously uninsured or underinsured. Several reports by the Institute of Medicine (IOM) have argued that the time is right for all nurses to function to their full capacity and that the barriers for advanced practice nursing need to be removed. Chapter 9 argues this is the "golden age" for APRNs. This chapter reviews the critical events that have sculpted the APRN policy role in influencing and creating legislation and discusses how to become an engaged citizen in directing change.

Chapter 14 has been revised and expanded and discusses health information technology (HIT) competencies for nurses and APRNs, as well as common information management resources that APRNs are using or likely to encounter in the near future. The chapter explores meaningful use as described in Health Information Technology for Economic and Clinical Health legislation and includes a discussion of select HIT controversies and failures.

All APRNs are scholars. APRNs should therefore be actively engaged in the scholarship of practice. Chapter 15 explores the multiple modalities that are incorporated into the scholarship of practice such as sharing tricks of the trade, completing quality improvement projects, collaborating with nursing researchers, and being an active member in professional organizations. The chapter highlights the tools to disseminate knowledge, which is critical for the scholarship of practice.

Woven throughout the text is the evolution of nursing education for APRNs in the context of the DNP. The future of APRN education will be the DNP as the norm rather than as the exception. The DNP-educated APRN will be able to bring to the table a broader knowledge base of population-based health care, organizational systems, leadership skills, utilization of best practices or evidence-based practice, and meaningful use of electronic information systems.

Material to accompany this book's content for qualified instructors is available from Springer Publishing Company by e-mailing textbook @springerpub.com.

As with previous editions, this text equips the APRN student. This edition continues to share the tools for success in the multidimensional advanced practice role.

Kathryn A. Blair
Michaelene P. Jansen

PART I: FOUNDATIONS OF ADVANCED NURSING PRACTICE

Linda L. Lindeke, Melissa Avery, and Kathryn W. White 1

OVERVIEW OF ADVANCED PRACTICE REGISTERED NURSING

Advanced practice registered nurses (APRNs) are at the forefront of the rapidly changing health care system, filling myriad roles in organizations where they provide cost-effective, high-quality care. APRNs are found in virtually every area of the American health care system: clinics, hospitals, community health, government, administration, policy making boards, and private practice. In addition, APRNs have expanded practice into international and trans-global arenas. They serve the most economically disadvantaged as well as the elite. APRNs are deans, educators, consultants, researchers, policy experts, and, of course, outstanding clinicians.

Advanced practice registered nursing is an exciting career choice with many opportunities and challenges. The challenges are sometimes related to health care reform that is polarized and responsive to rapidly evolving political influences. Prospective payment systems, decreased hospital stays, health inequities, and spiraling costs are daily APRN practice realities. Technology produces amazing diagnostic and treatment results; genetic research is unraveling complex pathophysiology; and sophisticated "big data" electronic infrastructures change the way information is gathered, stored, analyzed, and shared. Innovative care models are common and include home health care programs, integrated or complementary modalities, and retail clinics. These and other trends result in a rapidly changing health care system, ready for the influence and influx of APRNs.

Graduate education prepares APRNs to be key players in these complex systems. Midrange nursing theories provide strong conceptual foundations for APRN practice and nurse scholars. Nursing research uncovers scientific evidence for best practice, and research utilization skills enable APRNs to bring fresh ideas and proven interventions to health care consumers.

Complex reimbursement policies and mechanisms require that APRNs navigate reimbursement, management, and health policy regulations. Although APRNs were traditionally educated to provide advanced nursing care in specific clinics or hospital units, they now often work across system boundaries as they follow their patients through transitions of care. For example, APRNs care for patients in outpatient clinics, admit them to the hospital, assist in coordinating discharge plans, and collaborate with long-term care organizations, perhaps working with public health agencies to return their patients to their home communities. These new cross-system care models result in regulatory complexity for APRNs. They must be able to legally provide care across systems. Working across state lines results in even more issues because each state has its own laws and rules. In addition, each health care organization can interpret state and federal laws and regulations in its own professional staff policies. Organizations can be more restrictive than laws, but they cannot be less restrictive. Given considerable variations among practice environments, APRNs must be experts and proactive in the business and regulatory policies and processes. Staying current is best accomplished by participation in role-specific APRN professional organizations.

ADVANCED PRACTICE REGISTERED NURSING: THEN AND NOW

Advanced specialization of nurses beyond their formal entry-level education has a long and proud history of many innovative risk takers and key events. To capture that history and unify the advanced nursing specialists, the term *advanced practice registered nurse* (APRN) became the common umbrella term used to designate four specialty roles of nurses with formal postbaccalaureate preparation: certified nurse-midwives (CNMs), certified registered nurse anesthetists (CRNAs), nurse practitioners (NPs), and clinical nurse specialists (CNSs).

Nurse anesthetists and nurse-midwives organized nearly a century ago and were the first APRNs to develop national standards for educational programs, professional organizations, and certification. NPs and CNSs standardized their preparation, certification, and licensing incrementally in recent decades. Various scholars and professional organizations have documented the unique history of each APRN role.

A number of factors led nursing leaders to delineate these four APRN roles. A critical factor was obtaining legal status to be directly reimbursed for their nursing services, a gradual process first achieved by nurse-midwives more than 30 years ago and subsequently expanded through federal and state legislation for the other three roles. Reimbursement laws and regulations require that nursing be able to specify the qualifications of these reimbursable APRNs, which contributed to increased standardization of titling, education, and national certification.

Public protection was another factor that led to the delineation of the APRN roles. State boards of nursing are mandated by state legislatures to safeguard the public from unsafe practice, and over time, all states have implemented laws and regulations to ensure that nurses in the four roles have specific expertise and skills. Some states have accomplished this through a second-level licensure process. In other states, APRNs are regulated through title protection and scope of practice laws. In 2008, APRNs reached an agreement defining a desired national model of regulation for the United States. This agreement, the *Consensus Model for APRN Regulation: Licensure, Accreditation, Certification, and Education,* is known as the LACE model (APRN Consensus Work Group & National Council of State Boards of Nursing APRN Advisory Committee, 2008). By mid-2014, the LACE model had been enacted in 19 states through complex legislative initiatives (Kopanos, 2014). Most other states' APRN groups are working toward amending state nurse practice laws by adopting the LACE model of regulation.

A final factor influencing APRN standardization has been the adoption of national APRN curricular guidelines and program standards. These standards were developed by many specialty organizations and brought through negotiations to consensus by nursing organizations such as the American Association of Colleges of Nursing (AACN), the American Nurses Association (ANA), and the National Organization of Nurse Practitioner Faculties (NONPF). APRN educational standards have been endorsed by numerous nursing specialty organizations in the past decade and are used for national program accreditation.

Nursing's Scope and Standards of Practice (ANA, 2010) defines APRNs as having advanced specialized clinical knowledge and skills through master's or doctoral education that prepares them for specialization, expansion, and advancement of practice. Specialization is concentrating or limiting one's focus to part of the whole field of nursing. Expansion refers to the acquisition of new practice knowledge and skills, including knowledge and skills legitimizing role autonomy within areas of practice that overlap traditional boundaries of medical practice. Advancement involves both specialization and expansion and is characterized by the integration of theoretical, research-based, and practical knowledge that occurs as part of graduate education in nursing. This APRN definition, which is regulated by state and federal laws, does not include nurses with advanced preparation for administration, education, public health or research; those roles are considered "advanced nursing practice" and are not regulated, a fine but important legal distinction.

APRNs are educated within master's or doctoral nursing programs. Although CNSs have always required master's nursing degrees, in the past nurse-midwives, nurse anesthetists, and NPs were not all prepared in graduate nursing programs. Now, however, NPs must receive their education in graduate master's or clinical doctoral programs in nursing. CRNAs are prepared in graduate programs, although the master's degree does not necessarily have to be in nursing. Although the majority of CNMs are prepared in graduate nursing programs, some nurse-midwifery programs are located in health-related professional schools.

Because of their unique historical underpinnings, members of each APRN category have strong allegiance to their titles and their professional organizations. At times, this allegiance has been a barrier to the development of consistent language regarding APRN roles because each group has developed its own education, history, and titles. However, significant progress continues to be made in identifying commonalities.

Research-based practice (sometimes called evidence-based practice) is a key characteristic of APRN practice. Clinical doctoral nursing programs emphasize and expand the utilization of evidence-based practice, especially in terms of preparing APRNs to be organizational change agents.

Through a consensus-building process, the AACN formulated curricular elements for graduate APRN education (AACN, 2011), specifying the content of the graduate core curriculum and the advanced practice nursing core curriculum in master's programs (Exhibit 1.1). Practice doctoral nursing programs are based on the *Essentials of Doctoral Nursing Education for Advanced Practice Nurses* (AACN, 2006; Exhibit 1.2). The role-specific professional nursing organizations have further delineated specialized core competencies; documents are readily available on their websites and are frequently updated.

The core clinical content requires advanced health and physical assessment, advanced physiology and pathology, and advanced pharmacology (often referred to as the three Ps). These courses must be taught across the life span, with additional specific content required for students in each specialty area. For example, nurse-midwifery students need additional content on assessment of pregnant women and newborn infants, nurse anesthetist students require extensive content on anesthetic agents, and psychiatric/mental health students need additional content on antipsychotic medications.

Exhibit 1.1 ESSENTIAL ELEMENTS OF MASTER'S CURRICULUM FOR ADVANCED PRACTICE NURSING

    I. Background for Practice From Sciences and Humanities
    II. Organizational and Systems Leadership
    III. Quality Improvement and Safety
    IV. Translating and Integrating Scholarship Into Practice
    V. Informatics and Healthcare Technologies
    VI. Health Policy and Advocacy
    VII. Interprofessional Collaboration for Improving Patient and Population Health Outcomes
    VIII. Clinical Prevention and Population Health for Improving Health
    IX. Master's-Level Nursing Practice

Source: American Association of Colleges of Nursing (2011).

Exhibit 1.2 ESSENTIALS OF DOCTORAL EDUCATION AND COMPETENCIES FOR
ADVANCED NURSING PRACTICE

    I. Scientific Underpinnings for Practice
    II. Organizational and Systems Leadership for Quality Improvement
and Systems Thinking
    III. Clinical Scholarship and Analytical Methods for Evidence-Based
Practice
    IV. Information Systems/Technology and Patient Care Technology for
the Improvement and Transformation of Health Care
    V. Health Care Policy for Advocacy in Health Care
    VI. Interprofessional Collaboration for Improving Patient and
Population Health Outcomes
    VII. Clinical Prevention and Population Health for Improving the
Nation's Health
    VIII. Advanced Practice Nursing

Source: American Association of Colleges of Nursing (2006).

There are also professional ethics standards for APRNs. In addition to issues related to confidentiality and relationships, APRNs must provide support to patients and families in making ethical decisions related to treatment options (ANA, 2013). Although ethical issues appear to be more prominent in tertiary care settings, issues such as abuse and neglect are present in all settings. APRNs are frequently called on to work with professional colleagues, patients, and families to resolve ethical dilemmas.

All APRNs collaborate with other health professionals. Collaboration is a standard of ARPN care and is also referenced in state and federal law. Functioning on interdisciplinary teams or working in teams with other health professionals, APRNs need to clearly identify their unique contributions to patient outcomes. APRNs also collaborate with patients and their families in planning care and making decisions about the most acceptable treatments.

One emerging area of scholarship emphasizes APRN care outcomes (Kapu & Kleinpell, 2012), especially essential in this era of health care reform. A new term is *comparative effectiveness research* (CER), promoted by the Agency for Healthcare Research and Quality (AHRQ) and the Institute of Medicine (IOM). Given their history of cost-effectiveness, good patient satisfaction, and high-quality outcomes, APRNs should fare well in CER studies focused on APRN care models and outcomes. A critical review of relevant APRN outcomes research (Newhouse et al., 2011) is a milestone document that summarizes nursing effectiveness and APRN-sensitive indicators of care quality.

APRNs and Doctoral Education

The previous description of content in APRN education and professional standards demonstrates the complexity and depth of APRN preparation and practice. Some nurse leaders question whether APRNs can be fully prepared for their scope of practice in 2-year master's programs. This has prompted discussion of the feasibility of doctoral preparation being required for APRN practice (Edwardson, 2004).

Doctoral APRN education existed in nursing doctorate (ND) programs as early as the mid-1980s at Rush University, Case Western Reserve University, and the University of Colorado, all of which awarded ND degrees to students completing NP programs. These ND programs have now discontinued the ND degrees; they have been replaced by doctorate of nursing practice (DNP) degrees. The DNP is a new degree first advocated by the AACN and the NONPF. In October 2004, the nation's nursing deans attending AACN passed a resolution to move APRN education to a practice doctorate level by 2015. Although a recommendation rather than a mandate, much progress has been made in increasing the number of NPs with doctoral degrees in the past decade. More than 240 DNP programs were under way nationwide by early 2014 (AACN, 2014).

There are pros and cons related to the DNP degree. The increased time and cost for students is balanced by the increase in knowledge, skill, and prestige that this doctoral degree confers. Pharmacy, audiology, physical therapy, and psychology have doctoral education as their entry to practice. The practice community has quite quickly embraced the DNP preparation; however, whether employers will compensate DNP graduates at levels commensurate with their education is undecided. Physician reactions to the nursing practice doctorate has been mixed; for example, several states have implemented legislation that reserves the term *doctor* for physicians in clinical arenas. A joint dialogue statement eloquently points out that "Graduate educational programs in colleges and universities in the United States confer academic degrees, which permit graduates to be called 'doctor.' No one discipline owns the title 'doctor'" (Nurse Practitioner Roundtable, 2008). The DNP degree continues to be debated; regardless, the new degree is propelling APRN roles forward with new knowledge and abilities at a time when health care reform is at the forefront of the national conversation. Understanding each of the roles is essential.

Nurse Practitioners

NPs are registered nurses with master's or doctoral nursing preparation who perform comprehensive assessments, promote health, and treat and prevent illness and injury. In doing so they diagnose, develop differential diagnoses, and order and interpret diagnostic tests. They prescribe pharmacologic and nonpharmacologic treatments while providing care in primary, acute, and long-term care settings. NPs specialize in certain populations of patients and in areas such as family, adult/geriatric, pediatric, and psychiatric/mental health. NPs practice autonomously and in collaboration with other health care professionals as researchers, consultants, and patient advocates.

The role first developed in primary care settings. However, NPs now function in tertiary care, and specific competencies and examinations have been developed for acute-care NPs (NONPF, 2004). Health promotion and health maintenance are emphasized in all the ARPN nursing standards. Nurses have traditionally emphasized health promotion activities as being a key characteristic of the professional practice of nursing. Health promotion, whether it is for persons who have no specific illness or for persons who have chronic health problems, is critical in our current society. Implementation of care that focuses on health promotion also has been shown to be cost effective (Mundinger et al., 2000; Safriet, 1998). Horrocks, Anderson, and Salisbury (2002) noted that NPs offered more advice on self-care and management than did physicians, and they seemed to identify physical abnormalities more frequently. However, there was no difference in patient health outcomes between the NP- and physician-managed patient groups.

The NP movement began at the University of Colorado; Loretta Ford, PhD, RN, and Henry Silver, MD, both full professors, collaborated to launch a postbaccalaureate program to prepare nurses for expanded roles in the care of children and their families. Professors Ford and Silver (Ford, 1979) recognized that nurses had the ability to assess children's health status and define appropriate nursing actions. The purpose of the first NP demonstration project was to implement new roles to improve the safety, efficacy, and quality of health care for children and families (Ford, 1979). Although the project's initial focus was on children and families, Ford noted that she was confident that nurses could be educated to meet the health needs of community-dwelling persons across the life span. Nurses in the Colorado program received 4 months of intensive didactic education in which assessment skills and growth and development were emphasized. The nurses then completed a 20-month precepted clinical rotation in a community-based setting.

Following Colorado's lead, many schools initiated educational programs, admitting nurses with varying levels of educational preparation. The growth of the NP movement was facilitated by many studies through the years, such as those summarized in a meta-analysis by Brown and Grimes (1995). Over the years, NPs have demonstrated that they safely provide high-quality health care, and the NP role has expanded into many new practice areas (Martin, 2000; Mundinger et al., 2000; Newhouse et al., 2011). Although Dr. Ford's goal initially was to prepare NPs within master's programs, societal demand for NPs led to a proliferation of postbaccalaureate continuing education programs rather than graduate education (Ford, 1979, 2005). Federal funding for NP programs also prompted the initiation of numerous postbaccalaureate and graduate NP programs. The length of these early NP programs varied from a few weeks to 2 years, with many certificate programs being 9 to 12 months in length.

The proliferation of postbaccalaureate programs rather than graduate programs for the education of NPs was partially attributable to the resistance of graduate nursing programs to recognize NPs as being a legitimate part of nursing. A number of nursing leaders termed NPs "physician extenders" and did not view NP practice as "nursing." This lack of enthusiasm for NP education exhibited by numerous nursing leaders in the 1960s and 1970s may also have been fostered by the fact that the NP movement grew out of a collaborative nurse–physician effort rather than being solely initiated by nurses. The early NP curricula were viewed as being based on the medical model rather than a nursing framework, although that was not the focus of Dr. Ford's original NP curriculum, which emphasized child development and health promotion (Ford, 1979).

The NP domains and competencies were based on the work by Brykczynski (1989), Benner (1984), and Fenton (1985). The seven domains are (a) management of client health/illness status, (b) NP–patient relationship, (c) teaching/coaching function, (d) professional role, (e) management and negotiation of health care delivery systems, (f) monitor and ensure the quality of health care practice, and (g) culturally sensitive care (NONPF, 2006). Specific competencies are described for each domain. These domains are detailed and encompassing, indicating that APRN practice requires a broad range of knowledge and expertise. Recently, NONPF (2012) revised the domains for all NP programs and developed nine core competencies: scientific foundation, leadership, quality, practice inquiry, technology and information literacy, policy, health delivery system, ethics, and independent practice. NPs are prepared in a multitude of specialties, including acute care, adult health, family health, gerontology, pediatrics, psychiatry, neonatology, and women's health. Population-specific competencies have been elaborated and defined (NONPF, 2013).

The ANA, along with other organizations, has developed many types of practice standards, some broadly inclusive and others specialty focused (ANA, National Association of Pediatric Nurse Practitioners [NAPNAP], & Society of Pediatric Nurses [SPN], 2010). For example, the ANA, NAPNAP, and SPN created a joint document that outlines pediatric nursing competencies at both basic and advanced practice levels.

The American Academy of Nurse Practitioners (AANP, 2013) estimated that there were more than 190,000 NPs in the United States in 2013, 95% of whom were prepared with graduate degrees and 97% with national certification in their NP specialties. Many NPs assume positions that combine clinical practice with employment as educators, administrators, and policy makers or choose other employment.

After completing graduate education, NPs are eligible to sit for national certification examinations in their specialty areas. Certification is a mechanism for the nursing profession to attest to the entry-to-practice knowledge of NPs. The certification requirement has been adopted by third-party payers such as the Centers for Medicare & Medicaid Services (CMS) and by most state boards of nursing as a standard that assists in protecting the public from unsafe providers. Certification examinations are offered by a variety of bodies: the American Nurses Credentialing Center (ANCC), the AANP, the Pediatric Nursing Certification Board (PNCB), the American Association of Critical Care Nurses (AACCN), and the National Certification Corporation (NCC) for the obstetric, gynecologic, and neonatal specialties.

Changes in reimbursement laws, regulations, and policies that allow for direct reimbursement of NPs, the rapid increase in managed care as a mechanism to control health care costs, and the growing recognition of the significant contributions of NPs to positive patient outcomes have resulted in a rapid increase in the number of NP programs, particularly DNP programs. The American Association of Nurse Practitioners (AANP, 2013) estimated that 14,000 new NPs graduated in 2011–2012. APRNs who are savvy about ascertaining the gaps in health care and designing roles for themselves that are not merely physician-replacement roles are likely to be very successful in obtaining satisfactory employment.

Scope of practice is regulated by state laws and describes the legal boundaries of health professional practice. NPs practicing outside the designated scope of practice risk legal sanctions and potential liability (Klein, 2005). Changes in scope of practice reflect the dynamic evolution of NP roles. However, great variability exists regarding the regulation of acute and primary care NPs by individual states.

Relative to CNMs and CRNAs, NPs have a relatively short history in the health care delivery system. However, in this short period of time they have gained the respect of many health professionals and of their patients (Scherer, Bruce, & Runkawatt, 2007). Recently, television and lay publications have featured NPs and the significant contributions they are making to improving health. New areas of practice and settings for NPs continue to arise. In many instances, NPs have succeeded in caring for persons in rural areas, in inner cities, and for other vulnerable groups. NPs have established themselves as an integral part of the health care system.

Nurse-Midwives

Nurse-midwives are unique among APRNs because they are educated in two different professions. Midwifery is a profession in its own right; nursing is not a prerequisite to midwifery in many countries around the world. The American College of Nurse-Midwives (ACNM, 2004a) defines CNMs as individuals educated in the two disciplines of midwifery and nursing who complete a graduate degree program accredited by the Accreditation Commission for Midwifery Education (ACME) and pass the national certification examination of the American Midwifery Certification Board (AMCB). According to the ACNM (2004a), midwifery as practiced by CNMs and certified midwives (CMs)

> encompasses a full range of primary health care services for women from adolescence beyond menopause. These services include the independent provision of primary care, gynecologic and family planning services, preconception care, care during pregnancy, childbirth and the postpartum period, care of the normal newborn during the

first 28 days of life, and treatment of male partners for sexually transmitted infections. Midwives provide initial and ongoing comprehensive assessment, diagnosis and treatment. They conduct physical examinations; prescribe medications including controlled substances and contraceptive methods; admit, manage and discharge patients; order and interpret laboratory and diagnostic tests and order the use of medical devices. Midwifery care also includes health promotion, disease prevention, and individualized wellness education and counseling. These services are provided in partnership with women and families in diverse settings such as ambulatory care clinics, private offices, community and public health systems, homes, hospitals and birth centers. (p. 1)

Although the focus of midwifery care has historically been prenatal care and managing labor and birth, nurse-midwives are primary care providers for essentially healthy women. Nurse-midwives strongly believe in supporting natural life processes and not using medical interventions unless there is a clear need. This belief and others are reflected in the 2004 ACNM (2004b, p. 1) philosophy statement, which states that every person has a right to:

- Equitable, ethical, accessible, quality health care that promotes healing and health
- Health care that respects human dignity, individuality, and diversity among groups
- Complete and accurate information to make informed health care decisions
- Self-determination and active participation in health care decisions
- Involvement of a woman's designated family members, to the extent desired, in all health care experiences

Midwives also believe in:

- Watchful waiting and nonintervention in normal processes
- Appropriate use of interventions and technology for current or potential health problems
- Consultation, collaboration, and referral with other members of the health care team as needed to provide optimal health care (ACNM, 2004b)

Midwifery is a very old profession, mentioned in the Bible. The practice of midwifery declined in the 18th and 19th centuries, and obstetrics developed as a medical specialty. In 1925, Mary Breckinridge established the Frontier Nursing Service (FNS) in Kentucky and was the first nurse to practice as a nurse-midwife in the United States. She received her midwifery education in England and returned to the United States with other British nurse-midwives to set up a system of care similar to that which she had observed in Scotland. The FNS was begun to care for individuals who were without adequate health care. The nurse-midwives of the FNS provided maternal and infant care and effectively demonstrated quality care and significantly improved outcomes.

The first U.S. nurse-midwifery education program was started at the Maternity Center Association, Lobenstein Clinic, in New York City in 1932. The American College of Nurse-Midwives was incorporated in 1955. Nurse-midwifery practice grew slowly until the late 1960s and early 1970s, when the profession experienced increased acceptance and consumer demand increased for nurse-midwives and the kind of care they provided (Varney, 2015). There are more than 13,000 CNMs/CMs in the United States, and in 2012, they attended 313,846 births, or 7.9% of all births, 11.8% of vaginal births, and 30.4% of all out-of-hospital births in the United States (ACNM, 2014a). Nurse-midwives have direct third-party reimbursement and prescriptive authority in all 50 states (ACNM, 2014b).

In the 1970s, national accreditation of nurse-midwifery education programs and national certification of nurse-midwives was begun by ACNM. The ACME accreditation process is recognized by the U.S. Department of Education, and the certification process now conducted by the AMCB is recognized by the National Commission of Health Certifying Agencies.

The ACNM document, *Core Competencies for Basic Midwifery Practice* (ACNM, 2012), describes the skills and knowledge that are fundamental to the practice of a new graduate of an ACME-accredited education program. These competencies guide curricular development in midwifery programs and are used in the nationally recognized accreditation process. Competencies described in the document include professional responsibilities; the midwifery management process; and midwifery care of women, including primary care; preconception care; gynecologic care (including contraceptive methods); perimenopausal and postmenopausal care; prenatal, intrapartum, and postpartum care of the childbearing woman; and care of the newborn. Hallmarks of midwifery practice are also delineated.

Nurse-midwifery education began with certificate programs and has progressed to graduate education. There are presently 38 ACME-accredited programs in the United States. Most midwifery programs are in schools of nursing, but two are in university-based health-related professions schools. A direct-entry (nonnursing) route to midwifery education, using the same nationally recognized accreditation and certification standards, began in 1997 at the State University of New York (downstate campus). CM students are required to complete certain prerequisite health sciences courses, such as chemistry, biology, nutrition, and psychology, before beginning midwifery education. In addition, certain knowledge and skills common in nursing practice are required before beginning the midwifery clinical courses in the program (ACME, 2005). CMs are currently authorized to practice in five states (ACNM, 2014a). Certified professional midwives (CPMs), another category of direct-entry midwives who attend out-of-hospital births, are recognized in approximately half of the states and have a different scope of practice and regulation process than midwives who graduate from ACME-accredited programs.

Nurse-midwives in the United States have consistently demonstrated that their care results in excellent outcomes and client satisfaction among all women, including the large proportion of underserved, uninsured, low-income, minority, and otherwise vulnerable women for whom CNMs provide care. Births attended by CNMs and CMs occur primarily in hospitals; more than 98% of births in the United States occurred in hospitals in 2012, although the number of home and freestanding birth center births has been rising (MacDorman, Mathews, & Declercq, 2014). Past researchers have demonstrated fewer interventions, including lower caesarean birth rates, among CNM-attended births versus physician-attended births, as well as outcomes at least comparable to physician-attended births (Blanchette, 1995; MacDorman & Singh, 1998; Rosenblatt et al., 1997).

A systematic review and meta-analysis of midwifery care globally demonstrated that women receiving midwifery-led care experienced equivalent or better outcomes—including fewer episiotomies, less anesthesia use, reduced likelihood of preterm birth, and more spontaneous vaginal births—than those receiving other types of care (Sandall, Soltani, Gates, Shennan, & Devane, 2013). Another systematic review identified exclusively U.S.-based studies and found similar results, with equivalent or superior outcomes in initiating breastfeeding, operative and cesarean births, and perineal lacerations (Newhouse et al., 2011). From a policy perspective, midwifery care can be a cost-effective and sustainable approach to meeting society's women's health care needs (Renfew et al., 2014).

Over the nearly 90-year history of nurse-midwifery/midwifery in the United States, a strong base of support documented by research has been developed and is ongoing. The number of educational programs and practitioners has grown substantially. The passage of the Patient Protection and Affordable Care Act in 2010 resulted in a key provision sought by CNMs for nearly 20 years: the same reimbursement as physicians under Medicaid for providing the same service (Bradford, 2013). During this era of health care reform, as health care dollars continue to be carefully allocated and specific outcomes measured more closely, CNMs and certified midwives can be expected to play a more prominent role in providing quality primary health care to women.

Clinical Nurse Specialists

CNSs are leaders and experts in evidence-based nursing practice (National Association of Clinical Nurse Specialists [NACNS], 2014). They are registered professional nurses with graduate preparation earned at the master's or doctoral level. They may also be educated in a postmaster's program that prepares graduates to practice in specific specialty areas (Lyon, 2004; Lyon & Minarik, 2001). In 2000, 183 schools offered CNS master's programs, an increase from 147 programs in 1997 (Dayhoff & Lyon, 2001). The NACNS has developed curriculum recommendations for CNS education (NACNS, 2011) as well as competencies to reflect the *Essentials of Doctoral Education for Advanced Nursing Practice* (NACNS, n.d.). CNSs have traditionally worked in hospitals, but they now practice in many settings, including nursing homes, schools, home care, and hospice. NACNS's essential characteristics and essential core content for CNS programs are based on CNSs' spheres of influence: patients/clients and patients, nurses and nursing practice, and organizations/systems.

The CNS role has had a long history in the United States. The CNS role was developed after World War II. Before that time, specialization for nurses was in the functional areas of administration and education. Recognizing the need to have highly qualified nurses directly involved in patient care, the concept of clinical nurse specialists emerged. Reiter (1966) first used the term *nurse clinician* in 1943 to designate a specialist in nursing practice. The first master's program in a clinical nursing specialty was developed in 1954 by Hildegard E. Peplau at Rutgers University to prepare psychiatric clinical nurse specialists. That program launched the CNS role that has been an important player in the nursing profession and health care arena ever since, although the role has not been without controversy. Health care restructuring and cost-cutting initiatives in the 1980s and 1990s resulted in a loss of CNS positions in the United States. However, after increasingly frequent reports of adverse events in hospital settings in the 1990s (IOM, 1999; IOM Committee on the Quality of Health Care in America, 2001), it became apparent that CNSs were critical to obtaining quality patient outcomes (Clark, 2001; Heitkemper & Bond, 2004), with the result that CNSs are again seen as valuable professionals in many U.S. health care systems.

As with the NP movement, the availability of federal funds for graduate nursing education programs and the Professional Traineeship Program through Health Resources and Services Administration (HRSA) that provides stipends for students have played a role in the development of many graduate CNS programs.

The development and use of complex health care technology in the management of patients in hospitals and intricate surgical procedures has resulted in increasing acuity and complexity of patient care delivery. Thus, there is a need for nurses with advanced knowledge and expertise to be integrally involved in working with staff to assess, plan, implement, and evaluate care for these patients. Many hospitals have used CNSs as care coordinators and case managers in which they coordinate the care of patients with acute or chronic illnesses during their hospital stays and prepare them for discharge to their homes or other care facilities. CNSs have also been used as discharge planners working with staff to plan posthospital care for patients who have complex health problems (Naylor et al., 1994; Neidlinger, Scroggins, & Kennedy, 1987). Their importance in care coordination over the care continuum is only now being lauded, exemplified in the work of Naylor and colleagues, who reported that use of gerontologic CNSs as discharge planners resulted in fewer readmissions of elderly cardiac patients.

Since its inception, the CNS role has suffered from role ambiguity (Rasch & Frauman, 1996; Redekopp, 1997). Although the initial vision was for CNSs to be integrally involved in patient care for a specific patient population, they have assumed many other roles, such as staff and patient educators, consultants, supervisors, project directors, and more recently, case managers. Redekopp noted that it is difficult for CNSs to precisely describe their roles to others because their roles are continually evolving to meet the health needs of a changing patient population in an ever-changing health care system. Role ambiguity has made it difficult to measure the impact that CNSs have on patient outcomes. Thus, when budgetary crises have occurred in hospitals, CNSs have frequently had to advocate strongly to maintain their positions because outcome data to support the positive impact of their practice have either not been readily available or simply did not exist.

There are numerous CNS specialties and subspecialties: psychiatric/ mental health nursing, adult health, gerontology, oncology, pediatrics, cardiovascular, neuroscience, rehabilitation, pulmonary, renal, diabetes, and palliative care, to name a few. Numerous organizations offer certification examinations for CNSs. However, some organizations do not specify that master's degrees are required for certification in the specialty, causing confusion regarding the regulation and title of clinical nurse specialist. In the past, many CNSs have not sought third-party reimbursement, so they have not taken specialty CNS certification examinations. With changes in state nursing practice acts and the increase in third-party payment and prescriptive privileges for APRNs, the number of certified CNSs is now increasing. Controversy regarding CNS certification continues, however, because the examinations are not available in the many specialties that CNSs perform. Exemptions from state laws and regulations for CNSs have been provided by some states because of this lack of certification. To address this need, a core CNS certification examination is under development by the ANCC.

In the late 1980s and early 1990s, many discussions and debates took place around the merging of the CNS and NP roles (Page & Arena, 1994). Several studies were conducted comparing the knowledge and skills of these two advanced practice roles (Elder & Bullough, 1990; Fenton & Brykczynski, 1993; Forbes, Rafson, Spross, & Kozlowski, 1990; Lindeke, Canedy, & Kay, 1996). Research indicated that there were many similarities in the educational preparation of these two groups of APRNs. Many CNSs viewed the proposed merger as the demise of the CNS role. NPs were concerned that they would need to abandon the title of NP, a title that had become familiar to many patients and health professionals. A new organization, the NACNS, was formed to assist CNSs and to provide a vehicle to publicize the many contributions that CNSs have made and continue to make in providing quality patient care. The CNS role today is a dynamic and needed advanced practice nursing role, and many in the nursing profession anticipate that it will continue to exist for years to come.

Certified Registered Nurse Anesthetists

Nurse anesthesia practice traces its origins to the inception of surgical anesthesia, a major innovation that allowed for the development of surgery as a means of treatment for disease. Anesthesia in the late 1800s was hazardous and crude. There was not a good understanding of the pharmacologic and physiologic effects of anesthetic drugs, primarily diethyl ether and chloroform. These anesthetics were often delivered in a "careless manner" by a surgical resident fresh out of medical school who had little or no training in the effects of the anesthetic (Bankert, 1989, p. 22). This led to disastrous results for patients. Thus, some surgeons turned to religious Hospital Sisters who would devote their entire attention to the well-being of the patient during the delivery of the anesthetic. One of the Hospital Sisters, Sister Mary Bernard, was the first identified nurse that delivered anesthesia at St. Vincent's Hospital in Erie Pennsylvania in 1877 (Bankert, 1989).

The practice of utilizing nurses to deliver anesthesia spread rapidly through the Catholic and secular hospitals of the late 1800s and early 1900s. In 1912, a formal program of training in the delivery of anesthesia for nurses was developed in Springfield, Illinois, by Mother Magdalene Wiedlocher of the Third Order of the Hospital Sisters of St. Frances. This order of Hospital Sisters went on to establish St. Mary's Hospital in Rochester, Minnesota, that we now know as the origin of the Mayo Hospitals. These nurse anesthetists at St. Mary's Hospital became known as experts in the delivery of anesthesia who devoted their full attention and skill to the well-being of the patient receiving anesthesia. One nurse anesthetist in particular, Alice Magaw, stood out as an example of the diligent care delivered by nurse anesthetists. In addition to skillfully delivering anesthetics, Magaw recorded her work and published it in respected medical journals of the time. One such paper published in 1906 documented 14,000 anesthetics at St. Mary's Hospital "without a death directly attributable to anesthesia" (Bankert, 1989, p. 31). Magaw's legacy is honored in the motto of the American Association of Nurse Anesthetists (AANA): Safe and effective anesthesia care (AANA, n.d.-b).

Certified Registered Nurse Anesthetists (CRNAs) are

> registered nurses who have become anesthesia specialists by taking a graduate curriculum which focuses on the development of clinical judgment and critical thinking. They are qualified to make independent judgments concerning all aspects of anesthesia care based on their education, licensure, and certification. CRNAs are legally responsible for the anesthesia care they provide and are recognized in state law in all 50 states, the District of Columbia, Puerto Rico, and the Virgin Islands. (AANA, 2010)

Anesthesia care is delivered in collaboration with surgeons, podiatrists, dentists, radiologists, psychiatrists, cardiologists, and anesthesiologists in outpatient, inpatient, and office-based settings.

The CRNA scope of practice includes comprehensive anesthesia and pain care across the lifespan in many different settings. The scope includes:

1. Performing and documenting a preanesthetic assessment and evaluation of the patient, including requesting consultations and diagnostic studies; selecting, obtaining, ordering, and administering preanesthetic medications and fluids; and obtaining informed consent for anesthesia.
2. Developing and implementing an anesthetic plan.
3. Initiating the anesthetic technique which may include: general, regional, local, and sedation.
4. Selecting, applying, and inserting appropriate noninvasive and invasive monitoring modalities for continuous evaluation of the patient's physical status.
5. Selecting, obtaining, and administering the anesthetics, adjuvant and accessory drugs, and fluids necessary to manage the anesthetic.
6. Managing a patient's airway and pulmonary status using current practice modalities.
7. Facilitating emergence and recovery from anesthesia by selecting, obtaining, ordering, and administering medications, fluids, and ventilatory support.
8. Discharging the patient from a postanesthesia care area and providing postanesthesia follow-up evaluation and care.
9. Implementing acute and chronic pain management modalities.
10. Responding to emergency situations by providing airway management, administration of emergency fluids and drugs, and using basic or advanced cardiac life support techniques. (AANA, 2010b)

The CRNA may also have other responsibilities that could include administration and management activities, education, research, quality improvement, interdepartmental liaison, committee appointments, and oversight of other non-anesthesia departments.

Nurse anesthesia educational programs are offered at both the master's level and the clinical doctoral level. The Council on Accreditation of Nurse Anesthesia Educational Programs (COA) is the entity that accredits all nurse anesthesia educational programs regardless of the degree offered. This formal process of accreditation began in 1952 (Bankert, 1989). At this time, nurse anesthesia programs at the master's degree level are a minimum of 24 months in length and at the doctoral level, a minimum of 36 months. All nurse anesthesia educational programs must provide a minimum number of cases and a minimum curriculum that includes pharmacology of anesthetic agents and adjuvant drugs including concepts in chemistry and biochemistry (105 hours); anatomy, physiology, and pathophysiology (135 hours); professional aspects of nurse anesthesia practice (45 hours); basic and advanced principles of anesthesia practice including physics, equipment, technology and pain management (105 hours); research (30 hours); and clinical correlation conferences (45 hours); radiology; and ultrasound. In addition, the curriculum must include three (3) separate comprehensive graduate level courses in advanced physiology/ pathophysiology, advanced health assessment, and advanced pharmacology. Students must administer a minimum of 550 clinical cases that prepare them for the full scope of practice in a variety of clinical settings (COA, 2014). Completion of the nurse anesthesia educational program and the required cases qualifies the student to sit for the national certification examination (NCE).

Following publication of the America Association of Colleges of Nursing's initiative to move education of advanced practice nursing into doctoral frameworks by 2015, the AANA established a task force on doctoral education for nurse anesthetists in 2005. The task force recommended to the Board of Directors of the AANA that all nurse anesthesia educational programs be offered in a clinical doctoral framework by the year 2025 (AANA, 2007). The COA will not consider any new master's degree programs for accreditation beyond 2015. Students accepted into an accredited program on January 1, 2022, and thereafter must graduate with doctoral degrees (COA, 2014). Unlike other nursing advanced practice specialties, nurse anesthesia programs are not necessarily housed in schools of nursing. Of the 113 programs of nurse anesthesia accredited in the United States, 47 (42%) are in a variety of non-nursing academic units (COA Annual Report, 2013). These programs may offer the Doctorate of Nurse Anesthesia Practice (DNAP) degree. Wherever the educational program is housed, all nurse anesthesia educational programs must be accredited through the COA and the graduates must pass the national certification examination. Thus the public is assured that every nurse anesthetist has met a set of predetermined qualifications for entry into practice.

In 1986, the passage of the Omnibus Budget Reconciliation Act marked nurse anesthetists as the first group of advanced practice nursing professionals to be granted direct reimbursement for anesthesia and pain management services to Medicare enrollees. This paved the way for entrepreneurship and innovative practice settings for nurse anesthetists. In the 2013 AANA Practice Survey, 23.4% of respondents identified themselves as "independent contractors" (AANA, 2013). Furthermore, in 2001 the Center for Medicare and Medicaid Services (CMS) published its anesthesia care rule granting state governors the ability to opt out of the federal physician supervision requirement, thus allowing nurse anesthetists to work in collaboration with other healthcare providers without physician supervision (AANA, 2001). To date, 17 states have opted out of the CMS requirement for physician supervision of nurse anesthetists. In a recent study in the journal Health Affairs compared outcomes in states with physician supervision and those opt-out states. No harm was found when CRNAs delivered anesthesia without physician supervision (Dulisse & Cromwell , 2010).

Nurse anesthesia practice is remarkably varied and flexible. Nurse anesthetists function in fast paced trauma team settings in urban areas and in highly independent rural settings. Nurse anesthetists provide critically needed surgical and obstetric anesthesia, acute pain management, trauma stabilization, and, in some instances, chronic pain management for the rural communities they live in. Without the services of nurse anesthetists, many of these small rural hospitals would close (Siebert, Alexander, & Lupien, 2003) . Nurse anesthetists have served in the military in peace and on the battlefield in every armed conflict since the World War I, including the most recent conflicts in Iraq and Afghanistan (AANA, 2010a). Nurse anesthetists are a crucial part of the modern health care system today both in terms of quality of care and access to highly skilled affordable care. The education and training of nurse anesthetists position these advanced practice nurses to lead healthcare into the future.

INTERNATIONAL

Although the content in this chapter has focused on APNs in the United States, it is encouraging to see the continuing development of these roles in other countries. Midwifery, a profession often distinct from nursing, has a longer history internationally than in the United States. The International Confederation of Midwives, so named in 1954, has more than 116 midwifery organization members representing 102 countries (see www.internationalmidwives.org). The recent *Lancet Series on Midwifery* (2014) highlighted midwifery as " a vital solution to the challenges of providing high-quality maternal and newborn care for all women and newborn infants, in all countries" (Renfrew, 2014). Clinical specialization in nursing has existed in many countries for a very long time. For example, in the United Kingdom the NP role developed dramatically during the 1990s once the National Health Services recognized its legitimacy (Reverly, Walsh, & Crumbie, 2001). However, in other countries APNs are only beginning to develop programs and practices (Wang, Yen, & Snyder, 1995).

CONCLUSION

APRNs have made significant contributions to quality health care, particularly for vulnerable populations. If all Americans are to receive quality, cost-effective health care, it is critical that greater use be made of APRNs. Their advanced knowledge and skills, both in nursing and related fields make valuable contributions to the current and future health care system, especially in the task of meaningful health care reform. As the United States becomes more diverse, APRNs play key roles in providing culturally competent care. They assume leadership in developing new practice sites and innovative systems of care to enhance health care outcomes. A bright future awaits nursing and APRNs.

Acknowledgment

The author acknowledges the contributions of Mary Zwygart-Stauffacher, who contributed to this chapter in a previous edition.

REFERENCES

Accreditation Commission for Midwifery Education. (2005). *The knowledge, skills, and behaviors prerequisite to midwifery clinical coursework.* Washington, DC: Author.

Advanced Practice Registered Nurses Consensus Workgroup & APRN Joint Dialogue Group. (2008). *Consensus model for APRN regulation: Licensure, accreditation, certification, and education.* Retrieved from http://www.aacn. nche .edu/Education/pdf/APRNReport.pdf

American Association of Colleges of Nursing. (2006). *The essentials of doctoral education for advanced nursing practice.* Washington, DC: Author. Retrieved from http://www.aacn.nche.edu/DNP/pdf7Essentials.pdf

American Association of Colleges of Nursing. (2011). *The essentials of master's education for advanced practice nursing.* Washington, DC: Author.

American Association of Colleges of Nursing. (2014). *Doctor of nursing practice programs.* Retrieved from http://www.aacn.nche.edu/media-relations/fact-sheets/dnp

American Association of Nurse Anesthetists. (n.d.-a). *Certified registered nurse anesthetists at a glance.* Retrieved June 30, 2014, from http://www.aana.com/ ceandeducation/becomeacrna/Pages/Nurse-Anesthetists-at-a-Glance. aspx.

American Association of Nurse Anesthetists. (n.d.-b). *Who we are.* Retrieved June 30, 2014, from http://www.aana.com/aboutus/Pages/Who-We-Are.aspx.

American Association of Nurse Anesthetists. (2001). *Iowa becomes first state to opt out of federal anesthesia requirement.* Retrieved June 30, 2014, from http:// www.aana.com/newsandjournal/News/Pages/121301-Iowa-Becomes-the-First-State-to-Opt-Out-of-Federal-Anesthesia-Requirement.aspx.

American Association of Nurse Anesthetists. (2007). AANA position on doctoral preparation of nurse anesthetists. Retrieved June 30, 2014, from http://www. aana.com/myaana/AANABusiness/professionalresources/Documents/dtf_ posstatemt0707.pdf.

American Association of Nurse Anesthetists. (2010a). *History of nurse anesthesia practice.* Retrieved June 30, 2014, from http://www.aana.com/aboutus/ Documents/historynap.pdf.

American Association of Nurse Anesthetists. (2010b). *CRNA scope of practice.* Retrieved May 28, 2014, from http://www.aana.com/aboutus/Documents/ scopeofpractice.pdf.

American Association of Nurse Practitioners. (2013). *NP facts.* Retrieved from http://www.aanp.org/images/documents/about-nps/npfacts.pdf

American College of Nurse-Midwives (2004a). *Definition of midwifery practice.* Washington, DC: Author.

American College of Nurse-Midwives. (2004b). *Philosophy of the American College of Nurse-Midwives.* Washington, DC. Author.

American College of Nurse-Midwives. (2012). *Core competencies for basic midwifery practice.* Washington, DC: Author.

American College of Nurse-Midwives. (2014a). *CNM/CM-attended birth statistics in the United States.* Washington, DC: Author.

American College of Nurse-Midwives. (2014b). *Essential facts about midwives.* Washington, DC: Author.

American Nurses Association. (2010). *Nursing: Scope and standards of practice.* Washington, DC: Author.

American Nurses Association. (2015). *Code of ethics for nurses with interpretive statements* (2nd ed.). Washington, DC: Author.

American Nurses Association, National Association of Pediatric Nurses Practitioners, & Society of Pediatric Nurses. (2010). *Pediatric nursing: Scope and standards of practice.* Washington, DC: American Nurses Association.

Bankert, M. (1989). *Watchful care: A history of America's nurse anesthetists.* New York, NY: Continuum.

Benner, P (1984). *From novice to expert: Excellence and power in clinical nursing practice.* Menlo Park, CA: Addison-Wesley.

Blanchette, H. (1995). Comparison of obstetric outcome of a primary-care access clinic staffed by certified nurse-midwives and a private practice group of obstetricians in the same community. *American Journal of Obstetrics & Gynecology, 172*(6), 1868–1871.

Bradford, H. M. (2013). Women's health and maternity care policies: Current status and recommendations for change. In M. D. Avery (Ed.), *Supporting a physiologic approach to pregnancy and birth: A practical guide.* Ames, IA: Wiley-Blackwell.

Brown, S., & Grimes, D. (1995). A meta-analysis of nurse practitioners and nurse midwives in primary care. *Nursing Research, 44*, 332–339.

Brykczynski, K. (1989). An interpretive study describing the clinical judgment of nurse practitioners. *Scholarly Inquiry for Nursing Practice: An Interpretive Journal, 3*, 113–120.

Clark, A. (2001). What will it take to reduce errors in health care settings? *Clinical Nurse Specialist, 15*(4), 182–183.

Council on Accreditation of Nurse Anesthesia Educational Programs. (2004). *Standards for accreditation of nurse anesthesia educational programs, Revised May 2014.* Retrieved June 30, 2014, from http://www.aana.com/myaana/Accreditation/Documents/Standards%20for%20Accreditation%20of%20Nurse%20Anesthesia%20Education%20Programs%20_May%202014.pdf.

Council on Accreditation of Nurse Anesthesia Educational Programs. (2013). *Nurse anesthesia programs summary of 2013 annual report data.* Retrieved June 30, 2014, from http://www.aana.com/myaana/Accreditation/Documents/Summary%20of%20COA%20Annual%20Report%20Data%202013.pdf.

Dayhoff, N., & Lyon, B. (2001). Assessing outcomes of clinical nurse specialist practice. In R. Kleinpell (Ed.), *Outcome assessment in advanced nursing* (pp. 103–129). New York, NY: Springer Publishing.

Dracup, K. (2004). Peterson's nursing programs. Retrieved from http://www.petersons.com/nursing/articles/masters.asp?sponsor = 1

Dulisse, B, & Cromwell, J. (2010). No harm found when nurse anesthetists work without supervision by physicians. *Health Affairs* 29(8), 1469–1475.

Edwardson, S. (2004). Matching standards and needs in doctoral education in nursing. *Journal of Professional Nursing, 20*, 40–46.

Elder, R., & Bullough, B. (1990). Nurse practitioners and clinical nurse specialists: Are the roles merging? *Clinical Nurse Specialist, 4*, 78–84.

Fenton, M. (1985). Identifying competencies of clinical nurse specialists. *Journal of Nursing Administration, 15*, 31–37.

Fenton, M., & Brykczynski, K. (1993). Qualitative distinctions and similarities in the practice of clinical nurse specialists and nurse practitioners. *Journal of Professional Nursing, 9*, 313–326.

Forbes, K., Rafson, J., Spross, J., & Kozlowski, D. (1990). Clinical nurse specialist and nurse practitioner core curricula survey results. *Nurse Practitioners, 15*, 45–48.

Ford, L. (1979). A nurse for all settings: The nurse practitioner. *Nursing Outlook, 27*, 516–521.

Ford, L. (2005). Opinions, ideas and convictions for NPs' founding mother, Dr. Loretta Ford. *The American Journal for Nurse Practitioners, 9*(3), 31–33.

Heitkemper, M., & Bond, E. (2004). Clinical nurse specialists: State of the profession and challenges ahead. *Clinical Nurse Specialist, 18*(3), 135–140.

Horrocks, S., Anderson, E., & Salisbury, C. (2002). Systematic review of whether nurse practitioners working in primary care can provide equivalent care to doctors. *British Medical Journal, 324*(7341), 819–823.

Institute of Medicine (IOM). (1999). *To err is human: Building a safer health system.* Washington, DC: National Academy Press.

Institute of Medicine Committee on the Quality of Health Care in America. (2001). *Crossing the quality chasm: A new health system for the 21st century.* Washington, DC: National Academy Press.

Kapu, A., & Kleinpell, R. (2012). Developing nurse practitioner associated metrics for outcomes assessment. *Journal of the American Academy of Nurse Practitioners, 1*–8. doi:10.1111/1745-7599.12001

Klein, T. (2005). Scope of practice and the nurse practitioner: Regulation, competency, expansion, and evolution. *Topic in Advanced Practice Nursing eJournal, 7*(3), 1–10.

Kopanos, T. (2014). Celebrating mile markers. *The Journal for Nurse Practitioners, 10*(7), A13, A14.

Lindeke, L, Canedy, B., & Kay, M. (1996). A comparison of practice domains of clinical nurse specialists and nurse practitioners. *Journal of Professional Nursing, 13*, 281–287.

Lyon, B. (2004). What to look for when analyzing clinical nurse specialist statutes and regulations. *Clinical Nurse Specialist, 16*(1) 33–34.

Lyon, B., & Minarik, P. (2001). Statutory and regulatory issues for clinical nurse specialist (CNS) practice: Ensuring the public's access to CNS services. *Clinical Nurse Specialist, 15*(3), 108–114.

MacDorman, M. F. & Singh, G. K. (1998). Midwifery care, social and medical risk factors, and birth outcomes in the USA. *Journal of Epidemiology and Community Health, 52*(5), 310–317.

MacDorman, M. F., Mathews, T. J., & Declercq, E. (2014). *Trends in out-of-hospital births in the United States, 1990–2012. NCHS data brief, no. 144.* Hyattsville, MD: National Center for Health Statistics.

Martin, K. (2000). Nurse practitioners: A comparison of rural-urban practice patterns and willingness to serve in underserved areas. *Journal of the American Academy of Nurse Practitioners, 12*, 491–496.

Mundinger, M., Kane, R., Lenz, E., Totten, A., Tsai, W., Cleary, P., …, Shelanski, M. L. (2000). Primary care outcomes in patients treated by nurse practitioners or physicians: A randomized trial. *Journal of the American Medical Association, 283*, 59–68.

National Association of Clinical Nurse Specialist (NACNS). (2011). *Criteria for the evaluation of clinical nurse specialist master's, practice doctorate, and post-graduate certificate educational programs.* Retrieved from http://www.nacns.org/docs/CNSEducationCriteria.pdf

National Association of Clinical Nurse Specialists. (n.d.). *Organizing framework and CNS core competencies.* Retrieved from http://www.nacns.org/docs/CNSCoreCompetencies.pdf

National Association of Clinical Nurse Specialists. (2014). What is a clinical nurse specialist? Retrieved from http://www.nacns.org/html/cns-faqs1.php

National Center for Health Statistics. (2006). *Births: Final data for 2006.* Report available from National Center for Vital Statistics (Report No. 57-7). Hyattsville, MD: Author.

National Council of State Boards of Nursing. (2002). *Regulation of advanced practice nursing.* Retrieved from http://www.ncsbn.org

National Organization of Nurse Practitioner Faculties. (1995). *Advanced nursing practice: Curriculum guidelines and program standards for nurse practitioner education.* Washington, DC: Author.

National Organization of Nurse Practitioner Faculties. (2006). *2006 domains and core competencies of nurse practitioner practice.* Washington, DC: Author. Retrieved from http://www.nonpf.org/NONPF2005/CoreCompsFINAL06.pdf

National Organization of Nurse Practitioner Faculties. (2012). *Nurse practitioner competencies.* Retrieved from http://c.ymcdn.com/sites/www.nonpf.org/resource/resmgr/competencies/npcorecompetenciesfinal2012.pdf

National Organization of Nurse Practitioner Faculties. (2013). *Population focused nurse practitioner competencies: Family/across the lifespan, neonatal, pediatric acute care, pediatric primary care, psychiatric mental health and women's health/gender related.* Retrieved from http://c.ymcdn.com/sites/www.nonpf.org/resource/resmgr/competencies/populationfocusnpcomps2013.pdf

Naylor, M., Brooten, D., Jones, R., Lavizzo-Mourey, R., Mezey, M., & Pauly, M. (1994). Comprehensive discharge planning for the hospitalized elderly: A randomized clinical trial. *Annals of Internal Medicine, 120,* 999–106.

Neidlinger, S., Scroggins, K., & Kennedy, L. (1987). Cost evaluation of discharge planning for hospitalized elderly. *Nursing Economics, 5,* 225–230.

Newhouse, R. P., Stanik-Hutt, J., White, K. M, Johantgen, M., Bass, E. B., Zangaro, G., …, Weiner, J. P. (2011). Advanced practice nursing outcomes 1990–2008: A systematic review. *Nursing Economics, 29,* 230–250.

Nurse Practitioner Roundtable. (2008). *Nurse practitioner DNP education, certification and titling: A unified statement.* Washington, DC: Author.

Page, N., & Arena, D. (1994). Rethinking the merger of the clinical nurse specialist and the nurse practitioner roles. *Image: The Journal of Nursing Scholarship, 26,* 315–318.

Rasch, R., & Frauman, A. (1996). Advanced practice in nursing: Conceptual issues. *Journal of Professional Nursing, 12,* 141–146.

Redekopp, J. (1997). Clinical nurse specialist role confusion: The need for identity. *Clinical Nurse Specialist, 11,* 87–91.

Reiter, F. (1966). The nurse clinician. *American Journal of Nursing, 66,* 274–280.

Renfrew, M. J., Homer, C. S. E., Downe, S., McFadden, A., Muir, N., Prentice, T., & ten Hoope-Bender, P. (2014). Executive Summary. *The Lancet Series on Midwifery, 384,* 1–8.

Reverly, S., Walsh, M., & Crumbie, A. (2001). *Nurse practitioners: Developing the role in hospital settings*. Oxford, UK: Butterworth Heinemann.

Rosenblatt, R., Dobie, S., Hart, L., Schneeweiss, R., Gould, D., Raine, T. R., ..., Perrin, E. B. (1997). Interspecialty differences in the obstetric care of low-risk women. *American Journal of Public Health, 87*, 344–351.

Safriet, B. (1998). Still spending dollars, still searching for sense: Advanced practice nursing in an era of regulatory and economic turmoil. *Advanced Practice Nursing Quarterly, 4*, 24–33.

Sandall, J., Soltani, H., Gates, S., Shennan A., & Devane, D. (2013). Midwife-led continuity models versus other models of care for childbearing women. Cochrane Database of Systematic Reviews. Aug 21;8:CD004667.

Scherer, Y. K., Bruce, S. A., & Runkawatt, V. (2007). A comparison of clinical simulation and case study presentation on nurse practitioner students' knowledge and confidence in managing a cardiac event. *International Journal of Nursing Education, 4*(1), 1–14.

Siebert, E., Alexander, J., & Lupien, A. (2004). Rural nurse anesthesia practice: A pilot study. *AANA Journal, 72*(3), 181–190. Retrieved June 30, 2014, from http://www.aana.com/newsandjournal/Documents/181-190.pdf.

U.S. Department of Health and Human Services, Health Resources and Services Administration, National Center for Health Workforce Analysis. (2014). *Highlights From the 2012 National Sample Survey of Nurse Practitioners*. Rockville, Maryland: U.S. Department of Health and Human Services.

Varney, H. (2015). *Varney's midwifery*. Boston, MA: Jones & Bartlett.

Gail B. Katz

2

ADVANCED PRACTICE WITHIN A NURSING PARADIGM

The most important word in the title of advanced practice registered nurse (APRN) is the last one: *nurse*. Advanced education enables nurses to expand their knowledge base and expertise in nursing so that their practices differ not only from those of nurses with an associate's or bachelor's degree but also from those of other health professionals, particularly physicians or physician assistants. Nurses often underestimate the profound positive effect that their care can have on improving individual and population outcomes and the impact on quality of care. Florence Nightingale, in *Notes on Nursing* (1859/1992), noted that people in her day often thought of nursing as signifying "little more than the administration of medicines and the application of poultices" (p. 6). Efforts are still necessary to convey the full scope of nursing practice to other professionals and to the public so that nurses' contributions to positive health outcomes are understood, respected, valued, and reimbursed. So often the media have focused on the physical assessment skills, tasks, and prescriptive privileges of APRNs rather than on the distinctive and unique knowledge, education, abilities, and expertise that characterize advanced practice registered nursing practice.

As advanced practice nursing moves rapidly toward the practice doctorate as entry into practice, an excellent opportunity exists to reconceptualize how advanced practice nursing is taught in APRN programs. Burman et al. (2009) challenge educators to focus on health promotion and disease management, incorporating theories from a variety of disciplines to improve health behavior and change their pedagogies as doctorate of nursing practice (DNP) programs and curricula continue to develop. Chism (2013) supports the need for DNP curricula to focus on the leadership of chronic disease management and the care of our aging population.

WHAT IS NURSING?

Definitions of Nursing

For many years the nursing profession has sought to define nursing and to identify its scope of practice. It is critical that APRNs and those aspiring to this role have a clear understanding of what nursing is in order for them to provide a clear understanding of nursing's unique contributions to health care outcomes in their interprofessional interactions. Therefore, several of the many definitions of nursing that have been put forth over the years are reviewed.

Florence Nightingale (1859/1992) formulated one of the earliest definitions of nursing, which went beyond caring for ill patients. She emphasized the whole person, including diet and environment. The aim of nursing care, according to Nightingale, is to put the individual in the best possible condition so that nature can act upon the person. Nightingale's *Notes on Nursing,* although written 150 years ago, speaks to the substantive basis of nursing. Not only does Nightingale elaborate on interventions nurses can employ, she also underscores the necessity of thorough assessments before planning nursing care. Reading *Notes on Nursing* should therefore be a part of every APRN curriculum.

In Virginia Henderson's (1966) definition of nursing, emphasis is placed on the nurse collaborating with the individual to enhance the individual's health status. Henderson defined *nursing* as

> assisting the individual, sick or well, in the performance of those activities contributing to health or its recovery (or to a peaceful death) that he would perform unaided if he had the necessary strength, will, or knowledge. And to do this in such a way as to help him gain independence as soon as possible. (p. 15)

Henderson's definition contains many elements that constitute the substantive nature of nursing. Health promotion is a key component of her definition. In addition, the caring aspects of nursing are emphasized. Not all individuals will recover from their diseases or injuries. It is the nurse's role to assist the individual to achieve the goals he or she has established. Myss (1996, 2004) noted in her well-known works on healing that in curing modalities the individual is passive, but she argues that the individual must take an active role to be healed. APRNs can play a key role in assisting individuals in their healing process because APRNs are able to bring additional expertise to these interactions and to perform holistic health assessments. Henderson stresses helping the individual gain independence. Independence is a Western belief and may not be a value in all cultures. Thus, it is important for the nurse to ascertain the personal values of each individual and realize that independence may not be one of their preferences.

Nojima (1989), a Japanese nursing theorist, defined *nursing practice* as "a human activity carried out by nurses to help individuals organize their health conditions so that they are able to live optimally and realize their potential" (pp. 6–7). In her definition, the focus is on a person's quality of life. The partnership between the nurse and the individual is evident in Nojima's definition of nursing. With the advent of globalization, it is important to review the characteristics of nursing outside of Western medicine (Nojima, Tomikana, Makabe, & Snyder, 2003).

The American Nurses Association (ANA) has defined *nursing* as follows:

> Nursing is the protection, promotion, and optimization of health and abilities, prevention of illness and injury, alleviation of suffering through the diagnosis and treatment of human response, and advocacy in the care of individuals, families, communities, and populations. (ANA, 2010, p. 10)

Previously, the definition of nursing focused on persons and their responses to health problems, rather than specific illnesses. This definition of nursing developed in 2003, which emphasizes health promotion and optimal health, remains unchanged in current discussions of the ANA's *Social Policy Statement* (ANA, 2010). The focus on health differentiates nursing from the practice of medicine.

Despite the frequent reference to the ANA definition of nursing, many APRNs have encountered difficulty practicing from a nursing model. They have been seemingly forced to launch their practice within the medical model in part because of medical diagnoses used for billing and coding and in part because of the medical community's and the public's perception of APRNs. Although it is important to know the cause of a person's pain or stress, much of nursing care remains the same despite the cause. It has been encouraging to see the Agency for Healthcare Research and Quality (AHRQ) consider problems or responses, rather than disease entities, as the focus of practice guidelines. The AHRQ website (www.ahrq.gov) is an excellent resource for evidence-based practice and current clinical practices.

Advanced practice nursing builds on the competence of the professional nurse and is characterized by the integration and application of a broad range of theoretical and evidence-based knowledge (ANA, 2010). APRNs are prepared in one of the four roles: certified nurse-midwife, clinical nurse specialist, nurse practitioner, or certified registered nurse anesthetist. The APRN consensus model (2008) defines the *APRN* as a "provider that is certified in one of the four roles, educated in health promotion, assessment, diagnosis, management, pharmacotherapeutics, and direct care to individuals, populations, and communities" (Stanley, 2012, p. 244). Licensure, accreditation, certification, and education (LACE) should be consistent with role population (APRN Consensus Workgroup & APRN Joint Dialogue Group, 2008). Specialization within advanced practice focuses beyond the six populations (family/individual across lifespan, adult-gerontology, neonatal, pediatrics,women's health/gender related, psychiatric/mental health) and provides depth within a population. One of the most important aspects of specialization in nursing is that the distinct specialization is always a part of the whole field or discipline of professional nursing (ANA, 2010).

The APRN consensus model, LACE has stipulations that APRNs be educated within an accredited program with advanced pathophysiology, advanced health assessment, advanced pharmacology—the three Ps; complete a minimum of 500 clinical hours; and be nationally certified. The licensure of an APRN is "defined as a legal title and credentials to be granted to all advanced practice registered nurses meeting the definitional criteria. Boards of nursing are responsible for granting a second license to APRNs in all four roles" (Stanley, 2011, p. 248). Rounds, Zych, and Mallary (2013) further state that the LACE model is not only relevant to the national movement of improving nursing regulation but has been shown to improve the professional transition for APRNs. Safety is once again emphasized as the primary motivator for national regulation of advanced nursing practice (Rounds et al., 2013).

The ANA's *A Social Policy Statement* (2010) emphasizes the characteristics of nursing practice to include human responses, theory application, evidence-based nursing actions, and outcomes. These characteristics build the foundation for professional nursing (ANA, 2010). Within this model, nursing's professional scope of practice, code of ethics, specialization, and certification laid the base for professional nursing. Building on this base in a pyramid model are individual state's nurse practice acts, rules, and regulations. From this level, institutional policies and procedures guide nursing practice, with self-determination as the top level of the pyramid model. This model lays the foundation not only for professional nursing but for all its expanded roles and specializations.

Scope of Practice

Gaining more knowledge about the substantive basis of nursing is an essential component of APRN education. Scope of practice can be viewed in several ways. In fact, findings from the numerous studies undertaken to identify, describe, and classify the phenomena of concern to nurses have helped clarify our understanding of scope of practice. One way to determine scope of practice from a regulatory framework is to focus on population, with each APRN working within his or her specific practice population and his or her actual practice is determined by the APRN regulatory model. Other initiatives delineate the substantive basis of nursing. Two of these initiatives—nursing diagnoses and human responses—will be discussed further.

Nursing Diagnoses

Nursing diagnoses are one strategy nurses have used to describe phenomena for which nurses provide care. Since the First Nursing Diagnosis Conference in 1973, nurses within the North American Nursing Diagnosis Association International (NANDA-I) have worked to identify, describe, and validate individual problems and concerns that fall within the domain of nursing. Currently there are 235 approved or revised nursing diagnoses (NANDA-I, 2015). Continued efforts are necessary to identify and validate new diagnoses and to revise existing diagnoses. APRNs have provided and can continue to provide leadership in the nursing diagnosis movement.

NANDA-I diagnoses are grouped under nine functional patterns: exchanging, communicating, relating, valuing, choosing, moving, perceiving, knowing, and feeling. According to Newman (1984), it is important for nurses to determine changes in an individual's patterns. In approaching assessment in this manner, the focus is on the whole person rather than on specific diagnoses.

Nursing diagnoses have been widely accepted not only in the United States but also internationally (NANDA-I, 2015). As the first effort to develop a common language for nursing phenomena, and despite numerous criticisms, using such diagnoses assists nurses in focusing on those aspects of care for which nursing interventions can be identified and nurse-sensitive outcomes can be determined. APRNs therefore need to be familiar with both nursing and medical diagnoses.

In the United States, a number of projects to identify and classify nursing interventions have been initiated. The National Intervention Classification (NIC) has identified and classified more than 550 research-based nursing interventions (Bulechek, Butcher, Dochterman, & Wagner, 2013). A project identifying nursing outcomes links nursing diagnoses, nursing outcomes, and interventions (Johnson et al., 2005).

Human Responses

The ANA (2010) has delineated phenomena of concern to nursing. The identified phenomena were not meant to be exhaustive but rather exemplars of the types of concerns that fall within the purview of nursing. Human experiences and responses proposed by the ANA (2010) include promotion of health and wellness; promotion of safety and quality of care; care and self-care processes; physical, emotional, and spiritual comfort, discomfort, and pain; adaptation to physiologic and pathophysiologic processes; emotions related to the experience of birth, growth and development, health, illness, disease, and death; meanings ascribed to health and illness; linguistic and cultural sensitivity; health literacy; decision making and the ability to make choices; relationships, role performance, and change processes within relationships; social policies and their effects on health; health care systems and their relationships to access, cost, and quality of health care; and the environment and the prevention of disease and injury.

As with nursing diagnoses, these identified human responses assist APRNs in focusing on the health concerns and needs for the individual, population, or communities. Advanced practice nursing care is of primary importance in producing positive individual outcomes while focusing on health promotion, disease management, education, and wellness. Therapeutics for managing the human responses or assisting the person in managing them transcends medical entities. For example, despite various causes for sleep problems, nursing interventions, such as massage and music therapy, can be used successfully. Viewing nursing in the context of, and the perspective of, human responses helps all nurses organize the plan of care content from the nurse's point of view.

THE ART AND SCIENCE OF NURSING
The Art of Nursing

The art of nursing is integrally tied to the caring aspect of nursing. For many years, nursing was defined as both an art and a science. As nurses began to give more attention to establishing a scientific basis for nursing practice, they thereby gained greater acceptance in the scientific community and the art or caring aspect of nursing received less attention. In practice settings, for example, nurses focused more attention on the high technology used in caring for individuals with complex health problems. Nonetheless, the public has sustained its attachment and desire for caring interventions, such as massage, therapeutic touch, listening, guided imagery, and aromatherapy, to name a few. A number of reasons for which people seek nonpharmacologic complementary therapies have been proposed: (a) they wish to be treated as a whole person by health professionals; (b) they wish to be active participants in their care; (c) they desire that the treatment not be worse than the disease; and (d) they feel that Western health care does not meet all of their needs. Therefore, it is important that APRNs consider how they can integrate the art of nursing, which includes traditional and nontraditional nursing interventions, into their practice.

The essence of the APRN is the caring relationship with the patient. Through sharing knowledge and providing support through communication, caring, and relationship building, the APRN fosters health with patients and communities.

Caring is a critical element of nursing practice. Leininger (1990), Watson (1988), and Gadow (1980) have each put forth definitions of caring. Watson defined the art of caring as

> a human activity consisting of the following: a nurse consciously, by means of certain signs, passes on to others feelings he or she has lived through, realized or learned; others are united to these feelings and also experience them. (p. 68)

Newman, Sime, and Corcoran-Perry (1991) noted that the focus of nursing is "caring in the human health experience" (p. 3). The National Organization of Nurse Practitioner Faculties (NONPF) has identified patient- and family-centered care as a core competency (NONPF, 2012).

Caring requires that a nurse be competent in assessing and intervening. Benner (1998) noted that a caring attitude was not sufficient to make an action a caring practice. The practice must be implemented in an excellent manner in order to be viewed as caring. Caring and the art of nursing convey very similar meanings, but caring nurses also seek the scientific basis for their practice and continue to update their expertise and knowledge. APRNs possess the knowledge and ability to critique research about specific therapies and determine their applicability to specific individual populations.

In 1993 Schoenhoefer and Boykin proposed that the nursing process–based care models, including nursing diagnoses, did not truly address what nurses ought to be doing. Their grand theory of nursing has a framework based on caring that is specific to each nurse, person, and situation, requiring personal individual knowledge of each patient, as well as including empirical knowledge of each patient's situation. They acknowledge that all humans care and that nursing is a discipline that requires knowing and developing advanced nursing knowledge. Nursing is also a profession, in which nursing knowledge is applied and used in response to the individual's human needs while still being a dynamic, evolving, creative, and caring process (Schoenhoefer & Boykin, 1993; Zaccagnini & Waud White, 2014). APRNs are well prepared to practice from a theory-driven human caring basis. A theory-based advanced nursing practice defines and exemplifies many attributes of the APRN.

Hagedorn and Quinn (2004) proposed a *theory of primary caring* specific to the APRN that includes five domains: connection, consistency, commitment, community, and change. The domain *connection* describes the APRN's effectiveness based on relationship-centered caring with the patient, family, and community. *Consistency* describes the importance of evidence- and theory-based care in advanced nursing practice. *Commitment* describes how the nurse practitioner (NP) is committed to serve each patient and family to his or her best ability. *Community* illustrates the role of the NP in facilitating full access to health care for all persons and strives to meet unmet community health needs. The fifth domain, *change,* explains how APRNs introduce innovative models of health care and share decision making with patients.

Basic human needs are to be viewed as a whole person and cared for. It is the role of the APRN to support and assist the patient in being cared for in a holistic manner. APRNs incorporate the empiric aspects of medicine but practice within a nursing framework. The APRN's qualities and actions of presence, empowerment, reflection, listening, touch, empathy, humor, and knowing the community, as well as the APRN's ability to access care and to directly provide care, ensure patient satisfaction, and provide quality evidence-based outcomes (Hagedorn & Quinn, 2004).

The Science of Nursing

Significant progress has been made in developing the knowledge base that underlies nursing practice, revealing that nursing is characterized by both art and science (ANA, 2004). Although nursing is guided by standards of practice based on clinical evidence and research, additional research is always needed to further develop evidence-based practices so that APRNs will have a sound scientific basis from which to choose specific interventions for individuals or populations (ANA, 2010). The clinical guidelines developed by professional and governmental agencies—available through the National Guideline Clearinghouse—exemplify the work that has been done, and that continues to be done, in identifying "best practices" based on research findings. APRNs play a key role in helping nurses review research and develop clinical guidelines that incorporate existing knowledge bases.

THEORETICAL AND CONCEPTUAL MODELS

During the past 50 years, the nursing profession has given considerable attention to theoretical and conceptual models. This attention has served to differentiate nursing from other disciplines (Marrs & Lowry, 2009; Russell & Fawcett, 2005). However, nursing theories are not new in nursing. Nightingale (1859/1992) elaborated on the relationship of the environment to health and well-being. Numerous theoretical and conceptual models exist.

What relevance do nursing theories have to practice? Can't nurses merely practice nursing? Meleis (2011) noted that a theory articulates and communicates a mental image of a certain order that exists in the world. This image includes components, and these components inform a model or perspective that guides each nurse's practice. This model may be identical to one of the publicized nursing theories, or it may be based on a theoretical perspective from another discipline. In some instances, eclectic models are used in which nurses combine elements from established nursing theories or theories from other disciplines. New nursing theories continue to be developed. Of particular importance is the delineation of nursing theories that incorporate various cultural perspectives, because the Western philosophical perspective to date has not pervaded many of the existing theories.

There has been much discussion about whether one grand nursing theory is needed. Would the existence of a grand or meta-theory be advantageous to the progression of the profession and discipline? Riehl-Sisca (1989) stated that nursing has benefited from having a multiplicity of theories. The wide range of perspectives elaborated in these theories has helped nurses to more clearly define the nature of the discipline and profession, to evaluate various approaches that can be employed in practice, and to respect diversity as a positive element. Alligood and Marriner-Tomey (2005) identified seven theorists who have developed primary grand theories or conceptual frameworks for nursing: Johnson (1980), King (1971), Levine (1967), Neuman (1974), Orem (1980), Rogers (1970), and Roy (1984). Many other nurses have developed midrange theories or conceptual frameworks that have served as a basis for research and practice.

More recently, nurses have turned their attention to midrange theories. Midrange theories, which focus on a limited number of variables, are more amenable to empirical testing than are grand theories by definition. Examples of midrange theories include empathy (Olson & Hanchett, 1997), uncertainty in illness (Mishel, 1990), resilience (Polk, 1997), mastery (Younger, 1991), self-transcendence (Reed, 1991), caring (Swanson, 1991), and illness trajectory (Wiener & Dodd, 1993).

Duffy (2009) developed the quality-caring model, providing the APRN with a framework that emphasizes the less visible value of nursing—that is, caring. This is often the less obvious value, but one that guides practice, provides a foundation for quality care, improved outcomes, and patient satisfaction, and supports research. In her model, the evidence-based care environment in health care today is merged with the caring qualities and attributes of nursing. Caring values, attitudes, knowledge, and behaviors will guide and drive the process of the care plan and interventions, and will establish the foundation for strong relationships. The APRN patient–nurse relationship is primary and includes all interactions and interventions for which the APRNs are accountable and will implement autonomously. To be a successful APRN leader, collaborative relationships are necessary and include "those activities and responsibilities that nurses share with the members of the interprofessional healthcare team" (Duffy, 2009, p. 82).

Many nurses give little thought to the tenets that guide their practice; however, these philosophical underpinnings have a profound impact on the nature and scope of their practice. When APRNs have a theory-guided practice, they improve the care being provided by offering structure, efficiency in regard to continuity of care, and higher quality of care and improved health outcomes. The discipline of nursing, including professionalism, accountability, and APRN autonomy as a care provider, is supported with a nursing theory–guided practice. Often, an APRN practices and applies clinical decision making within a nursing framework but is not consciously aware of doing so. Nurses have an ethical and moral responsibility to practice nursing with a consciously defined approach to care. The theoretical or conceptual model used by a nurse provides the basis for making the complex decisions that are crucial in the delivery of high-quality nursing care. In this regard, Smith (1995) stated the following:

> The core of advanced practice nursing lies within nursing's disciplinary perspective on human-environment and caring interrelationships that facilitate health and healing. This core is delineated specifically in the philosophic and theoretic foundations of nursing. (p. 3)

Thus, nursing theory is an important component of APRN education. Nursing is a practice discipline, and theories achieve importance in relation to their impact on nursing care. Recently, attempts have been made to relate nursing theories to practice and to begin testing these theories. However, only minimal testing of these theories in practice settings has occurred. The number of theoretical nursing studies, particularly studies examining the efficacy of nursing interventions, is an indication of the apparent separation of theories and practice that has characterized much of nursing practice. As DNP programs continue to mature and develop, it is anticipated that the application gap between theories and practice will narrow.

The theoretical or conceptual framework that an APRN selects and uses has a major impact on the assessments that are made and the nature of the interventions that are chosen to achieve individual outcomes. Gordon (2007) and Johnson (1989) have noted the profound impact a nurse's theoretical perspective can have on a nursing practice. Gordon (1987) stated the following:

> One's conceptual perspective on clients and on nursing's goals strongly determines what kinds of things one assesses. Everyone has a perspective, whether in conscious awareness or not. Problems can arise if the perspective "in the head" is inconsistent with the actions taken during assessment. Information collection has to be logically related to one's view of nursing. (p. 69)

A conceptual model provides the practitioner with a general perspective or a mind-set of what is important to observe, which in turn provides the basis for making nursing diagnoses and selecting nursing interventions.

INCORPORATING NURSING INTO ADVANCED PRACTICE NURSING

Guaranteeing that APRNs view the provision of health care from a nursing perspective has implications for graduate curricula. The American Association of Colleges of Nursing (AACN, 2006) includes nursing theory as a component of its document *Essentials of Doctoral Education for Advanced Practice Nursing*. Students also need assistance in utilizing this theoretical content in their practice. Faculty and preceptors who model this approach for advanced practice nursing students are critical for helping them integrate theory into practice and to build bridges over the theory to practice gap that currently exists.

APRNs provide health care to many individuals and populations in diverse care environments and settings. APRNs have the opportunity to make major contributions to advance the nursing profession. By focusing on the nursing elements of health care, APRNs have the opportunity to demonstrate to the public and to policy makers the unique and significant contributions that nursing has on health outcomes. In using nursing frameworks rather than the medical model as the focus of practice, APRNs provide the public with a distinct and adjunctive model of care rather than a substitutive model (i.e., replacing physicians). APRNs may carry out activities that have traditionally been a part of medicine, but the manner, approach, style, and performance of these activities by APRNs need to be translated into the realm of nursing.

Acknowledgment

The author acknowledges the contributions of Michaelene Jansen to this chapter in the previous edition.

REFERENCES

Alligood, M. R., & Marriner-Tomey, A. (2005). *Nursing theory: Utilization and application.* St. Louis, MO: Mosby.

American Association of Colleges of Nursing. (2006). *Essentials of doctoral education for advanced practice nursing.* Washington, DC: Author.

American Nurses Association. (2004). *Nursing: Scope and standards of practice.* Washington, DC: Author.

American Nurses Association. (2010). *Nursing's social policy statement: The essence of the profession.* Washington, DC: Author.

APRN Consensus Workgroup & APRN Joint Dialogue Group. (2008). *Consensus model for APRN regulation: Licensure, accreditation, certification & education.* Retrieved from http://www.aacn.nche.edu/Education/pdf/APRNReport. pdf

Benner, P. (1998). *Nursing as a caring profession.* Paper presented at the meeting of the American Academy of Nursing, Kansas City, MO.

Bulechek, G. M., Butcher, H. K, Dochterman, J. M., & Wagner, C. (Eds.). (2013). *Nursing interventions classification (NIC)* (6th ed.). St. Louis, MO: Elsevier.

Burman, M. E., Hart, A. M., Conley, V., Brown, J., Sherard, P., & Clarke, P. N. (2009). Reconceptualizing the core of nurse practitioner education and practice. *Journal of the American Academy of Nurse Practitioners, 21,* 11–17.

Chism, L. (2013). *The doctor of nursing practice: A guidebook for role development and professional issues* (2nd ed.). Burlington, MA: Jones and Bartlett.

Duffy, J. (2009). *Quality caring in nursing: Applying theory to clinical practice, education and leadership.* New York, NY: Springer Publishing.

Gadow, S. (1980). Body and self: A dialectic. *The Journal of Medicine and Philosophy, 5,* 172–184.

Gordon, M. (1987). *Nursing diagnosis.* New York, NY: McGraw-Hill.

Gordon, M. (2007). *Nursing diagnoses* (11th ed.). Sudbury, MA: Jones and Bartlett.

Hagedorn, S., & Quinn, A. (2004). Theory-based nursing practitioner practice: Caring-in-action. *Topics in Advanced Practice Nursing e-Journal, 4*(4), 1–7.

Henderson, V. (1966). *Nature of nursing.* New York: Macmillan.

Johnson, D. E. (1980). The behavioral system model for nursing. In J. P. Riehl & C. Roy (Eds.), *Conceptual models for nursing practice* (2nd ed., pp. 207–216). New York, NY: Appleton-Century-Crofts.

Johnson, D.E. (1989). The nature of a science of nursing. *Nursing Outlook, 7*(4), 198–200.

Johnson, M., Bulechek, G., Butcher, H., McCloskey Dochterman, J., Maas, M., Moorehead, S., Swanson, E. (2005) *NANDA, NOC and NIC linkages* (2nd ed). St. Louis, MO: Mosby.

King, I. M. (1971). *Toward a theory of nursing.* New York, NY: Wiley.

Leininger, M. (1990). Historic and epistemologic dimensions of care and caring with future directions. In J. Stevenson & T. Tripp-Reimer (Eds.), *Knowledge about care and caring* (pp. 19–31). Kansas City, MO: American Academy of Nursing.

Levine, M. (1967). The four conservation principles of nursing. *Nursing Forum, 6*(1), 45–59.

Marrs, J. A., & Lowry, L. W. (2009). Nursing theory and practice: Connecting the dots. In P. G. Reed & N. C. Shearer (Eds.), *Perspectives on nursing theory* (5th ed, pp. 3–12). Philadelphia, PA: Lippincott Williams & Wilkins.

Meleis, A. I. (2011). *Theoretical nursing: Development and progress* (5th ed.). Philadelphia, PA: Lippincott Williams & Wilkin.

Mishel, M. H. (1990). Reconceptualization of the uncertainty in illness theory. *Image: Journal of Nursing Scholarship, 22,* 256–262.

Myss, C. (1996). *Anatomy of the spirit.* New York, NY: Three Rivers Press.

Myss, C. (2004). *Channeling grace in your every day life.* New York, NY: Free Press.

National Organization of Nurse Practitioner Faculties (NONPF). (2012). *Nurse practitioner core competencies.* Washington, DC: Author. Retrieved from https://c.ymcdn.com/sites/nonpf.siteym.com/resource/resmgr/competencies/npcorecompetenciesfinal2012.pdf

Neuman, B. (1974). The Betty Neuman health care system model: A total person approach to individual problems. In J. P Riehl & C. Roy (Eds.), *Conceptual approach to individual problems* (pp. 99–114). New York, NY: Appleton-Century-Crofts.

Newman, M. A. (1984). Looking at the whole. *American Journal of Nursing, 84,* 1496–1499.

Newman, M. A., Sime, A. M., & Corcoran-Perry, S. A. (1991). The focus of the discipline of nursing. *Advances in Nursing Science, 14*(1), 1–6.

Nightingale, F. (1992). *Notes on nursing.* Philadelphia, PA: Lippincott. (Originally published 1859).

Nojima, Y. (1989, May). *The structural formula of nursing practice: A bridge to new nursing.* Paper presented at the 19th Quadrennial Congress of the International Congress of Nurses, Seoul, Korea.

Nojima, Y., Tomikana, T., Makabe, S., & Snyder, M. (2003). Defining characteristics of expertise in Japanese clinical nursing using the Delphi technique. *Nursing Health Science, 5*(1), 3–11.

North American Nursing Diagnosis Association International (NANDA). (2015). *Nursing diagnoses: Definitions and classification 2015-2017* (10th ed). Ames, IA: Wiley-Blackwell.

Olson, J., & Hanchett, E. (1997). Nurse-expressed empathy, individual outcomes, and development of a middle-range theory. *Image—The Journal of Nursing Scholarship, 29,* 71–76.

Orem, D. E. (1980). *Nursing: Concepts of practice.* New York, NY: McGraw-Hill.

Polk, L. V. (1997). Toward a middle-range theory of resilience. *Advances in Nursing Science, 19*(3), 1–13.

Reed, P G. (1991). Toward a nursing theory of self-transcendence: Deductive reformulation using developmental theories. *Advances in Nursing Science, 13*(4), 64–71.

Riehl-Sisca, J. (1989). *Conceptual models for nursing practice.* Norwalk, CT: Appleton & Lange.

Rogers, M. (1970). *An introduction to the theoretical basis of nursing.* Philadelphia, PA: F.A. Davis.

Rounds, L., Zych, J., & Mallary, L. (2013). The consensus model for regulation of APRNs: Implications for nurse practitioners. *Journal of the American Associate of Nurse Practitioners, 25*(4), 180–185.

Roy, C. (1984). *Introduction to nursing: An adaptation model.* Englewood Cliffs, NJ: Prentice Hall.

Russell, G. E., & Fawcett, J. (2005). The conceptual model for nursing and health policy revisited. *Policy, Politics and Nursing Practice, 6*(4), 319–326.

Schoenhoefer, S. O., & Boykin, A. (1993). Nursing as caring: An emerging general theory of nursing. In M. E. Parker (Ed.), *Patterns of nursing theories in practice* (pp. 82–92). New York: National League of Nursing.

Smith, M. C. (1995). The core of advanced practice nursing. *Nursing Science Quarterly, 8*(1), 2–3.

Stanley, J. (2011). *Advanced practice nursing: Emphasizing common roles* (3rd ed.). Philadelphia, PA: F.A. Davis.

Swanson, K. M. (1991). Empirical development of a middle-range theory of caring. *Nursing Research, 40*, 161–166.

Watson, J. (1988). *Nursing: Human science and human care: A theory of nursing.* New York: National League for Nursing.

Wiener, C. L., & Dodd, M. J. (1993). Coping amid uncertainty: An illness trajectory. *Scholarly Inquiry in Nursing Practice, 7*(1), 17–30.

Younger, J. B. (1991). A theory of mastery. *Advances in Nursing Science, 14*(1), 76–89.

Zaccagnini, M., & Waud White, K. (2014). *The doctor of nursing practice essentials and new model for advanced practice nursing* (2nd ed.). Burlington, MA: Jones and Bartlett.

Jana Gail Zwilling

3

MULTIFACETED ROLES
OF THE APRN

Before delving into the various roles of the advanced practice registered nurse (APRN), the impact of the Patient Protection and Affordable Care Act (Public Law 111-148, 2010), and the Health Care and Education Affordability Reconciliation Act (Public Law 111-152) on the APRN role will be reviewed. These laws will be collectively referred to as the Patient Protection and Affordable Care Act (ACA) in this chapter. The ACA was signed into law on March 23, 2010. This comprehensive health care legislation is the biggest change in the United States health care system since the creation of Medicare and Medicaid programs in 1965. The ACA is anticipated to provide insurance coverage for an additional 32 million previously uninsured Americans. This new regulation has left the U.S. health care system in an uproar regarding reimbursement, access to care, and lack of health care providers. These new issues reflect that some major changes need to occur in the current system in order to cost-effectively provide care to an increased patient population. The changes associated with the implementation of the ACA have provided an opportunity for APRNs to remove legislative and regulatory barriers and become major players in the redesign of the health care system.

The implementation of the ACA (2010) has created a necessity for the doctorate of nursing practice (DNP)–prepared APRN. The DNP degree focuses on preparing APRNs not only for practice but also to be leaders in practice improvements. The DNP interprets original research into clinical application, health policy changes, and improvement of clinical outcomes with interdisciplinary collaboration (American Association of Colleges of Nursing [AACN], 2006). The ACA includes provisions for strengthening primary care, ensuring quality care, and reducing the costs associated with health care. DNP-prepared APRNs can use their practice background and systems thinking to initiate new processes and policies to better serve the potential increased number of patients. The public has also been enlightened to the role of the APRN in health care delivery via the Institute of Medicine's (IOM's) report on the future of nursing (Committee for the Robert Wood Johnson Foundation Initiative on the Future of Nursing, 2011). Whether it be the certified nurse practitioner (CNP) in an underserved area, the certified nurse-midwife (CNM) providing access to obstetric care, the certified registered nurse anesthetist (CRNA) providing a cost-effective solution to anesthetic care, or the clinical nurse specialist (CNS) maximizing the specialty care provided at the patient bedside, APRNs are poised to be forces of change in the future of health care.

Traditionally, the roles of the APRN have been clinically focused, as clinician, patient advocate, case manager, consultant, and collaborator, to name a few. Other roles have been underlying for many years, but more recently these have pushed into the limelight. These are the roles of leader, educator, researcher, and independent clinician. Ultimately, the APRN's foundation is that of a clinician—and always will be. With health care reform, we need to keep our clinical roots but must expand to best serve our patients and profession. This chapter will examine the various roles, focusing on incorporating them into the whole and consummate professional.

APRN ROLES

Several APRN nursing models have reviewed and researched roles for this growing profession. Hamric's integrative model of advanced nursing practice is a very comprehensive model that includes primary criteria for the APRN as well as central and core competencies (Hamric, Spross, & Hanson, 1996). Primary criteria included in this model are graduate education, certification in the specialty, and a focus on clinical practice. Core competencies referenced by Hameric et al. are direct clinical practice, collaboration, guidance and coaching, evidence-based practice, ethical decision making, consultation, and leadership. This model also incorporates outside elements affecting APRN practice. A framework for advanced practice nursing developed by Brown (1998, 2005) looked at the external issues, roles, APRN scope and competencies, as well as outcomes of APRN role. One model, the Strong Model of Advanced Practice (Ackerman, Norsen, Martin, Wiedrich, & Kitzman, 1996), is one of the few that has been tested for validity (Mick & Ackerman, 2000). This model has also been supported throughout the literature and used in other research, such as the development of a role-delineation tool by Chang, Gardner, Duffied, and Ramis (2012).

The Strong Model breaks down APRN roles by service parameters. These parameters include direct comprehensive care, support of systems, education, research, and publication and professional leadership. This model, with some modification, is used to further define APRN roles in this chapter.

Direct Care

Patient care is, and should remain, the priority of the APRN. Within this realm, several roles emerge, including patient advocate, educator to the patient and family, case manager, consultant, and collaborator. All these roles rely on APRNs using evidence-based practice as a basis for their care and decision-making processes. APRNs need to be staunch supporters of continued research and integrate these findings into practice. The continued advancement of health care depends on a culture of support for new and innovative ideas (Ackerman et al., 1996).

Patient Advocate

Advocacy for patients must remain fundamental to the practice of nursing. It is the underpinning of the nurse–patient relationship. *Advocacy* is defined as a way of being in a relationship that sees the patient as a whole human being in his or her experience with health and promotes the uniqueness of the patient (Nelson, 1998). Advocacy has progressed to being a guardian of the patient's rights and freedoms of choice. Although several other elements may be included in advocacy, a nurse's advocacy is guided by respect for the individual (Hameric, 2000; Nelson 1999).

Advocacy can be viewed from a variety of perspectives. Nelson (1998) maintains that advocacy includes legal advocacy, moral–ethical advocacy, substitutive advocacy, political advocacy, spiritual advocacy, advocacy for nursing, and advocacy for community health.

In legal advocacy, the nurse supports the patient's legal rights, such as informed consent or the right to refuse treatment. This may include ensuring that all patients have a copy of the institution's bill of rights. Moral–ethical advocacy requires that the nurse respect the patient's values and support decisions that are consistent with those values, such as decisions regarding abortion. In substitutive advocacy, if the patient is unable to express an opinion, the nurse should continue to respect the rights of the patient or surrogate and support any wishes that the patient may have previously expressed. In spiritual advocacy, the APRN ensures that the patient has access to spiritual support such as clergy and that the plan of care includes the spiritual aspects of care.

Advocacy must occur for all patients. APRNs should advocate for all patients to complete living wills and advance directives to make sure that health care issues are well documented and patient wishes are respected. On occasion, issues of patient competency may arise in areas such as substitutive advocacy and moral–ethical advocacy. When competency is a concern, the APRN must be familiar with laws governing competence, including criteria for the assessment of competence. At the same time, the APRN should be instrumental in establishing policies for direct action when a patient is judged incompetent. In such a case, the APRN must communicate the patient's expectations, if they are known, to the surrogate and/or the patient's family to support any requests and decisions to be made based on the patient's past recommendations. Because there can be confusion and conflict among family, friends, surrogates, and even health care professionals during these times, the APRN should have no reservation about convening family–patient conferences and implementing ethics committee evaluations if questions or controversies arise.

Advocacy carries a significant ethical dimension; therefore, principles of ethics can help to evaluate a nurse's effectiveness (Nelson, 1998). Pinch (1996) points out that some ethical principles may conflict. For example, the principle of autonomy (self-determination) could clash with distributive justice (fair, equitable distribution of goods or services) if the patient's decisions were to affect the community's greater need or safety. If a patient requested no treatment and is discharged with a dangerous communicable disease that may infect the community, or if a patient demanded resources that jeopardized the financial or medical resources of a community, the patient's autonomy may be at risk of being overshadowed by what is best for the majority. In maintaining advocacy, the APRN would need to be sure that there was, indeed, a conflict in distributive justice and no prejudices existed toward an individual or group.

Concerns exist regarding the ability of a nurse to be an advocate given our current health care systems and associated cost containment measures (Donagrandi & Eddy, 2000; Nelson, 1998; Watson, 1989). Is the APRN in a position to maintain advocacy despite the demands of the system? Nelson (1998) contends that the APRN can rise above these constraints. It is believed that the APN is in a unique position of influence through interaction with other team members, ensuring advocacy through policy formulation that directs patient care and through legislative involvement. It is also critical that the APRN be well versed in the areas of evidence-based practice, standards of care, ethics policies, accreditation criteria, nursing licensure regulations, and professional association standards that can help support an APRN's advocacy position.

Educator to the Patient and Family

Advanced practice nursing education makes the APRN an excellent resource for current knowledge in content areas, supportive resources, research findings, and the implementation of evidence-based practice. This is imperative when educating patients and their families. Today's health care consumers are very knowledgeable about their health and medical treatment. Assessment of this knowledge base is essential. Patients are using the Internet as a primary source of information. Some sources have information that is directed to health care professionals and is more likely to be reliable. The information that individuals gather is generated from a wide variety of Internet sources, such as chat rooms, blogs, non-evidence-based medical sites, or sites with medical opinions from nonmedical personnel. Information also comes from advertisements, brochures, newspapers, television, health kiosks, nontraditional care providers, and family and friends. This information can be skewed, inaccurate, or incomplete. The

APRN should take the time to access and review these sources to appraise the accuracy and reliability of the information that is being provided. Patients may experience fears or preconceived ideas regarding care strategies and inappropriate outcomes. These apprehensions can either motivate them to become very knowledgeable or to remain very uninformed about their health concern. Just as you might ask students for content references, the APRN should ask patients for their information sources.

The APRN needs to make a point of screening related health information made available by the health care organizations as well. Most printed educational content should be constructed at a fifth- to eighth-grade reading level. Background, color, and print format are all considerations. Many patients are overwhelmed simply by their diagnosis, much less their medication, treatment course, or plan of care. Printed information can be given to a patient to reinforce verbal information.

Case Manager

Case management is becoming a more common dimension of the APRN role with the enactment of the ACA. This role is greatly expanding with the implementation of more fixed or bundled reimbursement and inclusion of more patients with preexisting conditions. Health care organizations are looking to APRN case managers to coordinate the care of these individuals to reduce costs while providing comprehensive care. Coffman (2001) describes case management as a collaborative process promoting quality care and cost-effective outcomes to specific patients and groups. Umbrell (2006) outlines the value of an advanced practice trauma case manager in orchestrating a comprehensive plan to reduce fragmentation of care and better utilization of resources. The key features of the case manager as outlined by Benoit (1996) include (a) standardized resources for a length of stay for selected patient care, caregiver, and system outcomes; (b) collaborative team practice among disciplines; (c) coordinated care over the course of an illness; (d) job enrichment for the caregiver; (e) patient and physician satisfaction with the care; and (f) minimized costs to the institution.

Taylor (1999) initially described the two primary types of case management as (a) the patient-focused model, which supports the patient throughout the continuum of care and helps the patient access health care, and (b) the system-focused model, which involves the service environment and is structured for cost containment of a specific group of patients and use of critical pathways for cost-effective outcomes. However, Taylor advanced her model of comprehensive case management that incorporates elements of cultural competency, consumer empowerment, clinical framework, and multidisciplinary practice in addition to other activities of assessment, service, planning, plan implementation, coordination and monitoring, advocacy, and termination. The focus in health care is on patient empowerment and quality service based on process improvement, outcome measurements, and performance-based expectations. In the past, case management was associated with the utilization of clinical pathways to drive the plan of care—therefore focusing on process—but the focus since the early 2000s has been on outcome measures. Taylor asserts that this new model is optimal because it incorporates components of both patient and system models to ensure that the patient receives needed services.

Ethical concerns have persisted as to how APRNs who are active in nursing and case management can remain advocates for patients in the new accountable care organizations (ACO) and patient-centered medical home models. The disconnect is maintaining the five principles of ethical behavior while attempting to follow insurance, reimbursement, and other regulations that will come up as a result of this new legislation. The five principles include autonomy, beneficence, nonmaleficence, justice, and fidelity. These are basic principles we, as nurses, learn from the very beginning and need to bring forth these principles despite other overreaching pressures.

The utilization of APRNs as case managers has been advocated by multiple authors (Donagrandi & Eddy, 2000; Taylor, 1999). APRNs have enhanced capabilities in interdisciplinary coordination, advanced clinical decision making, autonomy, synthesis, and critical thinking. The APRN expertise would also be valuable in the development of outcome standards, communication and coordination among disciplines, and analysis of patient care trends. In addition, a focus on complex patient populations requiring extended lengths of stay or long-term care resources are very ably managed by the APRN (Abdellah, Fawcett, Kane, Dick, & Chen, 2005).

Consultant

Certainly consultation could be considered a primary vehicle for the dissemination of an APRN's expertise. Caplan (1970) notes that consultation can be described by the type of patient served, the type of activities requested in the consultation, the method of consultation (formal or informal) provided, and the relationship of the consultant to the organization (internal or external). Consultation is categorized in four ways: (a) patient-centered case consultation, (b) consultee-centered case consultation, (c) program-centered administrative consultation, and (d) consultee-centered administrative consultation. In relation to direct care we primarily look at patient-centered case consultation here.

Consultation requires much planning before the actual consultation meeting. Lippitt and Lippitt (1978) provide a six-phase guide that has been used in a variety of consultation situations: (a) contact and entry; (b) formulation of a contract and establishment of a helping relationship; (c) problem identification and diagnostic analysis; (d) goal-setting and planning; (e) action and feedback; and (f) contract completion, continuity, support, and termination.

In APRN practice, patient-centered consultation often uses an informal approach in phases (a) and (b) because of the casual nature and frequency of this type of consult in nurse-to-APRN interaction (Caplan, 1970). Although this informal approach can be educational and save time, Manian and

Janssen (1996) warn that the consultant and patient's care can be vulnerable to incomplete information and examination, especially if the consult is of a complex nature. It is always important to establish areas of responsibility for the consultant and consultee. The APRN who elects to function as a consultant must respect the confines of a consultant's practice and the authority that role assigns to others.

Consultation is a function into which the individual APRN must evolve. It is based on the APRN's knowledge, experience, and confidence. The beginning APRN will generally first serve in the area of direct practice and patient-centered consultations. Holt (1984) describes an evolution of development with many of the areas of consultation occurring much later in the professional development of the APRN. Certainly, the beginning APRN will need time in the application of newly acquired skills to be recognized as competent by others and to develop the personal confidence to provide expert consultation.

How the APRN consultant evolves will depend on the definition and parameters of the patient group, the framework of the consultant's practice, and the inherent rewards for maintaining consultation as part of the APRN practice. Over time, consultation should demonstrate growth, diversity, and mentorship as the practice is refined.

In the early years of practice, an APRN may choose to remain in a consultation area in which the parameters are those of a defined patient group with specific known problems. The APRN should always retain this patient-oriented consultation because it is a way to gain and explore new knowledge and a mechanism for implementing evidence-based practice.

Collaborator

Collaboration integrates the individual perspectives and expertise of various team members on behalf of providing quality patient care (Resnick & Bonner, 2003). Interdisciplinary collaboration has become a hot topic in today's health care environment. With escalating demands and the prospect of a rise in chronic illness, a cooperative effort among health care disciplines will be the most effective means to provide quality care.

One of the key messages in the IOM's report *The Future of Nursing* (2011) is, "Nurses should be full partners, with physicians and other health professionals, in redesigning health care in the United States" (p. 4). The ACA also emphasizes interdisciplinary collaboration as a means to provide cost-effective and comprehensive care. Matthews and Brown (2013) outline a collaborative health management model for effectively managing patients with chronic disease. This model includes the APRN, physician, registered nurse, medical assistant, pharmacist, social worker, mental health provider, and specialty consultants. The authors focus on goals of promoting patient self-management, preventive or proactive care, and close follow-up.

Unfortunately, there are varied thoughts about the definition of this collaborative process. Influences on these discrepancies include provider gender, level of professionalism, environment, and the traditional push for autonomy in the nursing field. Fast-paced clinical environments and traditional hierarchical roles contribute to poor communication across the disciplines. APRNs will need to lead the way to introduce the collaborative process as a professional behavior and best practice for the care of patients.

Systems Support

Within the paradigm of the health care system, the APRN needs to be a leader, a mentor, and a nursing advocate. These three roles ultimately support optimal and innovative patient care practices. The roles are so intertwined that it is difficult to dissect one from the others. This section presents the three as a cumulative role of leader.

The U.S. Army defines *leadership* as "the process of influencing people by providing purpose, direction, and motivation to accomplish the mission and improve the organization" (ADP, 2012, p. 1). There are many levels of both formal and informal leaders within the military structure. Some of these are by virtue of the position alone, which does not always constitute a good leader. Others, although not necessarily in a leadership position, clearly match the definition of a leader. An effective leader earns respect by setting the example, promoting an open and caring environment, being an inspiration to others, using resources wisely, and creating a strong and supportive team. The role of leader is relatively new and extremely important for the APRN. With the transition to DNP-prepared APRNs, the career field is now fully equipped to be the "tip of the spear" for change in our health care system.

The DNP-prepared APRN, although not a role in itself, contributes significantly to the advancement of APRNs in the leadership role. The AACN DNP essentials specifies two key components geared toward leadership. The first is "Organizational and Systems Leadership for Quality Improvement and Systems Thinking." The key here is emphasizing practice while working to improve health outcomes and patient safety on a practice-level or system-wide basis. The second essential relating to leadership is "Health Care Policy for Advocacy in Health Care." The DNP-prepared APRN has the capabilities to broaden the scope of nursing leadership and take on public and nursing profession policy issues (Ehrenreich, 2002).

The National Organization of Nurse Practitioner Faculties (NONPF) outlines nurse practitioner leadership with six core competencies: (a) initiating and guiding change, (b) fostering collaboration with multiple stakeholders, (c) using critical and reflective thinking, (d) advocating for improved access and cost-effective health care, (e) developing and implementing innovations, and (f) using effective communication (NONPF, 2011). The other APRN disciplines have similar competency statements. The CNS [clinical nurse specialist] Systems Leadership Competency has 13 issues addressed within the leadership scope, including system change, fiscal and budgetary decision making, evaluation of the effect of nursing, dissemination of outcomes of change, provision of clinically competent care by team, assessments performed at the systems level, and interdisciplinary collaboration (National Association of Clinical Nurse Specialists

[NACNS], 2010). The American Association of Nurse Anesthetists (AANA, 2013, p. 1) states, "Nurse anesthetists are innovative leaders in anesthesia care deliver, integrating progressive critical thinking and ethical judgment." The American College of Nurse Midwives (ACNM) delineates leadership competencies as professional responsibilities of the CNM. Some of the outlined responsibilities include knowledge of national and international issues and trends, support of legislation and policy initiatives, and knowledge of issues and trends in health care policy and systems (ACNM, 2012).

There are obviously varied levels of leadership. The APRN is well suited for this role at all levels, including clinical, system, community, national, and international. Clinically, the APRN is automatically placed in a leadership role as a result of preparation at the advanced level. The knowledge base of the clinician is the foundation of clinical leadership and ultimately of other echelons as well. As a knowledgeable clinician, the APRN can lead collaborative teams for the improvement of care delivery and outcomes. The health care system can also be an important arena for the APRN to lead. APRNs have a unique view of the patient, community, and health care system needs and thus can bring needed insight to the administration of hospitals, clinics, and other health care delivery formats. On the community, national, and international levels, the APRN can be involved and lead various professional organizations and influence health care policy. This is a very important area for APRNs to be involved. It can be very time-consuming and frustrating but ultimately very rewarding as APRNs advocate not only for improved health care but also for the nursing profession. APRNs make a huge impact not only at the bedside but also by using that clinical knowledge to induce change.

The IOM report *The Future of Nursing* (2011) emphasizes mentoring as an important part of the leadership role for APRNs. For example, APRNs can take the lead in fostering growth and promoting forward thinking in new or less-experienced nursing staff and APRNs. Some facilities or programs have introduced formal mentoring programs for nurse leaders. In these programs a senior nursing leader will partner with a newer nursing leader for a period of time to guide the newer nursing leader in his or her role (Bally, 2007). It has also been suggested that APRN education programs include more of a focus on leadership qualities. Superior leaders require not only a strong clinical background but also formal education on leadership models, behaviors, and communication in interpersonal and large scale formats (Adeniran, Bhattacharya, & Adeniran, 2012). Bedside mentoring would be the most effective for the majority of APRNs. However, in our fast-paced system, new trends are emerging. Mentoring can take place via e-mail, social networking sites, and blogs. Ultimately, however the relationship is carried out, it is most important to have a good rapport between the individuals and promote an open and caring environment for learning.

Advocacy for nursing directs the APRN to support other nurses in their professional growth and to contribute to the evolution of the nursing profession (Nelson, 1998). Nelson suggests that this is an opportunity for APRNs to facilitate and empower other nurses through leadership, education, and modeling standards for practice. APRNs are in a unique position of influence through interaction with other team members, ensuring advocacy through policy formulation that directs practice and through legislative involvement. In addition, APRNs are versed in the areas of evidence-based practice, standards of care, ethics policies, accreditation criteria, nursing licensure regulations, and professional association standards that can help to support an APRN's advocacy position.

Educator

The APRN has a wealth of experiences for developing standards for practice, strategies for use of equipment and procedures, assessment of patient issues and concerns, and evaluations of nursing staff capabilities and limitations. Advanced practice nursing education makes the APRN a resource for current knowledge in content areas, supportive resources, research findings, and implementation of evidence-based practice. When providing education to students and staff, APRNs can provide sound clinical examples that enhance the application of content. APRNs may find it helpful to seek assistance from their colleagues in academic settings when they are initially developing educational content. It takes considerable knowledge and skill to develop a sound teaching–learning plan.

Although isolated teaching events can be provided, a planned content series is most effective for ensuring learner outcomes and competencies. When planning for the dissemination, an assessment first needs to be completed to determine what knowledge is needed so that the APRN can focus the content. This may be guided through planned curriculum, observed problems in patient care, standards or protocols for practice, or common patient questions, to name a few. The assessment identifies what type of learner outcomes (competencies) are to be achieved.

When the assessment is complete, the APRN needs to develop content objectives to achieve these outcomes. Guidelines for the development of objectives were established by Bloom (1956), who divided objectives into three domains of learning: cognitive, affective, and psychomotor. Content objectives are used to guide the development of the learning tools, whether this be a one-on-one instruction, large live lecture, or online asynchronous format. The format needs to properly fit the learning audience to provide the optimal environment for achieving the prescribed outcomes. Demonstrating outcomes or competencies is consistent in evaluating whether learning has occurred. Identification could be done with a written test, skill demonstration, or return presentation of data. Support content such as handouts or video may also need to be developed. These, too, should reflect the level of learning being addressed. With staff, the APRN has the unique opportunity of continuing to work beside a staff member. In this way, a staff member can continue to pursue clarification and assistance, and the APRN can evaluate the staff member for his or her grasp of the information.

With regard to APRN education, there is a trend toward competency-based programs. This concept began in the 1970s and defines educational goals by precise and measurable descriptions of knowledge, skills, and attitudes the students should have at the culmination of their program (Savage, 1993). Competencies can generally be divided into three cores: APRN, role, and population. Each APRN organization and/or certifying body delineates these a little differently. NONPF approved the DNP as the entry level for NP practice in 2008 (NONPF, 2010a). Within this endorsement is a listing of "core competencies." NONPF states that it is more valuable to have successful achievement of these competencies than to be concerned strictly with the number of clinical hours performed (NONPF, 2010b). There are nine core competencies for the NP graduate regardless of population focus (NONPF, 2012). These include the topics of leadership, scientific foundation, quality, practice inquiry, technology and information literacy, policy, health delivery system, ethics, and independent practice. Released in 2013 are the specific competencies for each NP population focus area, including family across the life span, neonatal, acute care pediatric, primary care pediatric, psychiatric/mental health, and women's health/gender related.

The NACNS produced a similar document in 2010, listing comprehensive, entry-level competencies expected of graduate-level CNSs (NACNS, 2010). The competencies are reflective of all CNS specialty areas and are divided into three categories: direct patient care, consultation, and systems leadership. The Council on Accreditation of Nurse Anesthesia Educational Programs has recently approved *Trial Standards for Accreditation of Nurse Anesthesia Programs,* which is a practice doctorate standards document (CANAEP, 2014). The competencies for the CRNA specialty are very skill based. This recent document provides a guideline for minimum numbers of cases and clinical hours, as well as preferred number of cases. The cases are broken down into three categories: patient physical status, special cases, and anatomic categories. The variety of anesthesia methods and skill techniques are also addressed (CANAEP, 2014). CNMs have the *Core Competencies for Basic Midwifery Practice,* approved by the American College of Nurse-Midwives in 2012 (ACNM, 2012). This document outlines the midwifery management process as well as skills and professional responsibilities.

APRN programs are using the competencies outlined by their organizations in developing and monitoring their curricula. The core competencies for each type of APRN can be used as a baseline for new clinician performance. Some programs are even using these competencies as criteria for progression and graduation. The competency measures can include, but are not limited to, clinical portfolios, peer reviews, and examinations.

SUMMARY

For the APRN to fully participate in these roles, administration needs to be educated about the many aspects of the APRN's position and the benefits that accrue to patient care and the institution in supporting expanded

APRN practice. The APRN should market these capabilities to people and groups at all levels—from patients to legislators. Although providing direct patient care is valuable and rewarding, the APRN can continue to evolve and actually have greater effect in patient care, community and social health, and the development of nursing as a profession by pursuing advanced APRN roles. Whether the APRN works as part of a practice or in a separate position, the opportunity to function in these advanced roles will give the APRN personal satisfaction, enhance the care of patients, and contribute to the profession of nursing.

Acknowledgment

The author acknowledges the contributions of Mary Zwgart-Stauffacher to this chapter in the previous edition.

REFERENCES

Abdellah, L, Fawcett, J., Kane, R., Dick, K., & Chen, J. (2005). The development and psychometric testing of the Evercare Nurse Practitioner Role and Activity Scale (ENPRAS). *Journal of the American Academy of Nurse Practitioners, 17*(1), 21–26.

Ackerman, M. H., Norsen, L., Martin, B., Wiedrich, J., & Kitzman, H. J. (1996). Development of a model of advanced practice. *American Journal of Critical Care, 5*(1), 68–73. Retrieved from http://ezproxy.undmedlibrary.org/login?url=http://search.ebscohost.com.ezproxy.undmedlibrary.org/login.aspx?direct=true&AuthType=ip,url,uid,cookie&db=c8h&AN=1996014089&site=ehost-live

Adeniran, R. K., Bhattacharya, A., & Adeniran, A. A. (2012). Professional excellence and career advancement in nursing: A conceptual framework for clinical leadership development. *Nursing Administration Quarterly, 36*(1), 41–51. Retrieved from http://ezproxy.undmedlibrary.org/login?url=http://search.ebscohost.com.ezproxy.undmedlibrary.org/login.aspx?direct=true&AuthType=ip,url,uid,cookie&db=c8h&AN=2011413424&site=ehost-live

ADP 6-22, Army Leadership, 8/2012. Retrieved from http://armypubs.army.mil/doctrine/DR_pubs/dr_a/pdf/adp6_22_new.pdf

American Association of Nurse Anesthetists (AANA). (2013). *Scope of nurse anesthesia practice.* Retrieved from http://www.aana.com/resources2/professionalpractice/Documents/PPM%20Scope%20of%20Nurse%20Anesthesia%20Practice.pdf

American Association of Colleges of Nursing (AACN). (2006). *The essentials of doctoral education for advanced nursing practice.* Washington, DC: Author.

American College of Nurse Midwives (ACNM). (2012). *Core competencies for basic midwifery practice.* Retrieved from http://www.midwife.org/ACNM/files/ACNMLibraryData/UPLOADFILENAME/000000000050/Core%20Comptencies%20Dec%202012.pdf

Bally, J. (2007). The role of nursing leadership in creating a mentoring culture in acute care environments. *Nursing Economic$, 25*(3), 143–149. Retrieved from http://ezproxy.undmedlibrary.org/login?url=http://search.ebscohost.com.ezproxy.undmedlibrary.org/login.aspx?direct=true&AuthType=ip,url,uid,cookie&db=c8h&AN=2009611159&site=ehost-live

Benoit, B. C. (1996). Case management and the advanced practice nurse. In J. Hickey, R. Ouimette, & S. Venegoni (Eds.), *Advanced practice nursing. Changing roles and clinical application* (pp. 107–125). Philadelphia, PA: Lippincott.

Bloom, B. S. (Ed.). (1956). *Taxonomy of educational objectives.* New York, NY: David McKay.

Brown, S. J. (1998). A framework for advanced practice nursing. *Journal of Professional Nursing, 14*(3), 157–164. Retrieved from http://ezproxy.undmedlibrary. org/login?url=http://search.ebscohost.com.ezproxy.undmedlibrary.org/ login.aspx?direct=true&AuthType=ip,url,uid,cookie&db=c8h&AN=199804 8077&site=ehost-live

Brown, S. J. (2005). Direct clinical practice. In A. B. Hamric, J. A. Spross, & C. M. Hanson (Eds.), *Advanced practice nursing: An integrative approach* (3rd ed., pp. 143–185). Philadelphia, PA: Elsevier Saunders.

Caplan, G. (1970). *The theory and practice of mental health consultation.* New York: Basic Books.

Chang, A. M., Gardner, G. E., Duffield, C., & Ramis, M. A. (2012). Advanced practice nursing role development: Factor analysis of a modified role delineation tool. *Journal of Advanced Nursing, 68*(6), 1369–1379.

Coffman, S. (2001). Examining advocacy and care management in managed care. *Pediatric Nursing, 23*(3), 287–289, 304.

Committee for the Robert Wood Johnson Foundation Initiative on the Future of Nursing, at the Institute of Medicine. (2011). *The future of nursing: Leading change, advancing health.* Washington, DC: National Academies Press. Retrieved from http://thefutureofnursing.org/sites/default/files/Future %20of%20Nursing%20Report_0.pdf

Council on Accreditation of Nurse Anesthesia Educational Programs (CANAEP). (2014). *2014 trial standards for accreditation of nurse anesthesia programs: Practice doctorate.* Retrieved on from http://home.coa.us.com/accreditation/ Documents/Practice%20Doctorate%20Standards%20Trial%20Standards_ May%202014.pdf

Donagrandi, M. A., & Eddy, M. (2000). Ethics of case management: Implications for advanced practice nursing. *Clinical Nurse Specialist: The Journal for Advanced Nursing Practice, 14*(5), 241–249. Retrieved from http://ezproxy. undmedlibrary.org/login?url=http://search.ebscohost.com.ezproxy. undmedlibrary.org/login.aspx?direct=true&AuthType=ip,url,uid,cookie& db=c8h&AN=2000075215&site=ehost-live

Ehrenreich, B. (2002). The emergence of nursing as a political force. In D. Mason, D. Leavitt, & M. Chaffee (Eds.), *Policy & politics in nursing and health care* (4th ed., pp. xxxiii–xxxvii. St. Louis, MO: Saunders.

Hamric, A. B. (2000). Ethics. What is happening to advocacy? *Nursing Outlook, 48*(3), 103–104. Retrieved from http://ezproxy.undmedlibrary.org/ login?url=http://search.ebscohost.com.ezproxy.undmedlibrary.org/login. aspx?direct=true&AuthType=ip,url,uid,cookie&db=c8h&AN=2000057150& site=ehost-live

Hamric, A. B., Spross, J. A., & Hanson, C.M. (1996). *Advanced practice nursing: An integrative approach.* Philadelphia, PA: W.B. Saunders.

Holt, F. (1984). A theoretical model for clinical specialist practice. *Nursing and Health Care, 5,* 445–449.

Institute of Medicine (IOM). (2011). *The future of nursing: Leading change, advancing health.* Washington, DC: National Academies Press.

Lippitt, G., & Lippitt, R. (1978). *The consulting process in action.* LaJolla, CA: University Associates.

Manian, F., & Janssen, D. (1996). Curbside consultation. A closer look at a common practice. *Journal of the American Medical Association, 275*(2), 145–147.

Matthews, S. W., & Brown, M. A. (2013). APRN expertise: The collaborative health management model. *Nurse Practitioner, 38*(1), 43–48. doi:10.1097/01. NPR.0000423382.33822.ab

Mick, D., & Ackerman, M. (2000). Advanced practice nursing role delineation in acute and critical care: Application of the Strong model of advanced practice. *Heart & Lung, 29*(3), 210–221.

National Association of Clinical Nurse Specialists. (2010). Clinical nurse specialist core competencies. Retrieved from http://www.nacns.org/docs/CNS CoreCompetenciesBroch.pdf

National Organization of Nurse Practitioner Faculties. (2010a). Eligibility for NP certification for nurse practitioner students in doctor of nursing practice programs. In: *Clinical education issues in preparing nurse practitioner students for independent practice: An ongoing series of papers.* Retrieved from http:// c.ymcdn.com/sites/www.nonpf.org/resource/resmgr/imported/clinical-educationissuespprfinalapril2010.pdf

National Organization of Nurse Practitioner Faculties. (2010b). Clinical hours for nurse practitioner preparation in doctor of nursing practice programs. In: *Clinical education issues in preparing nurse practitioner students for independent practice: An ongoing series of papers.* Retrieved from http:// c.ymcdn.com/sites/www.nonpf.org/resource/resmgr/imported/ clinicaleducationissuespprfinalapril2010.pdf

National Organization of Nurse Practitioner Faculties. (2012). *Nurse practitioner core competencies.* Retrieved http://c.ymcdn.com/sites/www.nonpf.org/resource/ resmgr/competencies/npcorecompetenciesfinal2012.pdf

Nelson, M. (1998). Advocacy. In M. Snyder & R. Lundquist (Eds.), *Complementary/ alternative therapies in nursing* (3rd ed., pp. 337–352). New York, NY: Springer Publishing.

Nelson, M. (1999). Client advocacy. In M. Snyder & M. Mirr (Eds.), *Advanced practice nursing: A guide to professional development* (2nd ed., pp. 235–253). New York, NY: Springer Publishing.

Patient Protection and Affordable Care Act; HHS Notice of Benefit and Payment Parameters for 2012, 78 Fed. Reg. 15410 (March 11, 2013) (to be codified at 45 C.F.R. pts. 153, 155,156, 157, & 158).

Pinch, W. J. (1996). Ethical issues in case management. In D. L. Flarey & S. S. Blancett (Eds.), *Handbook of nursing case management: Health care delivery in world of managed care* (pp. 443–460). Gaithersburg, MD: Aspen Publishers.

Public Law 111-148. (2010). Patient Protection and Affordable Care Act.

Resnick, B., & Bonner, A. (2003). Collaboration: Foundation for a successful practice. *Journal of the American Medical Directors Association, 4*(6), 344–349. Retrieved from http://ezproxy.undmedlibrary.org/login?url=http://search. ebscohost.com.ezproxy.undmedlibrary.org/login.aspx?direct=true&AuthTy pe=ip,url,uid,cookie&db=c8h&AN=2004117379&site=ehost-live

Savage, L. (1993). *Literacy through a competency-based education approach.* Washington, DC: Center for Applied Linguistics.

Taylor, P (1999). Comprehensive nursing case management. An advanced practice model. *Nursing Case Management, 4*(1), 2–9.

Umbrell, C. E. (2006). Trauma case management: A role for the advanced practice nurse. *Journal of Trauma Nursing, 13*(2), 70–73. Retrieved from http://ezproxy. undmedlibrary.org/login?url=http://search.ebscohost.com.ezproxy. undmedlibrary.org/login.aspx?direct=true&AuthType=ip,url,uid,cookie& db=c8h&AN=2009370355&site=ehost-live

Watson, J. (1989). Transformative thinking and a caring curriculum. In E. O. Bevis & J. Watson (Eds.), *Toward a caring curriculum: A new pedagogy for nursing.* New York, NY: National League for Nursing.

Jana Gail Zwilling   4

ADVANCED PRACTICE NURSING WITHIN HEALTH CARE SETTINGS: ORGANIZATIONAL ROLES

The U.S. health care system has undergone a huge shift recently. These changes have and will continue to require the advanced practice registered nurse (APRN) not only to be clinically competent but also to have an understanding of the organizations in which care is presently being delivered. The APRN must have knowledge of and the ability to create the systems of care that will ensure the high-quality and cost-effective care needed in the future.

The economics of health care have become increasingly complex. In an attempt to achieve cost efficiencies, merging health care organizations have given birth to giant health care corporations. However, the goal of cost savings has not necessarily been consistently achieved. This is evidenced by ever-increasing health care costs and the percentage of the national budget being spent on health care today, with less than-ideal-outcomes for all citizens (Levit et al., 2003; National Center for Health Statistics, 2013).

THE U.S. HEALTH CARE SYSTEM

Health care delivery systems in the United States are unlike those of any other country in the world. Most other developed countries have national health insurance programs run by governments and financed through general taxes, so almost all citizens are entitled to receive health care. The United States has recently take steps toward a national health insurance program. The Patient Protection and Affordable Care Act (ACA) was signed into law in March 2010. As all laws do, it takes time to put processes in place and see the effects and outcomes of the new legislation. The initial year for individuals and families to sign up for health insurance as mandated by the ACA was 2014.

There are varying opinions regarding the health care reform law. For many, this law enables insurance coverage regardless of preexisting conditions or the ability to pay the insurance premiums. Other benefits of the new law include tax credits for small businesses to offer employee health coverage and the mandate that all coverage must include preventive services. There are some perceived drawbacks to the new health care legislation. Every individual is mandated to have some form of health insurance or will have to pay a fine. Also, the increasing costs of premiums needs to be considered, because insurance companies can no longer deny coverage and companies will need to raise rates to ensure coverage for everyone. Unfortunately, despite the increased premium costs, insurance reimbursement to health care providers has also decreased. This has created an environment of strategic health care implementation.

There is traditionally strong evidence that health insurance coverage improves access and quality of health and medical care, contributing to the overall health of individuals and their families. According to 2010 data from the National Hospital Ambulatory Medical Care Survey (NHAMCS, 2010a, 2010b):

- In emergency departments, the percentage of visits by patients who had some form of insurance coverage was 5 times higher that of uninsured visits.
- The number of patient visits to physician's offices was more than 20 times higher for individuals with private health insurance or Medicaid/Children's Health Insurance Program (CHIP) compared with those with no insurance.

An increasing number of Americans are gaining access to insurance coverage with the implementation of the ACA. In 2012, 45.5 million Americans, or 14.7% of the U.S. population, were underinsured or uninsured, including working-age adults (those aged 18–64; Cohen & Martinez, 2012; Kaiser Commission on Medicaid and the Uninsured, 2012). A Gallup poll in May 2014 revealed the rate of the uninsured had been reduced to 13.4% (Levy, 2014). These reports also show a narrowing in the inequity of coverage based on race and ethnicity, gender, and age. Uninsured persons are defined as persons without private health insurance, Medicare, Medicaid, State Children's Health Insurance Program (SCHIP) coverage, a state-sponsored or other government-sponsored health plan, or a military plan. Also included among the underinsured and uninsured are persons who have only Indian Health Service coverage or a private plan that pays for only one type of service, such as accidents or dental care (National Health Interview Survey, 2012).

The complexities of the various systems of care—which include nonprofit and proprietary organizations; large and small corporations; local, regional, and worldwide conglomerates; small and multisystem plans; multistate health care systems and payment mechanisms; and regulatory requirements—can be overwhelming to the new APRN. Few nurses have a strong background or experience in the organizational influences of health care. Content on the complexity of health care coverage has historically been minimal in nursing undergraduate education. This knowledge deficit is compounded by the fact that most nurses have limited experience with the organizational dimensions of health care coverage while they are employed as staff nurses (Ladden, Bednash, Stevens, & Moore, 2006).

What remains to be seen is the impact of increasing access on the health care system. Many believe this will cause a huge influx of patients needing care, thus overburdening an already short supply of primary care providers. Rationing of care has been discussed as a potential and negative outcome of this increased patient load (Robinson, Williams, Dickinson, Freeman, & Rumbold, 2012). This could mean long waits for nonemergent care and nonexistent elective services. A formal priority-setting approach has yet to be implemented on a large scale. Preventive care will become the focus, and nontraditional forms of health care delivery will need to be implemented (Cornelissen et al., 2014). The shortage of primary care physicians and the emphasis on preventive services create an opportunity for APRNs to have an impact on the health care delivery systems.

Organizational Influences

How does an understanding of these organizational influences affect the APRN's roles and functions? Many factors are involved, and these influences can clearly change during the tenure of the APRN's career. A beginning APRN needs to understand these organizations when selecting future employment and providing care to clients. As APRNs become more confident in their role as care providers, they can expand their roles as leaders and change agents to influence their organizations. To do so requires enhanced knowledge and skills in organizational design, systems, function, and complexity. Therefore, advanced knowledge in such fields as organizational behavior, cost analysis, risk management, patient satisfaction, safety, and quality are necessary to fully implement the role of the APRN. To ensure that the APRN is on the forefront of new and innovative care delivery practices, an understanding of the health care systems and organizations that are and should be in place where the APRN practices is a needed prerequisite.

Even though these rapidly changing health care system settings are ripe for innovation, the APRN may find it a daunting task to understand and negotiate them. Traditionally educated to provide advanced nursing care more closely aligned to a specific system or setting of care, the APRN is now faced with the challenge of a multisystem arena for care delivery. Understanding system issues has been identified as a necessary component of graduate education for nurse administrators and APRNs for many years, but the recommendation has not been fully embraced. As early as 1988, Lynn, Layman, and Englebardt (1998) identified the importance of incorporating such topics as leadership, financial management policies, health policy, and organizational culture and structure into course content in advanced practice educations programs.

The American Association of College Nurses (AACN) *Essentials of Doctoral Education for Advanced Nursing Practice* (AACN, 2006) identifies that advanced nursing practice includes an organizational and systems leadership component. This requires political skills, systems thinking, and business and financial expertise. In this environment of ongoing changes in the organization and financing of health care, this document asserts that it is imperative that all graduates of practice doctorate degree nursing programs have a keen understanding of health care policy, organization, and financing of health care. The purpose of this content is to prepare a graduate to provide quality cost-effective care, to participate in the design and implementation of care in a variety of health care systems, and to assume a leadership role in managing human, fiscal, and physical health care resources.

Analysis of Organizations

For the new APRN, understanding health care organizations is vital in determining the most appropriate place or setting for employment. The ability to understand an organization is based on several factors. Examples of questions APRNs should ask include:

- What is the organizational structure of the organization?
- What is the philosophical underpinning of the organization?
- What are the directions and goals of the organization?
- What are the culture and climate of the organization?

Organizational structure is one dimension that is important to understand. Historically, health care organizations have been structured in the more traditional hierarchical and bureaucratic organizational models. Many experts in organizational functioning believe that these traditional models will no longer work in the emerging health care arena. They have proposed that the new models need to be flat, innovative, nimble, and responsive to change. The health care organizations that will survive in the frenetic pace of today's world will promote greater flexibility and have the ability to deal with ambiguity and uncertainty (Porter-O'Grady & Malloch, 2007).

The APRN should evaluate the structure of the organization and how it will influence his or her ability to provide care and perform the various aspects of the APRN role. For instance, organizational structure clearly affects communication in a health care system and influences how and by whom decisions are made. The APRN should identify how many layers of the organization lie between the APRN and the person or persons who are responsible for making decisions that will affect the APRN's clinical decisions, the latitude of the APRN's daily practice, and the costs of care related to patient care. The APRN should understand the "official" organizational structure and recognize the "informal" lines of communication and decision-making networks.

Every organization has different philosophical underpinnings that frame the organization's direction for the future and give the APRN insight into how decisions will be made. An organization's mission, vision, values, philosophy, and organizational objectives are important. The mission of the organization describes the purpose for which that organization exists. The mission statement provides valuable information about the organization's direction and goals for the future. Mission statements allow the reader to understand what is meaningful to the organization, how that meaning may be measured, and clearly define the organization's reason for existing. They can also lead to an enhanced understanding of the ethics, principles, and standards for which the employees will be held accountable (Danna, 2011).

Mission statements should provide vision for the organization. The vision should be an image of the future, whereas value statements should bond people and set behavioral standards in the organization. The philosophy of the organization outlines values, concepts, and beliefs that establish the organization's care practices. Mission and vision statements can help a prospective employee understand the value placed on the clients and workers in an organization. Having a clear understanding of these foundational aspects of an organization can help inform the APRN about an agency's present and future goals and expected outcomes. For instance, an APRN who has a strong belief in providing care to all people regardless of their ability to pay or who has a strong belief in a certain ethical orientation is wise to identify that the organization being considered has values that are consistent with that person's belief system. Simply hoping that an organization promotes the same level of quality care that the individual APRN aspires to give or believing that all organizations are the same is naive and will affect whether the APRN will survive or strive in the practice setting.

A common method of analyzing health care organizations is to use a systems theory approach. The health care organization is considered an open system; it has permeable boundaries that are affected by the society in which it operates. Change in society forces internal change in the operation of an organization. The rapidity with which these changes have occurred recently is responsible for the chaotic situations in which many health care practitioners and administrators operate today (Yoder-Wise, 2006). Given the extraordinary complexity of these health care systems, an emerging field of science has been suggested as an alternative approach to understanding them (Plsek, 1999). This emerging field, termed *complexity science,* offers alternative leadership and management strategies for the chaotic, complex health care environment.

One method to evaluate an organization is to examine an organization's outcomes or its "organizational effectiveness." Danna (2011) provides a helpful listing of indicators to monitor organizational effectiveness. Those indicators include patient satisfaction with care; family satisfaction with care; staff satisfaction with work; staff satisfaction with rewards, intrinsic and extrinsic; staff satisfaction with professional development;

staff satisfaction with organization; and management's satisfaction with staff; community relationships; and organizational health. A malfunctioning organization would be reflected by such elements as focusing on the wrong elements of the operation, having too many meetings attended by too many people accomplishing little work, and having too many levels of administration, to name a few.

Healthy environments support meaningful work and provide an environment in which the APRN can excel and feel an important part of the team. The American Organization of Nurse Executives (AONE, 2009) has identified six critical factors to improve workplace initiatives, extracted from a study of workplace implementation and innovation. These factors are leadership development, empowered collaborative decision making, work design and service delivery innovation, a values-focused organizational culture, recognition and rewards systems, and professional growth and accountability.

Organizational Climate and Culture

All health care organizations have a climate and culture. Climate is described as the emotional states, feelings, and perceptions shared by the members of the organization. Climate can be described by such terms as positive or negative, hopeful or negative, trusting or suspicious, and competitive or nurturing. The APRN can influence the climate or be influenced by it. Climate can influence interactions and responses by patients and coworkers alike. It is a component of job satisfaction and enjoyment in one's work life. An organizational climate that is inconsistent with an APRN's preferred orientation can cause dissatisfaction and limit the ability to excel. However, the seasoned APRN can be pivotal in establishing the day-to-day climate in the practice setting.

An organization's social system, including its beliefs, norms, mission, philosophies, traditions, and values, make up its culture. It represents the perspectives, values, assumptions, language, and behaviors that have been effectively used by the members of the organization. Culture influences the formal and informal methods and styles of communication. When considering employment in an organization, an APRN should assess the culture and climate of an organization to assess whether it is an appropriate fit. The APRN may wish to practice with a specific population or within a specialty area. However, without an appreciation of the organization's climate and culture, the APRN may be unable to implement the changes and level of care he or she hopes to provide. Finding an organization that is consistent with the APRN's preferred culture and climate can provide a solid and more comfortable practice arena for an individual practitioner.

The Culture of Safety and Quality

Beginning in the 1980s and continuing with increased emphasis during the past decade, there has been a nationwide agenda to address the culture of safety and quality in health care organizations. National health care quality accreditation and regulatory agencies have taken major steps to enhance quality and safety by identifying evidence-based best practices and encouraging measurement and monitoring of these practices and care outcomes. The Joint Commission (formerly known as the Joint Commission on the Accreditation of Health Care Organizations [JCAHO]), the Institute of Medicine (IOM), the Agency of Healthcare Research and Quality (AHRQ), and the Centers of Medicare & Medicaid Services (CMS) of the U.S. Department of Health and Human Services (HHS) are just a few of the many organizations and agencies focused on enhancing health care quality and safety.

The IOM has identified safety concerns and problems with quality of care. It defines *quality* as "the degree to which health services for individuals and populations increase the likelihood of desired health outcomes and are consistent with current professional knowledge" (Lohr, 1990, p.21).

A series of IOM reports help illustrate how wide the quality chasm is and how important it is to close the gulf between our standards of high-quality care and the prevailing norm in practice. Two landmark reports released by the IOM, *To Err Is Human: Building a Safer Health System* (1999) and *Crossing the Quality Chasm: A New Health System for the 21st Century* (2001), moved the national dialogue, asserting that reform is not accomplished by simply addressing the issues around its margins. The third phase of the IOM's *Quality Initiative* focuses on setting the vision outlined in *Quality Chasm* into operation. This implementation is on three levels: environmental, health care organization, and interaction between clinicians and patients. Thus far, focus has been on the redesign of care delivery, reform of health professions' education, technology implementation, safety, and quality care that is accessible and cost-effective (IOM, 2001, 2003c, 2005, 2006).

The overall goal for the Quality and Safety Education for Nurses (QSEN) project (2012) is to meet the challenge of preparing future nurses who will have the knowledge, skills, and attitudes (KSAs) necessary to continuously improve the quality and safety of the health care systems in which they work. Using the IOM *Health Professions Education: A Bridge to Quality* (2003a) competencies, QSEN faculty and a national advisory board have defined quality and safety competencies for graduate-level nursing and proposed targets for the knowledge, skills, and attitudes to be developed in APRN programs for each competency (AACN, 2012). These competencies serve as a guide to curricular development for formal academic programs, transition to practice, and continuing education programs (Bargagliotti & Lancaster, 2007; Cronenwett et al., 2007).

CMS finalized its initiatives to develop quality measures of health care providers following the institution of the ACA in 2011. One of these initiatives is the "Pay for Reporting and Pay for Performance" standard. This standard outlines four quality measures that will be tracked, and provider reimbursement will be affected by the outcomes. These measures are tracked with a variety of methods, including patient surveys, claims calculation, electronic health record (EHR) review, and group practice reporting option (CMS, 2012).

The APRN should be aware of these outcome measures when considering a place of employment and use them as a mechanism to monitor the quality of services provided by their organization. There are now innumerable quality and safety initiatives nationwide, and astute APRNs will understand what is occurring in their place of employment and will help shape its practices to enhance quality. Several studies show APRNs' practices are already demonstrating high-level outcomes for patient satisfaction and chronic disease management (Boville et al., 2007; Dinh, Walker, Parameswaran, & Enright, 2012; Green & Davis, 2005). Continued positive outcomes will propel APRNs to be the exemplary model of quality health care.

SUMMARY

The APRN of today and tomorrow will need to address organizational and system issues. Although it may seem daunting in our changing health care landscape, APRNs must develop the knowledge to analyze organizational variables and the skills and abilities to enhance quality and safety. The APRN must be a leader and change agent instrumental in creating the care delivery systems that will be needed in the future.

Acknowledgment

The author acknowledges the contributions of Mary Zwygart-Stauffacher to this chapter in a previous edition.

REFERENCES

American Association of Colleges of Nursing. (2006). Essentials of doctoral education for advance practice nursing. http://www.aacn.nche.edu/publications/position/DNPEssentials.pdf

American Association of Colleges of Nursing. (2012). QSEN Education Consortium. *Graduate-level QSEN competencies: Knowledge, skills, and attitudes.* Retrieved from http://www.aacn.nche.edu/faculty/qsen/competencies.pdf

American Organization of Nurse Executives. (2009). http://www.aone.org

Bargagliotti, L., & Lancaster, J. (2007). Quality and safety education in nursing: More than new wine in old skins. *Nursing Outlook, 55*(3), 156–158.

Boville, D., Saran, M., Salem, J., Clough, L., Jones, R., Radwany, S., & Sweet, D. (2007). Perspectives in ambulatory care. An innovative role for nurse practitioners in managing chronic disease. *Nursing Economic$, 25*(6), 359–364.

Centers for Medicare & Medicaid Services. (2012). *Guide to quality performance standards for accountable care.* Retrieved from http://www.cms.gov/Medicare/Medicare-Fee-for-Service-Payment/sharedsavingsprogram/Downloads/ACO-Guide-Quality-Performance-2012.PDF

Cohen, R.A., & Martinez, M.E. (2012). Health insurance coverage: Early release of estimates from the national health interview survey, 2012. Retrieved from http://www.cdc.gov/nchs/data/nhis/earlyrelease/insur201306.pdf

Cornelissen, E., Mitton, C., Davidson, A., Reid, C., Hole, R., Visockas, A., & Smith, N. (2014). Determining and broadening the definition of impact from implementing a rational priority setting approach in a healthcare organization. *Social Science & Medicine, 114*, 1–9. doi:10.1016/j.socscimed.2014.05.027

Cronenwett, L., Sherwood, G., Barnsteiner, J., Disch, J., Johnson, J., Mitchell, P., …, Warren, J. (2007). Quality and safety education for nurses. *Nursing Outlook, 55*(3), 122–131.

Danna, D. (2011). Organizational structure and analysis. In L. Roussel (Ed.), *Management leadership for nurse administrators* (6th ed.). Boston, MA: Jones and Bartlett.

Dinh, M., Walker, A., Parameswaran, A., & Enright, N. (2012). Evaluating the quality of care delivered by an emergency department fast track unit with both nurse practitioners and doctors. *Australasian Emergency Nursing Journal, 15*(4), 188–194. doi:10.1016/j.aenj.2012.09.001

Green, A., & Davis, S. (2005). Toward a predictive model of patient satisfaction with nurse practitioner care. *Journal of the American Academy of Nurse Practitioners, 17*(4) 139–148.

Institute of Medicine. (1999). *To err is human: Building a safer health system.* Washington, DC: National Academy Press.

Institute of Medicine. (2001). *Crossing the quality chasm: A new health system for the 21st century.* Washington, DC: National Academy Press.

Institute of Medicine. (2003a). *Health professions education: A bridge to quality.* Washington, DC: National Academies Press.

Institute of Medicine. (2003b). *Key capabilities of an electronic medical record.* Washington, DC: National Academies Press.

Institute of Medicine. (2003c). *Patient safety: Achieving a new standard for care.* Washington, DC: National Academies Press.

Institute of Medicine. (2005). *Performance measurement: Accelerating improvement.* Washington, DC: National Academies Press.

Institute of Medicine. (2006). *Medicare's quality improvement organization program: Maximizing potential.* Washington, DC: National Academies Press.

Kaiser Commission on Medicaid and the Uninsured. (2012). *The uninsured and the difference health insurance makes.* Kaiser Family Foundation. Retrieved from http://www.kff.org/uninsured/upload/1420-14.pdf

Ladden, M., Bednash, G., Stevens, D., & Moore, G. (2006). Educating interprofessional learners for quality, safety, and systems improvement. *Journal of Interprofessional Care, 2*, 497–505.

Levit, K., Smith, C., Cowan, C., Lazenby, H., Sensenig, A., & Catlin, A. (2003). Trends in U.S. health care spending. *Health Affairs, 22*, 154–164.

Levy, J., (2014). Gallup *Well-being. U.S. Uninsured rate drops to 13.4%.* Retrieved from: http://www.gallup.com/poll/168821/uninsured-rate-drops.aspx

Lohr, K. N. (Ed). (1990). *Medicare: A strategy for quality assurance* (Vol 1). Washington, DC: National Academy Press.

Lynn, M., Layman, E., & Englebardt, S. (1998). Nursing administration research priorities, a national Delphi study. *Journal of Nursing Administration, 15*, 7–11.

National Center for Health Statistics. (2013). *Health, United States, 2006: With chartbook on trends in the health of Americans.* Hyattsville, MD: Department of Health and Human Services.

National Health Interview Survey. (2012). Early release of selected estimates based on data from the January-June 2012 national health interview survey. Retrieved on February 2, 2015 from: http://www.cdc.gov/nchs/data/nhis/earlyrelease/earlyrelease201212_01.pdf.

National Hospital Ambulatory Medical Care Survey. (2010a). 2010 emergency department summary tables. Retrieved from http://www.cdc.gov/nchs/data/ahcd/nhamcs_emergency/2010_ed_web_tables.pdf

National Hospital Ambulatory Medical Care Survey. (2010b). 2010 outpatient department summary tables. Retrieved from http://www.cdc.gov/nchs/data/ahcd/nhamcs_outpatient/2010_opd_web_tables.pdf

Plsek, P. (1999). Innovative thinking for improvement of medical systems. *Annals of Internal Medicine, 131,* 438–444.

Porter-O'Grady, T., & Malloch, K. (2007). *Quantum leadership: A textbook of new leadership.* Sudbury, MA: Jones and Bartlett.

Quality and safety education for nurses. (2012). Retrieved from http://www.qsen.org

Robinson, S., Williams, I., Dickinson, H., Freeman, T., & Rumbold, B. (2012). Priority-setting and rationing in healthcare: Evidence from the English experience. *Social Science & Medicine, 75*(12), 2386–2393. doi:http://dx.doi.org.ezproxy.undmedlibrary.org/10.1016/j.socscimed.2012.09.014

Yoder-Wise, P. (2006). *Leading and managing in nursing* (4th ed.). St. Louis, MO: Mosby.

Kathryn A. Blair   **5**

INTERPROFESSIONAL COLLABORATIVE TEAMS AND EDUCATION: ROLES FOR THE APRN

The current health care system struggles with rising costs of care with little improvement in patient outcomes. The existing system focuses on the patient seeking care for a problem. This reactive model of care does not engage a variety of health care professionals, resulting in a lack of continuity of care (Nuño, Coleman, Bengoa, & Sauto, 2012) and new ways of engaging families and patients in ways that facilitates behavior change (Kilgore & Langford, 2010; Nuño et al., 2012). As articulated in the 2003 Institute of Medicine (IOM) *Health Professions Education: A Bridge to Quality*, the present-day system of health care fails to translate research into practice, apply technology to enhance care and reduce errors, and fully utilize the available resources (IOM, 2003). The failure to use nurses to their full capacity was repeated in the IOM's *The Future of Nursing* (2010) document. This report recommended that nurses be full partners, with physicians and other health professionals, in redesigning health care in the United States. The current system continues to fail to use advanced practice registered nurses (APRNs) to their full capabilities, and the present-day model of care encourages underuse and/or overuse of resources, suboptimal care, inefficiencies, rising expenditures, and provider and patient dissatisfaction.

With the Patient Protection and Affordable Care Act (ACA), approximately 22 million Americans gained health care coverage resulting in access issues specifically a significant shortage of providers (Busen, 2014). Predictions suggest that 40,000 primary care physicians and more than 250,000 APRNs (nurse practitioners, clinical nurse specialists, nurse-midwives, and nurse anesthetists) are needed to provide care to the new enrollees (Brooten, Youngblut, Hannan, & Guido-Sanz, 2012).

Mitchell et al. (2012) reported that Medicare patients may see multiple physicians yearly (at least two primary care providers and five specialists). This number does not include other professionals involved in the patient's care, such as pharmacists, nurses, physician assistants, APRNs, social workers, dietitians, and chiropractors. Most of these professionals are working in isolation, addressing a specific problem. If a provider engages other professionals in patient care, the typical pattern is parallel or consultative and not integrated or collaborative. This model of care encourages duplications of services and fragmented care.

One proposed solution to address the shortage of health care providers, rising health care cost, errors, and suboptimal/fragmented care is the utilization of "teams." Team-based health care has been defined as care provided by two or more health care professionals who have different skills and expertise and who work together on common goals to provide quality patient-centered care (Mitchell et al., 2012). This definition could be expanded beyond health care providers to include non–health care professionals such as administrators, community leaders, and others.

If team care is important, then what kind of team? There exist several forms of teams: disaster teams; teams in the acute care setting caring for critically ill patients; community-based teams that care for people in their homes; office-based care teams; and teams that include the patient, family members, and supporting health care providers (Mitchell et al., 2012). Other teams are defined by their structure: multidisciplinary, transdisciplinary and interprofessional, or interdisciplinary. *Interdisciplinary* and *interprofessional* are interchangeable terms. Given the recent trend for promoting interprofessional collaboration, the term *interprofessional* will be used in place of *interdisciplinary*. Multidisciplinary team members assume a hierarchal role that is governed by professional identities. Transdisciplinary team members cross disciplines, and individual expertise blurs roles of team members. This team model is not often seen in health care. Interprofessional team member roles are synergistic and interdependent, characterized by open communication, collaboration, and leadership that is task driven (Youngwerth & Twaddle, 2011). When there is effective communication and collaboration in an interprofessional team, then members are empowered to take a leadership role based on their expertise for the patient's problem. The interdisciplinary collaborative team model promotes active engagement and joint decision making (Lapkin, Levett-Jones, & Gilligan, 2013).

As early as 2001 the authors of the IOM report *Crossing the Quality Chasm: A New Health System for the 21st Century* argued that patient safety, quality care, and cost containment are bundled in interprofessional collaborative teams (ICTs). If ICTs are necessary for improving health care, what are the fundamental principles guiding these teams? Researchers examining ICTs have identified six core competencies necessary for interprofessional collaborative practice that is patient-centered: (a) knowledge and skills for team functions, (b) communication, (c) leadership, (d) cooperation and negotiation for conflict resolution, (e) understanding and strength in one's professional role, and (f) appreciation of professional role of others (MacDonald et al., 2010; Patrician et al., 2012). The Interprofessional Education Collaborative Expert Panel (2011) classified four competency domains: values and ethics, roles and responsibilities, interprofessional communication, and team and teamwork. The committee argues that these domains must be incorporated into professional identity for ICTs to function.

Composition of the ICT is another topic for exploration. Although the primary members of a health care team are identified as a physician and primary care nurse, other health care professionals such as pharmacists, social workers, psychologists, and dietitians are included depending on the needs and goals of the patient (Sayah, Szafran, Robertson, Bell, & Williams, 2014). The question to be addressed is whether physician participation is necessary in all teams. As the APRN role continues to evolve, the answer may be no. This is not to be construed as marginalizing the physician's role but rather to highlight that there may be instances where the APRN is the primary provider of care or directly responsible for the care of a particular patient independent of a physician.

What remains elusive is when and where the ICTs are necessary. The day-to-day care for minor acute illnesses does not require ICT… or does it? When conceptualizing ICT on a macro level, then ICTs are necessary for all aspects of care. This might encompass system operations, population-based models of care, standards of practice, evidence-based practice models, and quality improvement projects. On a micro level, or the process of delivering care to the individual patient, the ICTs may be indicated for patients with chronic, complex health care issues, when minor illnesses are later defined as more complex than originally thought, or when instituting preventive services.

BARRIERS FOR ICTs

Professional barriers for ICTs include the classic physician-driven model as the leader of the team. The recent introduction of medical homes by the Accountable Care Organization promotes this concept of a physician-driven team model. This model dissuades the integration of interprofessional collaborative teams into the health care system. Other barriers to collaboration are related to differences in each discipline's professional orientation and funding sources (Gagliardi, Dobrowb, & Wright, 2011). Traditional hierarchical roles, power sharing and ownership of specific knowledge, technical skills, and clinical territory between professions produce interdisciplinary conflict (Brooten et al., 2012; Munro, Kornelsen, & Grzybowsk, 2013; Youngwerth, & Twaddle, 2011).

Systems factors such regulatory issues and billing practices have been cited as barriers for ICTs (Munro et al., 2013; Weinstein, Brandt, Gilbert, & Schmitt, 2014). Yet another confounding variable is the current reimbursement system. There is no compensation for providers when a patient is not seen; therefore, the work of the team is often not reimbursed (Gaboury, Bujold, Boon, & Moher, 2009), resulting in a disincentive to form teams. In academic centers, adding ICT concepts and incorporating interprofessional collaborative team education (ICTE) into existing curricula and enabling students from different disciplines to practice in teams has been challenging without administrative support (Youngwerth & Twaddle, 2011).

Role confusion has been recognized as a common barrier for effective ICTs. The ambiguity between roles is particularly troublesome for those professions with overlapping roles (i.e., APRNs and physicians).

Professional Socialization

The greatest barrier for ICT is *professional socialization*. Professional socialization is the developmental stage when a student learns about the profession from historical and social perspectives and incorporates the values and attitudes of that profession.

Although many health care professionals are members of the health care team, nurses and physicians play a central role given the status of medicine and the number of nurses. "Given the centrality of the nurse–physician relationship within healthcare, and the importance of collegiality to professional and organizational outcomes, promoting interprofessional respect and collaboration between nursing and medicine is of critical importance" (Price, Doucet, & McGillis-Hall, 2014, p. 106).

Traditionally, medicine remains at the top of the health care hierarchy, with all other health care professions deemed as second best (Price et al., 2014). Physicians assume a superior role in patient care decision making based on medical education and socialization. Historically, physician education prepares physicians for independence and autonomy. Ultimately this socialization discourages cooperation and interdependence.

Nurses are viewed as relying on physicians for direction; however, with the advent of academic degrees and training, increasing technology, and increasing health care complexity, nurses have expanded their scope of practice. The failure to educate the public and other health care providers has resulted in the APRN appearing second rate to the physician. "True collaboration between the two professions will remain elusive until nurses cease to attribute their knowledge to physicians, recognizing collective decision making and authority, effectively ending this historical game" (Price et al., 2014, p. 105).

With closer examination of the historical perspective of both professions, the roles of physicians were reflective of the roles of women and men. Several social changes have occurred over the past 50 years, such as the improved status of women and the advanced practice nursing options, and have contributed to a more collegial relationship between physicians and nurses. Unfortunately, "nurses are subordinate to not only medicine, but organizational structures as well" (Price et al., 2014, p. 106).

APRNs' expansion of practice and the development of doctorally prepared clinical nurses can and will challenge preconceived notions of professional practice. Without regulatory support through legislation and regulatory policies, the notion of APRNs being second best will persist. In addition to regulatory changes, health care organizations, communities, and educational institutions need to embrace interprofessional collaboration as the norm rather than the exception to providing the best patient care.

Solutions: Roles for APRNs

To address the professional barriers, APRNs must begin to unravel the confusion around nursing knowledge, skills, and roles. Nurse educators and nurses, including APRNs, need to clearly articulate what they know and do to increase nurses' visibility and participation in the design of an interprofessional health care system. Unifying the conflicting views among nurse scholars and educators regarding the relationship of nursing knowledge to practice will add additional clarity (Sommerfeldt, 2013).

With the expansion of the nursing role, the pervasive notion that medicine is superior to nursing is beginning to change. The belief that only nurses function within a caring, nurturing, and holistic model while physicians function within a scientific-based model is no longer true. The time has come to recognize that the practice of medicine and nursing (specifically the APRN role) has a great deal of overlap and the roles complement one another rather than compete against each other. With the continued evolution of the APRN role and the doctorate of nursing practice (DNP), these old viewpoints and models of practice are being challenged (Price et al., 2014).

APRNs need to challenge the early professional socialization by educating the public about the role and functions of the APRN. The school system can be one venue. When local schools have career days, the APRN can articulate the uniqueness of nursing and advanced practice nursing so that when students think about health care careers, nursing will be the first choice and not the second choice if they cannot get into medical school.

Using the media to foster public education is critical. In 2002, the Johnson & Johnson Corporation sponsored commercials about nursing. Although these commercials increased public awareness about the profession, they did little to emphasize the depth of nursing education, skills, and scope of practice. The commercials focused on "Dare to care" or nursing historical roots of being a "caring "profession.

Becoming involved in local health policies is another way to reach the public. The key is to become visible. APRNs need to engage legislators, insurance companies, industry stakeholders, and other stakeholders in facilitating the change in attitudes about nursing. If APRNs sit at the sidelines and wait for someone else to do the work, they will remain "second best."

To address systems barriers the APRN is in a pivotal position to facilitate the changes necessary to redesign the health care system such that ICTs can work. APRNs can foster partnerships among stakeholders (patients, families, and community leaders) to foster support for ICT health care initiatives; can become involved in legislative activities to change federal and state regulations regarding reimbursement and scope of practice issues; can work with technology experts to design information systems that support ICTs; and can develop a better understanding of how to encourage team-work through asynchronous health care delivery (Djukic, Fulmer, Adams, Lee, & Triola, 2012; Kuziemskya & Varpiob, 2011; Nuño et al., 2012).

With the increased use of health information systems as a tool in pro-viding care, APRNs can collaborate with information technology experts in the development and design of health information systems (HISs) to support collaborative care delivery (Kuziemskya & Varpiob, 2011). The redesign of HISs needs to incorporate communication mechanisms that interface with patients and families, communities, and other health care providers. This can facilitate asynchronous collaborative team efforts.

Reconceptualizing the APRN role as the liaison between and among team members (Légaré et al., 2011) and as the coordinator of care will clarify one function of the APRN within the team. The APRN is the glue that holds the team together. This does not mean always assuming the leadership role but rather keeping the patient/family connected with the entire team.

APRNs can participate in or conduct research examining team factors that promote optimal performance in applied clinical practice (Andreatta & Marzano, 2012). With this information, APRNs can work with educators to design ICTE programs as well as role model behaviors that contribute a functioning ICT that meets the needs of the patient without increasing cost by decreasing duplication of services and improving patient outcomes.

Interprofessional Collaborative Team Education: Role of the APRN

A variety of organizations have argued that fostering ICTs begins with ICTE. As articulated earlier, most health care professionals are educated in silos, interfacing little with other professions. The incorporation of ICTE into curricula challenges the status quo, blurs professional boundaries, and requires involvement of individual stakeholders (Lawlis, Anson, & Green-field, 2014). In other words, to implement ICTE, there must be support from the top down. Unless the leadership, academicians, and regulatory authorities are willing to support the initiative, ICTE will not be initiated or sustained as part of the curricula and clinical learning environment (Missen, Jacob, Barnett, Walker, & Cross, 2012; Schmitt, Gilbert, Brandt, & Weinstein, 2013).

The components of ICTE programs are many. Some of the elements, such as professional and personal responsibility and accountability, are already embedded in existing curricula. Others, such as mutual trust and respect, interprofessional communication, and coordination, are key for a successful ICTE program (Bridges et al., 2011) and may need expansion in existing curricula. Although the didactic portion is important, the actual operationalizing of these behaviors is critical.

Aligning medical, nursing, and other professional schools curri-cula (didactic and/or clinical experiences) is a daunting task; however, using simulations and other technology to facilitate the ICT learning and experience has been used with some success (Djukic et al., 2012; Liaw, Zhou, Ching Lau, Siau, & Wai-chi Chan, 2014). Most students' attitudes about ICTE were positive, whether they participated face-to-face or via asynchronous web-based activities. Most students believed the experience was useful in helping them understand the roles of various professions and in improving their communications skills. The evidence of these learning experiences translating into sustainable practice is inconclusive (Lapkin et al., 2013).

For ICTE to be implemented and sustained in academic centers, leadership among educators, health care professionals, and regulatory authorities must be incorporated into the planning as well as the implementation. From a student perspective, the ICTE must not be perceived as an "add-on" to curricula that are already full. Threads of communication, collaboration, joint decision making, conflict resolution, and role realignment from profession-centered care to patient-centered care (Veerapen & Purkis, 2014) should be woven into the existing courses and should have didactic experiences that enable the student to operationalize these concepts. The clinical setting is a great opportunity to apply these concepts into practice. This can be done in the direct clinical experiences or through simulation.

The APRN can play a role in designing the threads as an academician, practicing clinician, or team member (role modeling). Research suggests that role-modeling behaviors are as important as knowledge (Pollard, Miers, & Rickaby, 2012).

Introducing the concept of ICTE begins in school but continues in the workplace. Incorporating ICTE in the workplace is an example of "learning by doing" (Brennan, Olds, Dolansky, Estrada, & Patrician, 2014; Kuipers, Ehrlich, & Brownie, 2014). Novice practitioners (whether physicians or APRNs) struggle with roles and skills after graduation; however, continued work in this area will indirectly facilitate sustainability. When systems adopt ICTs as a mode of operation, the players will practice in ICTs.

For decades, health care scholars have discussed the role of ICTs in health care delivery systems while educational researchers examined the processes of ICTE. Although the literature is filled with research in both domains, little has been done to institute ICT in clinical practice or to incorporate ICTE in curricula.

Today's APRNs and those in the future will be responsible for determining the role of ICTs in the future health care system. If nurses and APRNs fail to become engaged in the discussion about health care reform and the structure and function of ICTs, they run the risk of being overlooked and irrelevant (Sommerfeldt, 2013). The future of nursing's contributions to ICTE and ICTs will depend on the participation of current and future nurses, especially APRNs, in the discussions about health care reform. The time is right for the development of new models of care through creating ICTs, remodeling academic nursing education curricula, and incorporating ICTE as a thread or theme; it is time for nursing as a profession to assume a major role in reconstructing health care.

REFERENCES

Andreatta, P., & Marzano, D. (2012). Healthcare management strategies: Inter-disciplinary team factors. *Current Opinion in Obstetrics and Gynecology, 24,* 445–452. doi:10.1097/GCO.0b013e328359f007

Brennan, C. W., Olds, D. M., Dolansky, M., Estrada, C. A., & Patrician, P. A. (2014). Learning by doing: Observing an interprofessional process as an interprofessional team. *Journal of Interprofessional Care, 28*(3), 249–251. doi:10.3109/1356 1820.2013.838750

Bridges, D. R., Davidson, R. A., Odegard, P. S., Ian, V., Maki, I. V., & Tomkowiak, J. (2011). Interprofessional collaboration: Three best practice models of interprofessional education. *Medical Education Online, 16,* 6035. doi:10.3402/meo.v16i0.6035

Brooten, D., Youngblut, J. M., Hannan, J., & Guido-Sanz, F. (2012). The impact of interprofessional collaboration on the effectiveness, significance, and future of advanced practice registered nurses. *Nursing Clinics of North America, 47,* 283–294. doi:10.1016/j.cnur.2012.02.005

Busen, N. H. (2014). An interprofessional education project to address the health care needs of women transitioning from prison to community reentry. *Journal of Professional Nursing.* doi:10.1016/j.profnurs.2014.01.002

Djukic, M., Fulmer, T., Adams, J. G., Lee, S., & Triola, M. M. (2012). NYU3T: Teaching, technology, teamwork: A model for interprofessional education scalability and sustainability. *Nursing Clinics of North America, 47,* 333–346. doi:10.1016/j.cnur.2012.05.003

Gaboury, I., Bujold, M., Boon, H., & Moher, D. (2009). Interprofessional collaboration within Canadian integrative healthcare clinics: Key components. *Social Science & Medicine, 69,* 707–715. doi:10.1016/j.socscimed.2009.05.048

Gagliardi, A. R., Dobrowb, M. J., & Wright, F. C. (2011). How can we improve cancer care? A review of interprofessional collaboration models and their use in clinical management. *Surgical Oncology, 20,* 146–154.

Institute of Medicine (IOM). (2001). *Crossing the quality chasm: A new health system for the 21st century.* Washington, DC: National Academies Press.

Institute of Medicine (IOM). (2003). *Health professions education: A bridge to quality.* Washington, DC: National Academies Press.

Institute of Medicine (IOM). (2010). *The future of nursing: Leading change, advancing health.* Washington, DC: National Academies Press.

Interprofessional Education Collaborative Expert Panel. (2011). *Core competencies for interprofessional collaborative practice: Report of an expert panel.* Washington, DC: Interprofessional Education Collaborative. Retrieved from http://www.aacn.nche.edu/education-resources/ipecreport.pdf

Kilgore, R. V., & Langford, R. W. (2010). Defragmenting care: Testing an intervention to increase the effectiveness of interdisciplinary health care teams. *Critical Care Nursing Clinics of North America, 22,* 271–278. doi:10.1016/j.ccell.2010.03.006

Kuipers, P., Ehrlich, C., & Brownie, S. (2014). Responding to health care complexity: Suggestions for integrated and interprofessional workplace learning. *Journal of Interprofessional Care, 28*(3), 246–248. doi:10.3109/13561820.2013.821601

Kuziemskya, C. E., & Varpiob, L. (2011). A model of awareness to enhance our understanding of interprofessional collaborative care delivery and health information system design to support it. *International Journal of Medical Informatics, 8,* 150–160. doi:10.1016/j.ijmedinf.2011.01.009

Lapkin, S., Levett-Jones, T., & Gilligan, C. (2013). A systematic review of the effectiveness of interprofessional education in health professional programs. *Nurse Education Today, 33*, 90–102. doi:10.1016/j.nedt.2011.11.006

Lawlis, T. R., Anson, J., & Greenfield, D. (2014). Barriers and enablers that influence sustainable interprofessional education: A literature review. *Journal of Interprofessional Care, 28*(4), 305–310. doi:10.3109/13561820.2014.895977

Légaré, F., Stacey, D., Pouliot, S., Gauvin, F. P., Desroches, S., Kryworuchko, J., … Graham, I. D. (2011). Interprofessionalism and shared decision-making in primary care: A stepwise approach towards a new model. *Journal of Interprofessional Care, 25*, 18–25. doi:10.3109/13561820.2010.490502

Liaw, S. Y., Zhou, W. T., Ching Lau, T. C., Siau, C., & Wai-chi Chan, S. (2014). An interprofessional communication training using simulation to enhance safe care for a deteriorating patient. *Nurse Education Today, 34*, 259–264. doi:10.1016/j.nedt.2013.02.019

MacDonald, M. B., Bally, J. M., Ferguson, L. M., Murray, B.L., Fowler-Kerry, S. E., & Anonson, J. M. (2010). Knowledge of the professional role of others: A key interprofessional competency. *Nurse Education in Practice, 10*, 238–242. doi:10.1016/j.nepr.2009.11.012

Missen, K., Jacob, E. R., Barnett, T., Walker, L., & Cross, M. (2012). Interprofessional clinical education: Clinicians' views on the importance of leadership. *Collegian, 19*, 189–195. doi:10.1016/j.colegn.2011.10.002

Mitchell, P., Wynia, M., Golden, R., McNellis, B., Okun, S., Webb, C. E., … Von Kohorn, I. (2012). Core principles and values of effective team-based health care. Discussion Paper, Institute of Medicine, Washington, DC. Retrieved from http://www.iom.edu/tbc

Munro, S., Kornelsen, J., & Grzybowsk, S. (2013). Models of maternity care in rural environments: Barriers and attributes of interprofessional collaboration with midwives. *Midwifery, 29*, 646–652. doi:10.1016/j.midw.2012.06.004

Nuño, R., Coleman, K., Bengoa, R., & Sauto, R. (2012). Integrated care for chronic conditions: The contribution of the ICCC Framework. *Health Policy, 105*, 55–64. doi:10.1016/j.healthpol.2011.10.006

Patrician, P. A., Dolansky, M., Estrada, C., Brennan, C., Miltner, R., Newsom, J., … Moore, S. (2012). Interprofessional education in action: The VA quality scholars fellowship program. *Nursing Clinics of North America, 47*, 347–354. doi:10.1016/j.cnur.2012.05.006

Pollard, K. C., Miers, M. E., & Rickaby, C. (2012). "Oh why didn't I take more notice?" Professionals' views and perceptions of pre-qualifying preparation for interprofessional working in practice. *Journal of Interprofessional Care, 26*, 355–361. doi:10.3109/13561820.2012.689785

Price, S., Doucet, S., & McGillis-Hall, L. (2014). The historical social positioning of nursing and medicine: Implications for career choice, early socialization and interprofessional collaboration. *Journal of Interprofessional Care, 28*(2), 103–109. doi:10.3109/13561820.2013.867839

Sayah, F. A., Szafran, O., Robertson, S., Bell, N. R., & Williams, B. (2014). Nursing perspectives on factors influencing interdisciplinary teamwork in the Canadian primary care setting. *Journal of Clinical Nursing.* doi:10.1111/jocn.12547

Schmitt, M. H., Gilbert, J. H., Brandt, B. F., & Weinstein, R. S. (2013). The coming of age for interprofessional education and practice. *The American Journal of Medicine, 126*(4), 284–288. doi:10.1016/j.amjmed.2012.10.015

Sommerfeldt, S. C. (2013). Articulating nursing in an interprofessional world. *Nurse Education in Practice, 13,* 519–523. doi:10.1016/j.nepr.2013.02.014

Veerapen. K., & Purkis M. E. (2014). Implications of early workplace experiences on continuing interprofessional education for physicians and nurses. *Journal of Interprofessional Care, 28*(3), 218–225. doi:10.3109/13561820.2014.884552

Weinstein, R. S., Brandt, B. F., Gilbert, J. H., & Schmitt, M. H. (2014). Bridging the quality chasm: Interprofessional teams to the rescue? [Editorial] *American Journal of Medicine, 126*(4), 276–277. doi:10.1016/j.amjmed.2012.10.014

Youngwerth, J., & Twaddle, M. (2011). Cultures of interdisciplinary teams: How to foster good dynamics. *Journal of Palliative Medicine, 14*(5), 650–654. doi:10.1089/jpm.2010.0395

Kathy J. Wheeler, Lorna L. Schumann,
Gene Harkless, Catherine G. Ling, Beverly Bird,
and Patricia Maybee

6

GLOBAL HEALTH: DYNAMIC ROLES FOR THE APRN/APN

Never doubt that a small group of thoughtful, committed citizens can change the world. Indeed, it is the only thing that ever has.

—Margaret Mead

Advanced practice nursing is on a rapidly unfolding evolutionary path globally, dictated by need, vision, and opportunity. The need for cost-effective quality health care providers is universal. Technology and communications have allowed global connections, thus effectively making the world small. Educational systems and methods have concurrently evolved. Individuals and organizations involved in health care delivery have seen and learned from each other at a pace not seen before. Patients, people, and providers have continued and, in some instances, accelerated transitory movements, relocating regionally and internationally. These factors have resulted in several occurrences regarding the role of the advanced practice registered nurse (APRN): (a) the advanced practice role is emerging and evolving in many countries; (b) those in the advanced practice role need to understand the global community in order to serve, educate, and treat that community; and (c) the migration of people has created global communities that can be served by APRNs.

GLOBAL APRN ROLES AND TRENDS

One of the most confusing aspects of advanced practice nursing pertains to the titling, definitions, and interpretations of the various APRN roles throughout the world. Only recently has the United States settled on consistent terms and definitions through the *Consensus Model for APRN Regulation: Licensure, Accreditation, Certification, and Education* (APRN Consensus Work Group & National Council of State Boards of Nursing APRN Advisory Committee, 2008). The APRN Advisory Committee, through the consensus model, settled on the global term *advanced practice registered nurse* (APRN). The consensus model further delineated four roles: certified registered nurse anesthetist (CRNA), certified nurse-midwife (CNM), clinical nurse specialist (CNS), and certified nurse practitioner (CNP). APRNs in the United States are to be educated in one of these four roles but must also be educated in one or more of six population foci: the family/individual across the life span; adult-gerontology; pediatrics; neonatology; women's health/gender related; or psychiatric/mental health. The consensus model is broader than merely setting titles—its underlying purpose was to create a document that "defines APRN practice, describes the APRN regulatory model, identifies the titles to be used, defines specialty, describes the emergence of new roles and population foci, and presents strategies for implementation" (p. 4). The model is still in the process of implementation in U.S. states and territories.

Just as the United States has struggled over titles, terms, and role interpretations, the same can be said of advanced practice nursing outside the United States. Many countries have chosen to recognize and encourage expanded roles for nurses beyond that of registered nurse, having done so uniquely and with great variety. The International Council of Nurses (ICN) reports that 70 countries have or are developing advanced practice roles for nurses. In 2002 the ICN defined an APN as a registered nurse who has acquired the expert knowledge base, complex decision-making skills, and clinical competencies for expanded practice, the characteristics of which are shaped by the context and/or country in which he or she is credentialed to practice. A master's degree is recommended for entry level. This term, *advanced practice nurse* (APN), is the commonly accepted international term. Despite the definition, defining characteristics, competencies, and scopes of practice, there is tremendous variation in titles, education, credentialing, policies, recognition, and support worldwide. A 2008 Web-based survey identified 13 different titles for APNs in countries recognizing advanced practice. The same survey also showed the following in respondent countries: 71% had some sort of APN education, 50% cited the master's degree as the primary credential, 72% had formal recognition of the role, and 48% had licensure or renewal requirements (Pulcini, Jelic, Gul, & Loke, 2009). Although showing tremendous advancement of the role, these data establish a clear need for some uniformity of role underpinnings.

A meeting was convened in 2014 to discuss APN practice around the globe as the importance for improved access to cost-effective, quality care in parts of the world where the APN role is absent or underutilized was recognized. The meeting brought together 30 health leaders from around the world. Attendees included representatives from the ICN, multiple universities, multiple ministries of health, the Organization for Economic Co-operation and Development (OECD), the Commission on Graduates of Foreign Nursing Schools (CGFNS), and other health organizations. The first recommendation of the report focused on removing the barriers to practice for APNs. These barriers are identified by the Global APN Nursing Symposium as follows:

• Lack of defined role for APNs
• Inconsistent educational and training standards

- Inconsistent or unnecessary regulation
- Unstable health care funding from government or third-party payers

Key findings were summarized as follows:

- APNs have the potential to play a much larger role in improving the health of people worldwide.
- Different nations are in different stages of developing their nursing workforce, and opportunities for advanced nursing practice vary significantly from country to country.
- Countries where APNs have a well-defined role and greater practice authority have increasingly used nurses to improve access to primary and preventive health care.
- APNs have been successfully deployed in both developed and developing countries to improve health.
- APNs around the globe have worked with governments, consumer groups, funders, investors, and business leaders to create innovative programs and interventions that improve people's health.
- APNs can be a cost-effective solution to existing health care access and quality problems, but additional data are needed to fully evaluate and capture the value of their services.

Based on these issues, the group recommended the following:

- Standardize the definition of the APN role.
- Improve the educational curricula for APNs while respecting each country's unique cultural and political context.
- Increase access to primary and preventive health care services by removing policy barriers that prevent APNs from practicing to the full extent of their education and training.
- Reform health care funding mechanisms to allow for APN-based practice models.
- Collect data and share information on APN quality and outcomes in a variety of countries/settings.

The full results of this meeting are detailed in the *2014 Global Advanced Practice Nursing Symposium—The Future of Nursing Across the Globe* document (Hansen-Turton, 2014).

Although the role will evolve according to unique regional issues, there are commonalities, such as the universal need for cost-effective quality care, APRNs can meet the need, and support for APRNs is through the development and maintenance of polices that provide the education, practice, and research frameworks.

BROADER GLOBAL TRENDS AND NEEDS

To prepare for a global experience, the APRN should understand the political, social, economic, and health care trends. Bass (2011) provided a comprehensive listing of megatrends to consider, detailed in Table 6.1. Megatrends

TABLE 6.1 Megatrends

Health	Education	Government and Society
• Longer life* • Healthier life* • Chronic is normal	• Better educated* • Distance education the norm	• Flattening world • Pockets of instability
Demographics	**Food and Agriculture**	**Environment**
• Older consumer	• Stable currently but linked to environment	• Business measure • Need to know
Economy	**Transportation**	**Energy**
• Water as currency	• Security challenged • Infrastructure affected • Tight economics	• Oil important, not king
Science and Technology	**Work**	**Business**
• Bandwidth is distance • Context is king	• Automation of *normal* • Skills gap and need for reskilling • Technology-enhanced employees	• New competitors • Competition everywhere
Security	**Religion**	**Law**
• Hacking is free	• Expanding impact	• Relative stability

*Not all the world may participate.
Source: Bass (2011, p. 1).

are defined as high-level trends that generally operate broadly, outside of industry and geography. Of interest to APRNs are the predictions of longer, healthier lives; disease as the norm; water as an economic factor; and distance education as the future. On this last issue, APRNs have been leaders, educating providers while maintaining quality outcomes. This has happened within regions and nations—can the process be duplicated globally?

Recently, the global health care megatrends have been elaborated. These megatrends are technological advances, personalized medicine, the demand for evidence-based medicine, increased influence by payers, over treatment decisions in emerging economies, aging populations, rising costs, global pandemics, environmental challenges that overwhelm the current system, nonphysician providers, the growing role of philanthropy, prevention, and medical tourism becoming the next big business opportunity (Dillon & Prokesch, 2014).

To celebrate its 100th anniversary the ICN (2002b) released the *Guidebook for Nurse Futurists* in 2002, listing societal, health, and nursing trends, detailed in Table 6.2. Although developed in 2002, the list is still valid today.

One trend that should be examined further is "population growth." The United Nations (2013) estimates the world's population will reach 9.6 billion by 2050. The prediction suggests populations in developed regions

TABLE 6.2 International Council of Nurses (ICN): Trends Affecting the Future of Nursing

TRENDS IN THE LARGER SOCIETY	HEALTH TRENDS	NURSING TRENDS
Information Technology	**Economic-Driven Health Care Reform**	**Nursing Education Changes**
• Rapid advances occur in information technology. • Communication worldwide is improved via international networks and advanced language translation. • Problems of information security and privacy need to be considered.	• Financial pressures exist to limit the costs of health care. • Health care is being restructured, with nurses increasingly being recognized as full partners in cost-effective health care delivery. • Economics conflicts with the needs of patients.	• Budget-constrained governments are less committed to supporting nursing education. • Inflexible nursing programs are out of touch with service needs and increasingly irrelevant to nursing practice. • Visionary and experienced nurses go into schools to teach and serve as mentors. • Nurses receive higher and broader education.
Social Change/Unrest	**Use of Technology in Caring**	**Advances in Nursing**
• Cooperation and embracing of diversity is what society increasingly expects of itself. • Political and social unrest, stresses from rapid change increase. • Fundamentalism, split between rich and poor, terrorism increase.	• More money goes to high tech. • High-tech drives our high touch. • Nurses humanize the use of technology and never forget the importance of personal caring and touch.	• Nurses are leading the health promotion effort throughout the world. • Nurses become the entry point into the health care system. • Internet-enabled technology helps nurses establish a strong research base for improving clinical practice.
Globalization	**Research and Development of New Therapies/Techniques**	**Turmoil in the Nursing Profession**
• Globalization of commerce and exchanges of information create greater prosperity and mutual understanding. • There is less of a nation-state orientation, more sense of global identity. • Economic problems are contagious in an interconnected global economy.	• Causes of cancer and AIDS are discovered. • Research focuses increasingly on problems of the poor, such as malnutrition, malaria, and water contamination.	• There is a shortage of nurses at the bedside with downsizing of the nursing profession. • Untrained personnel work as *nurses* worldwide. • International nursing organization specialization increases.

(continued)

TABLE 6.2 International Council of Nurses (ICN): Trends Affecting the Future of Nursing *(continued)*

TRENDS IN THE LARGER SOCIETY	HEALTH TRENDS	NURSING TRENDS
	• Developments in genomics take health care to a higher stage of customized care in which therapeutic selection is increasingly tailored to individual genetics. • The number of available, effective therapeutic agents increases dramatically.	
Environmental Hazards	**Empowerment of the Consumer**	**Working Environment for Nurses**
• Environmental problems have severe health effects and retard development in several nations (e.g., habitat destruction, topsoil loss, pollution, climate change, and water shortages and contamination). • Global adoption of *green* manufacturing and other environmentally advanced technologies reverses ecosystem-ruining effects. • Sustainable development principles are adopted throughout the world.	• People take a more active role in their personal health. • Health professionals are expert consultants for self-managed care. • People are empowered through technology: home testing and monitoring, online access to health information.	• Nurses are stressed, working with declining resources in settings where they often feel in competition with other health care providers. • Strikes and unrest over salary and working conditions are common. • Better pay and conditions are sought. • Effective global standards for nurses' working conditions are sought.
Changing Demographic/ Disease Patterns	**Focus on Community Health**	**Regulation and Governance of Nursing**
• Older populations world-wide place a burden on health systems. • Many cities in the South have populations of poor, unemployed, uneducated young people who are angry and violent. • Unmanageable urbaniz-ation causes public health breakdowns. • Immigration stresses society.	• There is a growing emphasis on delivering community-oriented health care. • Healthy community building becomes a major focus of public policy. • Breakdown of community and the resulting increases in crime, violence, and clinical depression are leading causes of morbidity and mortality.	• Self-regulation has given way to state or agency regulation. • Self-regulation is firmly established, and cre-dentialing plays a large role.

(continued)

TABLE 6.2 International Council of Nurses (ICN): Trends Affecting the Future of Nursing (*continued*)

TRENDS IN THE LARGER SOCIETY	HEALTH TRENDS	NURSING TRENDS
• AIDS, other new plagues, and antibiotic-resistant diseases spread. • New kinds of antibiotics limit the spread of new and old diseases.		
	Culture/Class and Its Relationship to Health	**Nursing Relationships With Other Health Professions**
	• Health status becomes more class-oriented. • Health for All strategies are pursued. • Scientific and technological advances create a widening gap where high-tech care is available to the affluent but not to others.	• Tensions between nursing and other health professions play out in educational and clinical settings. • Linkages between nursing and other health specialty groups increases. • Nursing is fully integrated into interdisciplinary health teams in all areas—health education, research, clinical care, management, and policy development.
	Rise of Alternative Medicine	
	• Hierarchical medicine has changed to comprehensive care interdisciplinary teams including alternative providers and nurses. • The most effective combination of various alternative approaches and conventional health care is now widely known and available. • The growth of medically pluralistic societies with effective evaluation of treatment outcomes provides more tools for people to improve their health.	

Source: ICN (2002b; pp. 13–16).

will remain unchanged; however, in 49 of the least developed regions, population growth is expected to double. More than half of these countries will be in Africa. This is significant because these areas struggle with limited resources and health care delivery.

The predicted population explosion can be explained by increased life expectancy. A variety of improved conditions in the world have led to a steady increase in life expectancy in developed and developing countries. By 2045–2050 the global life expectancy will likely be 76 years, and by the end of the century, it is thought life expectancy will be 89 years in developed countries and 81 years in developing countries (United Nations, 2013). With increased life expectancy comes issues. For example, there will be more wheelchairs and walkers than baby carriages in portions of Europe, there will be fewer family caretakers and income-earning adults to support the aging populace, and people will expect better health than their parents and grandparents (Massachusetts Institute of Technology, 2014).

However, despite the expectation of improved health, the reality will likely be more individuals with chronic disease. With ever-increasing diseases, such as obesity, diabetes, hypertension, and cardiovascular disease, this issue becomes even more significant as developing countries attempt to deal with increasing numbers of people with these noncommunicable diseases while still struggling with significant communicable disease (Anjana et al., 2011).

Another trend is the reorientation of health care systems toward primary care. The 2008 World Health Organization (WHO) *World Health Report—Primary Health Care, Now More Than Ever* cited shortcomings in the ability of health systems to meet health goals (WHO, 2008). These include disjointed systems that have focused specialization in wealthy countries, single-disease agendas in poor countries, and an absence of holistic delivery of health care. To that end, the report made four recommendations: universal health coverage, people-centered services, healthy public policies, and leadership from businesses, the private sector, and communities for health.

Another trend is the availability of health care workers. In 2006 the WHO issued the *World Health Report—Working Together for Health* (WHO, 2006), which was devoted to an assessment of the global health workforce. The report disclosed an estimated shortfall of 4.3 million doctors, nurses, midwives, and ancillary health workers worldwide. Most of the shortfall will be in sub-Saharan Africa, but there will also be critical shortages in Central and South America, Southeast Asia, and the Eastern Mediterranean, detailed in Table 6.3.

Table 6.3 demonstrates disparities—for instance, sub-Saharan Africa has only 4% of the total health workforce but 25% of the world's burden of disease. The report goes on to discuss solutions, such as recruitment, education, pay, resources, worker input, lifelong learning, and technology. The report also discussed the problems of migration of health care workers and the importance of balancing choice of individuals to pursue work as needed against the backdrop of health care need, putting retention strategies in place, and working with richer countries to adopt responsible

TABLE 6.3 Estimated Shortages of Doctors, Nurses, and Midwives by WHO Regions

WHO REGION	NUMBER OF COUNTRIES		IN COUNTRIES WITH SHORTAGES		
	Total	**With Shortages**	**Total Workforce**	**Estimated Shortage**	**Percentage Increase Required**
Africa	46	36	590,198	817,992	139
Americas	35	5	93,603	37,886	40
Southeast Asia	11	6	2,332,054	1,164,001	50
Europe	52	0	NA	NA	NA
Eastern Mediterranean	21	7	312,613	306,031	98
Western Pacific	27	3	27,260	32,560	119
World	192	57	3,355,728	2,358,470	70

WHO, World Health Organization. *Source:* WHO (2006).

recruitment. This last issue is a particular responsibility of the United States, United Kingdom, Canada, and Australia, as they are the primary recipients of medical migration workers (Zackowitz, 2014). To assist with this issue, O'brien and Gostin (2011) recommend the following:

- Address the health worker shortage in the United States.
- Develop a plan to address the global health worker shortage.
- Provide global leadership in addressing the global health worker shortage.
- Reform U.S.–global health assistance programs in partner countries.
- Increase financial assistance for global workforce capacity development.
- Increase the number of health workers being trained in the United States.
- Empower an appropriate agency to regulate recruiters of foreign-trained health workers. (pp. 4–7)

The Institute of Medicine's (IOM's) *The Future of Nursing: Leading Change, Advancing Health* reiterates many of these same points:

- Promote targeted educational investment in foreign-educated nurses in the U.S. nursing force.
- Promote baccalaureate education for entry into practice in the United States.
- Harmonize nursing curricula.
- Add global health as a subject matter to undergraduate and graduate nursing curricula.
- Establish a national system that monitors and tracks the inflow of foreign nurses, their countries of origin, the settings in which they work, and their education and licensure.

- Create an international body to coordinate and recommend national and international workforce policies. (Nichols, Davis, & Richardson, 2011)

World leaders agreed on the millennium development goals (MDGs), eight goals and multiple measureable targets aimed at solving some of the most demanding problems of the time (United Nations, 2014). Every single goal, directly or indirectly, affects global heath. Anyone who provides or plans care for patients and populations needs to be familiar with the goals:

1. Eradicate extreme poverty and hunger.
2. Achieve universal primary education.
3. Promote gender equality and empower women.
4. Reduce child mortality.
5. Improve maternal health.
6. Combat HIV/AIDS, malaria, and other diseases.
7. Ensure environmental sustainability.
8. Develop a global partnership for development.

Significant progress has been made toward goal achievement, particularly poverty reduction, improved access to water, reduction in infectious disease, reduction in disparities of education, and increased participation of women in policy. At the same time more effort is needed to accomplish nutrition and mortality goals. (For the full report, see United Nations, 2014.) The effort now is moving toward sustainable development goals (SDGs), with stakeholders creating an ongoing development agenda.

A last trend is the controversial topic of global warming or climate change. Regardless of views, most agree that some recent weather events will likely recur and have profound effects on health. Warmer temperatures, warmer waters, melting ice caps, and elevations in sea level are thought to lead to hurricanes, insect migration, zones of increased humidity, and zones of drought. These directly affect health and exposure to disease, cause significant damage to lands and crops, and impair economies attempting to provide for people (Kai, 2011).

Agencies Involved in the Global APRN Experience

Numerous agencies are involved in nursing and APRN issues and function across borders and nations. The ICN has been guiding nursing since 1899 with a mission "to represent nursing worldwide, advancing the profession and influencing health policy" (ICN, 2014, para. 1). In 2000, the ICN and American Association of Nurse Practitioners (AANP; formerly the American Academy of Nurse Practitioners) created the International Nurse Practitioner/Advanced Practice Nursing Network (INP/APNN). This network is considered a primary global resource for APRNs and those interested in advancing the role (AANP, 2014).

WHO has also worked on nursing issues such as education, governance, retention, and migration of nurses but has not been as involved with advanced nursing. Much WHO work has been devoted to workforce development of midwifery, rather than nurse midwifery. Similarly, the International Confederation of Midwives has done the same.

Other nursing organizations well known for supporting nursing around the world are Sigma Theta Tau International (STTI), the American Association of Nurse Practitioners (AANP), and the National Organization of Nurse Practitioner Faculties (NONPF). Currently STTI is working with world health leaders on the Global Advisory Panel on the Future of Nursing (GAPFON), which has been tasked to create a global nursing voice that will improve global health. STTI (2014) has been supportive to APRNs through grants, support of research initiatives, continuing education, conferences, and numerous publications, and AANP and NONPF assist APRNs educators to network, communicate, publish, and share common concerns related to international work.

Several organizations have influenced the standards of APRN practice and education in the United States. Although nations choose to self-determine if or how the APRN role develops, many use the same documents. Table 6.4 provides a partial listing of influential documents.

TABLE 6.4 Documents With Potential International Influence

American Association of Nurse Practitioners	• Clinical Outcomes: The Yardstick of Educational Effectiveness • Nurse Practitioner Cost-Effectiveness • Nurse Practitioner Curriculum • Quality of Nurse Practitioner Practice • Scope of Practice for Nurse Practitioners • Standards of Practice for Nurse Practitioners
American Association of Colleges of Nursing	• The Essentials of Baccalaureate Education for Professional Nursing and Tool Kit • The Essentials of Master's Education in Nursing (2011) • The Essential of Master's Education for Advanced Practice Nursing (1996) • The Essentials of Doctoral Education for Advanced Nursing Practice (2006)
National Organization of Nurse Practitioner Faculties (NONPF)	• Multiple examples of competencies for nurse practitioners available on the NONPF website. Intended for entry into practice, the competences are numerous, population-specific and separately include those for both master's and doctoral levels.
American College of Nurse Midwives	• Faculty Degree Requirements • Mandatory Degree Requirements for Entry Into Midwifery Practice • Midwifery Education • Midwives Are Primary Care Providers and Leaders of Maternity Care Homes

(continued)

TABLE 6.4 Documents With Potential International Influence *(continued)*

American Association of Nurse Anesthetists	• Scope of Nurse Anesthesia Practice (2013) • Standards of Nurse Anesthesia Practice (2013) • Quality of Care in Anesthesia
National Association of Clinical Nurse Specialists	• Clinical Nurse Specialist Core Competencies (2010) • Position Statement on the Importance of the CNS Role in Care Coordination (2013) • Impact of the Clinical Nurse Specialist Role on the Costs and Quality of Health Care (2013)

Recently, certification organizations are beginning to examine educational programs and to certify some APRNs who go to schools outside the United States. Given the variability of roles and education of international APRNs, there is little migration of APRNs across borders. Currently the Commission on Graduates of Foreign Nursing Schools (CGFNS) is working on an APRN education comparability tool to address the underlying issues. These issues are problems confronting APRNs from other countries coming to the United States to practice, nurses entering U.S. APRN programs, and the APRN role enactment in their home country (Schober, 2011). At some point the process of accrediting APRN schools outside the United States may become desirable.

Preparing the APRN for Global Experiences

International advanced practice nursing partnerships have become a popular method of exchanging nursing knowledge in that they provide a forum for access to international practice experiences and a forum for research in international health care issues. In today's global health care environment, APRNs educated in global health are prepared to network with international multidisciplinary health care providers to develop and deliver quality care. These partnerships have included long-term work assignments and medical brigades (previously called missions) of varied lengths, most with the goal of developing sustainable health care access. How this goal is carried out depends on the needs and plans of the supporting partners and may vary by time of year, current needs of the partner, and the political climate.

Aside from international experiences that occur in the United States, many health care providers are willing to volunteer on both short- and long-term undertakings outside the United States. World disasters like the 2010 Haiti earthquake that created catastrophic damage have prompted the need for increasing emergency medical relief and continuing sustainable medical work. Nongovernmental organizations (NGO) have teams who arrive regularly to provide sustainable help for this nation.

Ethics and Responsibilities: Approach to Care

A critical foundational element for any international experience involves the development of appropriate ethical and cultural approaches by involved health care. Ethical practice involves respectfully approaching those in need, treating them fairly and equitably, and thoughtfully approaching human rights (Hunter & Crabtree, 2010). A culturally competent health system is "one that acknowledges and incorporates—at all levels—the importance of culture, assessment of cross-cultural relations, vigilance towards dynamics that result from cultural differences, expansion of cultural knowledge, and adaptation of services to meet culturally unique needs" (Batancourt, Green, Carrillo, & Owusu, 2003, p. 294). Chase and Hunter (2010) describe *cultural competence* as a skill that can be learned and emphasize that the APRN should be not only culturally competent but culturally responsive, defining that as someone capable of relating in an ethnorelativistic, not ethnocentric, fashion. With an ethnorelativistic approach, the APRN provides care centered on the values and perspectives of the patient and the community. Resources to educate and assess those skills can be obtained through the National Center for Cultural Competence, assessable at http://nccc.georgetown.edu/index.html. They also emphasize that the APRN be not only culturally competent but culturally responsive, defining that as someone capable of doing what has been described in an ethnorelativistic, not ethnocentric, fashion. With an ethnorelativistic approach, the APRN provides care centered on the values and perspectives of the patient and the community.

A related issue pertains to the ethics and cultural sensitivity surrounding the level of participation in global experiences—short term (1 day to 1 month) versus long term (1 month to 2 years) versus permanent (2 years or more). APRNs have participated at all levels. The controversy stems from concerns that any effort without proven benefits to the patient or community is not ethical. Although patients who receive corrective lenses, are cured of an infection, or have a completely decayed tooth pulled may value the intervention, some want the measure of value to be based on level of sustainability. Martiniuk, Manouchehrian, Negin, and Zwi (2012) cited that benefits of short- and long-term medical brigades included transferring medical knowledge, helping communities convey their plight, and giving communities hope that problems might be solved. Negatives included problems of sustainability (unless that was specifically countered), limited relations with nearby health care systems, and lack of data analysis. The authors recommended the following to optimize global efforts: cross-cultural dialogue and efforts, determined efforts toward efficacy, transparency, and coordination with existing organizational programming. These are clear messages to any APRN considering such work or evaluating a program before joining.

Fulbright Programs and Project HOPE

Two organizations with long histories of providing high-quality opportunities for international nursing experience are the Fulbright Program and Project HOPE. The older Fulbright Program offers U.S. nursing professionals, educators, and scholars the opportunity to study, teach, and/or conduct research abroad through the Fulbright U.S. Scholar Program and the Fulbright Specialist Program. These are competitive programs that are open to most academic disciplines. The Fulbright initiative was spearheaded by Senator William J. Fulbright as a way to promote peace and mutual understanding at the close of World War II. Funding began in 1946, and now its programs are active in more than 155 countries. The Fulbright Scholar Program publishes the grant opportunities each spring with an application deadline of August 1. Many grant applications require a letter of invitation, so it is helpful to review the online catalogue early, speak with the Fulbright staff about the grant specifics, and communicate with the host institution about obtaining an invitation letter. The Scholar Program funds travel and a generous living stipend. These grants may be for teaching, research, or a teaching–research combination, and the time commitment (3 to 12 months) is specified in the grant opportunity. In contrast, the Fulbright Specialist Program offers an opportunity for experienced professionals and academics to collaborate on projects defined by the non-U.S. institution for 2 to 6 weeks. Travel and in-country costs are covered. However, the Fulbright Specialist Program does not fund activities such as direct patient care requiring a nursing license. See www.cies.org for more detail on the Fulbright programs.

Project HOPE, founded in 1958, began with a peacetime-deployed hospital ship and now provides land- and ship-based global nursing practice and education experience. Opportunities include but are not limited to 4- to 8-week ship-based nursing practice as well as 6-month teaching opportunities in countries such as China and project-based work, including implementing a tuberculosis (TB) control program in Tajikistan. Details can be found on the Project HOPE website, www.projecthope.org and Facebook site. For most volunteer positions the individual is expected to pay his or her own travel expenses and their daily living expenses.

Health Care Medical Brigades

Emerging health care needs such as Ebola, severe acute respiratory syndrome (SARS), and Middle East respiratory syndrome (MERS) require global partners working together to develop strategies to treat and prevent the spread of these diseases. The term *health care* is used to designate an interdisciplinary approach to deliver care internationally. An interdisciplinary team of health care individuals is needed to improve overall health care. A well-rounded team is composed of physicians, nurses, APRNs, dentists, health educators, nutritionists, social workers, pharmacists, physical therapists, occupational therapists, counselors, and students from all disciplines.

Countries such as the United States, Canada, Switzerland, Germany, England, and Australia have large numbers of NGOs and universities that send out health care teams regularly for the purposes of providing direct patient care, supervised experiences for students, and opportunities to network on research and education. Table 6.5 lists volunteer international health care websites and information to assist in planning a medical brigade.

Pretravel Preparations

Pretravel preparation should begin at least a year in advance. In preparing for a trip, the team leader should review online information about the

TABLE 6.5 Volunteer International Websites/Information to Assist in Planning

U.S. State Department Travel Warnings and Consular Information Sheets—provides country-by-country information relevant to health, safety, visa and entry requirements (travelers may be unable to board planes if they do not have the necessary visa), medical facilities, consular contact information, drug penalties, etc. http://travel.state.gov/travel/cis_pa_tw/tw/tw_1764.html

CIA Publications and Factbooks—includes among its sections World Factbook (provides a wealth of information on virtually all countries), Handbook of International Economic Statistics, CIA Maps and Publications Released to the Public. www.cia.gov/cia/publications

Centers for Disease Control and Prevention (CDC)—provides information for foreign travel and recommended immunizations. www.cdc.gov

Ford Foundation—is one of the largest U.S. foundations active in national and international health. www.fordfound.org

Hesperian Foundation—publishes low-cost, practical books for use in all aspects of international health practice at the community level. www.hesperian.org

Library of Congress Country Studies—provides detailed information on many of the countries of the world prepared by the Federal Research Division of the Library of Congress. The site has an impressive search engine that can search across the database for any combination of words, ranks the hits in order of closeness to your search terms, and then provides links to the desired text. http://lcweb2.loc.gov/frd/cs/cshome.html#toc

Teaching Aids at Low Cost—lists and distributes many health-related teaching aids that are provided in low-cost format and often in multiple languages for use by health care providers and patients in developing countries. www.talcuk.org

World Health Organization—http://www.who.int/topics/travel/en/

American Council for Voluntary International Action—is a consortium of more than 150 nonprofit organizations working worldwide in health, educational development, and other related fields. It is a source of jobs and volunteer resources. The site includes hotlinks to all of its members. www.interaction.org

Doctors Without Borders USA—is the famous French-originated organization (Medecins Sans Frontieres) that sends fully qualified health professionals into some of the most challenging parts of the world. Because they do not have job descriptions contracted for nurse practitioners, nurse practitioners function in the role of nurses. www.msf.org

Foundation of Integrated Education and Development (FUNEDESIN)—is a clinical rotation program that provides clinical experiences in the Amazon region of Ecuador. It is open to all levels of students and health professionals in the fields of medicine and nursing. Further information can be found on the website. (http://www.funedesin.org). The application pack can be requested by e-mailing clinic@funedesin.org.

Global Health: Making Contacts—contains a gold mine of international health resources and projects, including job opportunities. It provides links with a long list of governmental and nongovernmental agencies and organizations, people, academic institutions, and organizational directories relevant to health. The sections are conveniently grouped according to major mission, affiliation, type, etc. www.globalhealth.pitt.edu

(continued)

TABLE 6.5 Volunteer International Websites/Information to Assist in Planning *(continued)*

Global Service Corps—provides short- and long-term opportunities to volunteer in health, education, and environment projects in Kenya, Costa Rica, and Thailand. www. globalservicecorps.org

International Foundation for Education and Self-Help (IFESH)—provides assistance and opportunities for service much in the fashion of the U.S. Peace Corps. The primary focus is sub-Saharan Africa. Through its International Fellows Program (IFP), the Foundation has provided 9-month overseas internships for Americans who are graduate students or recent college and university graduates. Fellows are placed with development-focused organizations working overseas. www.ifesh.org

International Healthcare Opportunities Clearinghouse—provides listings of organizations with Internet links of online resources, courses, and books on international health, as well as information about how to get funding. It has a search engine that can locate organizations according to diverse search criteria and provides links to home pages of organizations where available. http://library.umassmed.edu/ihoc/

International Health Medical Education Consortium (IHMEC)—provides information about courses, curricula, annotated websites, foreign language study courses, and other materials useful for faculty and students interested in international health. Go to the Resources section of the IHMEC home page. www.globalhealtheducation.org

International Medical Corps (IMC)—is a private, nonsectarian, nonpolitical, humanitarian relief organization established in 1984 by volunteer U.S. physicians and nurses. The home page lists IMC's programs and job openings for doctors, nurses, and other health professionals. www.internationamedicalcorps.org

MPA International—is a nonprofit Christian relief and development organization, promoting the total health of people living in the world's poorest communities. www.map.org

Medical Missions Foundations—has multiple opportunities. www.mmfworld.org

Direct Relief—has many opportunities in the United States and abroad. www.directrelief.org

Humanitarian Medical Relief—has more than 60 possibilities for volunteer service and includes a link to Flights for Humanity, a nonprofit Christian organization that flies patients to medical centers for treatment. http://humanitarianmedical.org

International Health Database under the American Medical Association—has numerous opportunities. http://ama-assn.org//ama/pub/about-ama/our-people/member-groups-sections/medical-student-section/opportunities/internation-health-opportunities.page

Volunteer Humanitarian Opportunities—contains more than 40 opportunities for volunteer service. www.projects-abroad.org

Heal the Nations Christian Medical Missions—focuses on India and Uganda. www. mtghouse.org

American Medical Resources Foundation—donates used, but fully functional, medical equipment to hospitals serving the poor worldwide. www.amrf.com

Hearts in Motion (HIM)—is a nonprofit, nondenominational agency that focuses on the needs of less fortunate children and families. Each trip runs about 10 days and costs about $1,000 for airfare and lodging. http://www.heartsinmotion.org/index.php

(continued)

TABLE 6.5 Volunteer International Websites/Information to Assist in Planning *(continued)*

International Volunteer Work in India–Delhi—as Mark Twain recounted in *Following the Equator,* India is "the land of dreams and romance, of splendor and rags, of palaces and hovels, the country of a hundred nations and a hundred tongues." www.crossculturalsolutions.org

Monitoring Freedom—Human Rights Around the World—includes expatriate resources and resources for Americans fleeing America. Allows users to search the largest expatriate database of embassies, international jobs, and offshore financial services websites. www.escapeartist.com/jobs/overseas1.htm

International Grants and Funders—provides international grants and funders. www.grantspace.org

Global Volunteer Network—is a resource for those interested in volunteering. www.globalvolunteerntwork.org

Doctors of the World, USA: Volunteer/Recruitment—offers a wide array of opportunities for health professionals to contribute to ongoing efforts to alleviate suffering and help improve human rights around the world. http://doctorsoftheworld.org/get-involved/volunteer/

Healing Touch International: Clinics—is a listing of Healing Touch Clinics that are open to the public. Some clinics are by appointment only, and payment is by donation. Clinic choice can be made on the website. www.healingtouchinternational.org

The Medical Foundation, About Us—History—discusses the work of the Medical Foundation for the Care of Victims of Torture, which began more than 25 years ago under the auspices of the Medical Group of Amnesty International. www.freedomfromtorture.org

Mercy & Truth Medical Missions—desires to serve the public as much as possible. Mercy & Truth Medical Missions is a fee-for-service clinic. www.mercyandtruth.com

Global Health Outreach—organizes short-term medical group missions. Christian Medical & Dental Association, under Medical Missions tab. www.cmdahome.org

Medical Education International—medical education teams with Christian Medical & Dental Association, under Medical Missions tab. www.cmdahome.org

Northwest Medical Teams International—provides contact information under AERDO tab. www.aerdo.org/members/organizations/northwest_medical_teams.html

Heal the Nations—provides Christian Medical Missions links, a list of volunteer health care organizations, both Christian and secular. www.healthenations.com/links.html

United States Agency for International Development (USAID)—provides economic and humanitarian assistance. www.usaid.gov

Christian Connections for International Health—promotes international health. Has a job search section. www.ccih.org

"Nuestra Senora de Guadalupe"—based in Ecuador, organizes short-term medical missions into the remote areas of the Amazon basin. The Mission at Guadalupe also has a clinic that is looking for providers for longer terms. www.guadalupe-ec.org

(continued)

TABLE 6.5 Volunteer International Websites/Information to Assist in Planning *(continued)*

American Baptist Churches in the U.S.A International Ministries (ABC)—goals are theological eduction, evangelism, economic development, education, and health. http://internationalministries.org

International Medical Volunteer Association—provides information about volunteering and links to various international organizations. www.imva.org

Doctors for Global Health—a private, not-for-profit organization promoting health, education, art, and other human rights throughout the world. www.dghonline.org

University of Washington—provides information on overseas medical opportunities. www.globalhealth.washington.edu

University of Kentucky—offers weeklong medical brigades three times each summer at permanent UK clinic in Santo Domingo, Ecuador. www.uky.edu/international/shoulder_to_shoulder

American Medical Student Association—strives to extend the scope of our members' medical education through institutes, international exchanges and career development opportunities. www.amsa.org/global/ih/ihopps.cfm

MAP/Reader's Digest International Fellowships—a global Christian health organization that partners with people living in conditions of poverty to save lives and develop healthier families and communities. www.map.org

Save the Children—focuses on outreach efforts related to maternal, newborn, and child health. www.everybeatmatters.org

host country/sponsor, especially data related to finances and bringing medications and supplies. If the brigade is outside the United States, the State Department warnings specific to the country should be reviewed. Networking and developing a relationship with the host country/sponsor may require an initial visit to determine the needs. Issues such as requirements of the host country/sponsor for current provider licenses, medications, and supplies that are approved by the country/sponsor should be determined early in the pretravel period. Transportation and lodging will also need to be worked out with the host. One country (Burundi) requires visa applications be submitted a letter of invitation from the people with whom the volunteer is staying or documentation of hotel reservations.

There are a variety of ways team members may fund their trip expenses. Some pay the total amount out of pocket. Others will rely on fund-raisers to support all or part of the team's expenses. Some organizations do a one-third method, when the individual pays a third, the organization pays a third, and the last third is from donations or fund-raiser activities (Samaritans Now, 2014).

Funding needs to be discussed at one of the early team meetings—finances can become a source of friction in the group. Airline tickets are the most costly budget item. Some airline companies will provide group rates and allow extra baggage for free. Airlines request contact at least 60 days in advance to set up the team trips.

Team members frequently ask how much cash they should bring. In many cases, it depends on the economy of the host county. For example, costs in Thailand are higher than those in Guatemala.

Many countries (e.g., Ecuador, Guatemala) require preapproval for medications, and the expiration date on medications must be at least 6 months into the future. The preapproval requires listing expiration dates, names of the pharmaceutical company that produced the medication, and quantities of the medications. All documents must be notarized. Table 6.6 lists pharmaceutical organizations that will provide medications to health care teams. Some organizations require a physician's signature. If ordering medications outside the United States, for instance, from Action Medeor in Germany, U.S. Customs and Border Protection will need to be contacted for a list of brokerage firms that will support bringing the medications into the United States for transport to the host country. Some companies allow APRNs to purchase low-cost medications, and others require a physician or pharmacist to do the purchasing. This requirement is based on state regulation of the involved APRNs. Another source to review is www.who.int/medicines/areas/access/sources_prices/international_medicine_price_guidesprice_lists.pdf.

Some university pharmacy departments compound medications for interdisciplinary faculty/student medical brigades or assist in purchasing and packaging of medications. Some pharmaceutical companies will donate over-the-counter medications. Good sources of over-the-counter medications are APRN conferences. At the end of the conference, companies are willing to donate their remaining products. Table 6.7 provides a list of recommended medications for a trip. Occasionally, there is a request from the host administrator for a specific medication—for example, something to treat hyperthyroidism.

Team Meetings

Team meetings are essential to building a strong cohesive team. The meetings should include discussion of cultural traditions and behaviors; boundary setting; cultural differences and cultural sensitivity; and issues of dealing with extreme poverty, serious illnesses, abuse, and starvation. Illicit drug use and drunkenness are not acceptable behaviors on a medical brigade trip. Other issues to address are flights and lodging, itinerary, work schedules, local regional health issues, and practical tips for the trip. See Tables 6.8 to 6.13 for trip preparation materials.

The team should plan at least one or two tourist activities, such as sightseeing to the Taj Mahal and the Red Fort in the Delhi area. Shopping is also a fun experience for most team members, so selecting a hotel close to a shopping area is recommended.

Setting Up a Medical Camp

The host country/sponsor organization selects the sites for the camps and arranges the overall setup. For example, when working in the slums of New Delhi, the host rents tents that can be used in areas for slums that do not have school buildings. In some countries, established clinics, schools,

TABLE 6.6 Medical Brigade Pharmaceutical Resources

Agency	Website	Phone or E-mail/ Contact Person	Application	Pharmaceutical Supplier	Comments
Cross Link International	www. crosslinkinternational. net/RequestsFor CrossLink.shtml	(703) 534-5465	www.crosslink international.net/ App.shtml		Receiving agency must be a Christian faith–based organization.
Brother's Brother Foundation	www.brothersbrother. org/medical.htm	ccramer@ brothersbrother.org; Chris Cramer		Yes, and small trays of basic surgical instruments	Most medications are good for 4–6 months. No cost for medications and shipment in the United States.
Catholic Medical Mission Board	www.cmmb.org/What/ medical_shipments.htm#	ktebbett@cmmb.org	www.cmmb. org/pdfs/ HealingHelpMedical MissionsApp.pdf		Requires submission of an online application.
MAP	http://www. map.org/site/ PageServer?pagename =travel_Forms	(800) 225-8550 or online contact: www.map.org/site/ Survey?SURVEY_ ID=1320&ACTION_ REQUIRED=URI_ ACTION_USER_ REQUESTS	www.map.org/ site/DocServer/ MAP_Travel_Pack_ Program_All_Forms. pdf?docID=4781		Requires submission of an online application.
Kingsway Charities	www.kingswaycharities. org/index.php/ our-charity/ supply-request/	(800) 321-9234			Receiving organization must be Christian faith–based.
Vitamin Angels	www.vitaminangels. org/contact-us	(805) 564-8400			Not for short-term medical teams.

Globus Relief	www.globusrelief.org/partneringwithglobusrelief	Christopher Dunn, chdunn@globusrelief.org		Yes and medical equipment	They try to make pharmaceuticals below cost.
medWish International	www.medwish.org/handcarryinfo.html	(216) 692-1685 or info@medwish.org	www.medwish.org/handcarryinfo-app.html	No, only medical supplies	
Project Cure	http://projectcure.org/get-assistance	patricebaker@projectcure.org	www.projectcure.org/get-assistance/medical-kits#application	Yes	Most medications provided will only have 3 months remaining on their dating.
FAME	www.fameworld.org/home.aspx?iid=14334	(317) 358-2480 or medicalmissions@FAMEworld.org			Must be a faith-based organization.
International Aid	www.internationalaid.org/Health_Products.html	healthproduct@internationalaid.org		Yes, and lab-in-a-suitcase (www.internat-ionalaid.org/Lab-In-A-Suitcase_files/LIS%20Brochure%20New.pdf)	Need to complete online application.
Action Medeor	www.medeor.org	Inge.ricken@medeor.de	info@medeor.de	Yes	Product catalogue: http://medeor.de/en/medeor-market-en/price-indicator.html

(continued)

TABLE 6.6 Medical Brigade Pharmaceutical Resources *(continued)*

Agency	Website	Phone or E-mail/ Contact Person	Application	Pharmaceutical Supplier	Comments
World Medical Relief	www.world medicalrelief.org/	info@world medicalrelief.org, Carolyn Racklyeft	www.world medicalrelief.org/	Yes	Accommodates medical brigade teams with pharmaceuticals. Medications do not usually have a year before expiring but such medications can be purchased at lower cost. Need to fill out an online application.
Americares	www.americares.org/ whatwedo/mop/	cmarion@ americares.org, Cia Marion	www.americares.org/ whatwedo/mop/ mopapplication.pdf	Yes	Most medications are short-dated (3–6 months out), but they do have a few longer-dated medications. Suggest a $200 donation.
Blessings International	www.blessing.org	Fax number for ordering is (918) 250-1281	www.blessing. org/wp-content/ uploads/2012/09/ Blessings-Instructions. pdf	Yes	First-time users must fax a copy of their check for the estimated amount of the order with their application form.
Direct Relief International	www.directrelief.org	SJohnson@ directrelief.org	www.directrelief. org/wp-content/ uploads/Volunteer Application2013.pdf	Has medication and supplies for volunteers on disaster relief.	Participates in disaster relief worldwide.

Heart-to-Heart International	www.hearttoheart.org		https://hearttoheartinternational.wufoo.com/forms/heart-to-heart-international/	Yes	Physicians, optometrists, dentists, podiatrists, and pharmacists can apply for a standard Ready Relief pack of medications or a custom order.
Interchurch Medical Assistance	www.interchurch.org	(877) 241-7952 or (410) 635-8720	imainfo@imaworldhealth.org	They have medicines and supplies for their own projects. They run their own programs in Haiti, South Sudan, Dominican Republic, Congo, Tanzania, and Indonesia.	They deliver prepacked medicine and supply boxes to treat up to 1000 patients.
Project HOPE	www.projecthope.org	(800) 544-HOPE	Application to be a volunteer for Project HOPE can be found at https://projecthope.csod.com/ats/careersite/JobDetails.aspx?id=35	They have medication and supplies for their own country.	Project HOPE has worked in more than 120 countries.

Developed by Colleen Strand; modified by Lorna Schumann; reproduced with permission.

TABLE 6.7 Recommended Medications for International Medical Brigades

Analgesics, antipyretics, nonsteroidal antiinflammatory drugs (NSAIDs)	Antiinflammatory drugs
Anesthetics	Antimalarial drugs
Antiallergics	Cardiovascular drugs
Antiamoebic drugs	Dermatologic preparations, disinfectants
Antiasthmatic drugs, antitussives	Diuretics
Antibacterials, antifungals, antiviral drugs	Gastrointestinal drugs
Antidiabetics	Laxatives
Antidiarrheal drugs	Ophthalmologic preparations
Antiepileptics	Psychotherapeutic agents
Antihelminthics, antifiliarial drugs	Vitamins and food supplements

TABLE 6.8 Short-Term Health Care Mission Team Leader Responsibilities

1. Begin planning the trip a year in advance. Decide on the type of project, dates, and location. Work with host country/sponsor team members to plan the medical brigade and determine the needs of the people.

2. Solicit application for team members and select a team. Interview and select team members about 6 months in advance so that they can request time off work.

3. Develop a budget that includes air flights, all transportation, housing, and food. Share the information with the team. Develop a plan for financing the trip.

4. Set up a schedule for team meetings and posttrip debriefing. The first meeting should cover issues such as waivers, trip insurance, cultural sensitivity, appropriate behaviors for the trip, what to do in case of illness, how to obtain passports (if needed), how to obtain visas (if needed), needed immunizations, the approximate cost of the trip, and any issues the team members may have.

5. The team leader is responsible for coordinating medications and supplies to be taken on the trip. Each team member should pack the medications and supplies he or she is taking and make a list to give to the team leader. The number of bags allowed and the weight of the bags are determined by individual airlines. Some airlines allow only one checked bag free; others will allow up to three. Other luggage will need to be paid for, usually $25 to $75 per bag.

6. The team leader and host country/sponsor leader are responsible for the daily activities and debriefing activities. Should a team problem occur, the team leader and host country/sponsor leader should work together to resolve the issue.

7. Plan a posttrip debriefing meeting to discuss issues that occurred on the trip and since returning home. This meeting may need to take place on the last evening the team is together—some teams are composed of team members from other countries.

TABLE 6.9 Recommendations of What to Take for Medical Brigades to Developing Countries

Lightweight (silk?) sleeping bag for warm climates—spray with DEET and put in zip lock bag for penetration of the DEET into the material Miranda@nznature.co.nz ($2 NZ = $1 US)	Nonsteroidal antiinflammatory drug (NSAID) of choice (carry on the plane)—helps with jet-lag
Aluminum foil blanket for warmth, if needed	Clothes pins and roll of heavy string or lightweight rope
Mosquito net and repellant containing DEET (not in pressurized spray can)—recommend spraying suitcase and clothing with DEET before travel	Duct tape, colored (can help visualize bags or brigade items)
Citron wrist/ankle band to ward off mosquitos (effective for 400 hours)	Otoscope/ophthalmoscope (battery powered for places where there is no electricity)
	A ready-to-go bag that has stethoscope, blood pressure cuff, otoscope, ophthalmoscope, pens, urine dip sticks, scissors, duct tape, O_2 saturation monitor (inexpensive from Amazon.com), Doppler (relatively inexpensive from Amazon.com), reliable thermometer, etc.
Sunscreen	Flashlight or headlight (frees hands to fight off the elements), backpack (one that will carry water bottles)
Ciprofloxacin (enough for 3 days), for diarrhea, or use when starting to run a fever—is not effective in all countries	Belly pack—keep passport (in a zip lock bag) and money in your pack
Pepto-Bismol tablets (chew 2 before each meal)	Passport must be in a safe place at all times!
Imodium AD	Hat and lightweight rain poncho
Toilet paper, one roll—others may be purchased in country	Lightweight clothing that dries fast or scrubs—work well for seeing patients. What is worn depends on the culture. In India, females on the team wear the traditional dress of shalwar kameez and dupatta. Avoid wearing shorts and tank tops.
Nutritious snacks	Tennis shoes or boots with socks—recommended to protect from insect bites
Chocolate that will not melt	Colored photocopy of passport to give to the team leader
Personal medicines	Lightweight long-sleeve and long-leg pajamas with tight cuffs—keeps the mosquitoes and other insects off the skin

(continued)

TABLE 6.9 Recommendations of What to Take for Medical Brigades to Developing Countries *(continued)*

Language dictionary and medical language dictionary	Leatherman or other knife in *checked bag*
Gifts for people who help and children (stickers, blow-bubbles, inexpensive toys—chosen according to age and safety)	Country-specific electrical adapter plugs and voltage converters, if needed. For information: www.rei.com/learn/expert-advice/world-electricity-guide.html
Water bottle—bottled water usually can be bought in country	Extra batteries of standard sizes—in-country batteries may not be reliable
Flip-flops or Chacos for the shower	Locks for suitcase—not for use on flights but to use when working or away from them for the day
Towel, washcloth, and soap; hand wipes	Camera, extra camera batteries if battery-dependent camera
Toiletries (inexpensive shampoo or conditioners, if expensive Customs may inspect)	Learn to adapt and do without for a short time—think: patience, perseverance, and stamina

TABLE 6.10 Pretravel Safety Precautions

Review online travel recommendations:

- From the host country's embassy and other reliable resources

- Immunizations and medications (available at www.cdc.gov)

- Review State Department travel warnings (available at http://travel.state.gov/travel).

- Notify the State Department of trip purpose/travel itinerary (http://travel.state.gov or 888-407-4748).

- Collect team member licenses and colored copies of team member's signed passports/visas.

- Prepare a team emergency kit.

- Set up two or three team meetings. A conference call may be helpful using www.freeconferencecall.com.

TABLE 6.11 Travel Preparations

Documents	Passport	Application is available at http://travel.state.gov/passport Cost: $140 (adult first-time passport book and card) + $25 execution fee. Expedited services are an additional $60. Should not expire within 6 months after return to United States.
	Visa(s)	May be required by individual country; check http://travel.state.gov/visa/ to determine visa requirements. Cost: Varies, but often around $150 to $200, when added to cost of FedEx, new photos, and the visa itself.
	Immunization record	Some countries require verification of specific immunizations (especially yellow fever) to enter the country. Immunizations can be expensive for first-time trip members. The receiving country may require a photocopy of the yellow fever immunization when applying for a visa. Information is available at http://wwwnc.cdc.gov/travel/default.aspx.
Travel Arrangements	Flights	Flights can be arranged online, but commonly used travel sites (e.g., Travelocity, Cheap Flights, Expedia) are often unable to book international travel to more remote settings. Help may be obtained from a travel agent or the airline. Consider choosing airlines that add frequent flyer miles based on connecting flights with partner airlines. An example is Delta/KLM/Kenya airlines to Nairobi. An excellent site for host country maps is www.WHO.int/maps.
	Lodging	Hotels or other lodging facilities may not accept credit cards; other hotels may not accept *all* credit cards. If going to a malaria-endemic country, a bed net or net sleeping bag and mosquito repellant may be recommended. Recommendations of prophylactic medications can be reviewed at www.cdc.gov/travel. If air-conditioning is available, sleeping quarters need to be kept as cold as possible.
	Food/water	Familiarity of types of food that will be available is helpful; if food security is a potential problem, bringing protein bars, trail mix, and water purification tablets may be necessary. A quality water filter is the Pre-Mac travel well "Trekker" (www.shop.eri-online.com).

(continued)

TABLE 6.11 Travel Preparations *(continued)*

Health Care	Medications	The Yellow Book 2014 from the CDC (http://wwwnc. cdc.gov/travel/page/yellowbook-2014-home. htm) is a comprehensive resource for health risks and recommendations for every country, including medications. The Yellow Book is also available for Android and iOS mobile devices. The iTunes store has a Yellow Book app for iPads and iPhones. In-country medications, if available, may not be correctly formulated or may be contaminated. They may also be expensive. One Zofran ODT is $5 in Ecuador.
		When possible, enough medication (regularly taken medications and any prophylactic medications) to last the entire trip should be brought; some countries may require copies of prescribed medications, especially controlled substances; consider over-the-counter medications for pain, fever, nausea/ vomiting, diarrhea, constipation, cuts/scrapes, and insect bites. The team leader should obtain an emergency kit.
	Bed nets	These provide protection in malaria-endemic countries.
	Insurance coverage	Health insurance out-of-network coverage needs to be checked; evacuation insurance (e.g., www.medexassist. com) needs to be considered. Medicare/Medicaid does not provide coverage outside the United States.
Communication	Itinerary	All participants should carry a paper copy of the itinerary. An additional copy of the travel itinerary (flight, hotel, ground transportation) should be left with someone at home. Flight departures should be confirmed the day before traveling back to the United States.
	In-country contacts	The names and numbers of in-country contacts should be left with someone at home; include country codes as part of the phone number.
	Cell phones	Cell phone and data access can be expensive when used internationally; coverage and charges should be checked before departure to avoid huge bills upon return; purchase of an in-country cell phone is another option, with a SIM card to which more air time can be added as needed. Downloading WhatsApp to a smartphone for free text messaging when WiFi is available may be useful. Phone providers should be notified of travel outside the United States and may need details of the trip itinerary.

TABLE 6.11 Travel Preparations *(continued)*

Money	ATM cards	Money exchange should be done before leaving the country. Banks can help with this process. ATM machines are becoming more available in developing countries, but it cannot be assumed one will be available in all locations; PIN number should be four numbers (many foreign ATM machines do not have letters, just numbers). Use of debit cards can be a problem; it is often safer to use credit cards. The card provider needs to be contacted before leaving; otherwise, the card may be terminated or useless. Special debit cards can be purchased for travel (e.g., Contour card). These can be thrown away when the balance is gone. Use outside the United States needs to be verified.
	Traveler's cheques	Although fairly obsolete in many developed countries, traveler's cheques may still be used in some less developed settings.
	Credit cards	In developing countries, many businesses (hotels, restaurants, shops) do not accept credit cards; if intending to use credit cards, the credit card company will need to be notified of travel plans.
	Cash	All participants need to bring a certain amount of cash, exchanged as described earlier. In addition to personal expenses, there are always opportunities to help others (e.g., obtaining an oxygen tank for a young adult with tetralogy of Fallot). A working understanding of local currency is important to avoid overpaying or underpaying or being short-changed; there are smartphone apps that will help clarify currency exchanges. Cash should be carried in a money belt or belly pack. Some countries (e.g., Thailand) have a better exchange rate for larger bills.

TABLE 6.12 Packing Suggestions

Checked Luggage	Airline luggage limits need to be reviewed. Frequent flyer programs allow three free bags for Elite members.
	Unnecessary personal items (e.g., expensive jewelry/equipment) need to be left at home. Personal medical equipment without batteries may be checked. Expensive personal or other medical equipment with batteries will need to be in carry-on bags.
	Pack:
	Water filter, if bottled water will not be available (www.eri-online. com/ ERI_Equipment.html)
	Clothing appropriate for the weather and culture
	DEET

(continued)

TABLE 6.12 Packing Suggestions *(continued)*

	Itemized list of medications and supplies
	Gifts for hosts and children
	Towel and washcloth
Carry-on Luggage	Lightly packed, there may be limits of 10 kg.
	Include:
	Extra change of clothes (in case luggage gets lost or delayed)
	Toiletries
	Travel documents
	Personal medications and medical equipment
	Belly pack
	Cell phone

TABLE 6.13 Airline, Hotel, and Transportation Safety

Airline Safety	If there are unusual items being transported, the airline needs to be checked with in advance.
	Unruly passengers need to be avoided.
	Passport needs to be carried on the body.
Hotel Safety	Rooms between the second and sixth floors are recommended.
	Hotel business card should be carried in a wallet/belly pack, with the wallet in a front pocket.
	The hotel escape plan should be reviewed.
	Clothes, wallet, and shoes should be kept in the same place for emergency exiting.
	Participants should be observant and avoid crowds.
	Room safes are not safe.
Transportation Safety	Gasoline shortages are not uncommon in resource-poor settings; it is important to verify that your transport has enough gasoline to complete journeys.
	Some modes of transportation are relatively unsafe (e.g., mini-buses). In some countries (e.g., Guatemala), public buses are not safe.
	Some cities have very high rates of traffic accidents, particularly after dark.

or churches/temples can be used for the camp. Occasionally, setup may be under a tree.

Setup needs to include a patient check-in station (a triage nurse and interpreter) as the gatekeeper area for the flow of patients. Table 6.14 provides a list of common diseases seen in Central and South America. A similar analysis can be made for any region or country in order to prepare.

TABLE 6.14 Common Diseases/Disorders Exemplar—Central and South America

Burns/trauma/work injuries	Eye
Shoulder, neck, back, and leg pain	Conjunctivitis
	Cataracts
	Glaucoma
	Blindness
	Pterygium
	Pinguecula
Cardiac	**Fungal infections**
Hypertension	Vaginal: vulvar candidiasis
	Feet
	Oral
	Skin
	Tinea versicolor
Ear, nose, throat (ENT)	**Gastrointestinal conditions**
Cerumen impaction	Parasites: pinworms, amoebas, *Giardia*
Otitis media	Gastritis
Otitis externa	Peptic ulcers
	Diarrhea/constipation
Endocrine	**Genitourinary**
Type 2 diabetes	Urinary tract infections
Hypothyroidism	Benign prostatic hyperplasia
	Prostatitis
	Bacterial vaginosis
	Irregular menstrual cycles
	Pregnancy
	Chloasma

(continued)

TABLE 6.14 Common Diseases/Disorders Exemplar—Central and South America *(continued)*

Musculoskeletal problems	Other infectious diseases/ mosquito-borne diseases
Arthritis: osteoarthritis and rheumatoid	
Post trauma pain	Sexually transmitted infections
Back pain	Dengue fever
Myalgias	Malaria
	Chikungunya (Africa/India/Caribbean)
Neuropsychologic conditions	**Respiratory diseases**
Depression	Colds
Headaches	Chronic cough
Seizures	Bronchitis
Peripheral neuropathy	Asthma
	Pneumonia
	Environmental allergies
Nutritional disorders	**Skin**
Malnutrition	Rashes
Dehydration	Scabies
Anemia	Infections
Hyperhidrosis resulting from lack of B vitamins	

Many organizations have developed forms for recording patient identification information, vital signs, allergies, current medications, significant medical history, and a list of problems the patient wants treated. Teams will need to consider limiting the number of problems they can deal with per patient because there are often many people waiting to be seen. Occasionally, providers are faced with unknown diagnoses.

Although individuals usually queue up on the basis of first come, first serve, or the sickest first, there is often crowding and claiming rank and status. On a medical mission in a Delhi slum, a Mercedes pulled up, and an elegantly dressed woman went to the front of the line. No one seemed to be bothered by this, except the team members.

Referrals/Transfer to the Hospital

Before opening the clinic, organizers need to check with hosts about referrals and transferring patients to the hospital. In some countries individuals refuse to go to the hospital because of bad care and high mortality rates. These individuals may also become angry that the team is unable to resolve their problems. The host country/sponsor administrator is the best person to deal with these issues.

Home Visits

Team members may be asked to do a home visit on an individual who cannot come to the clinic or who is dying. For safety, it is best that several members of the team accompany the interpreter. Culturally, this is often a very positive experience for the team members because they have the opportunity to experience what the individuals deal with on a daily basis. Wound care may require daily visits.

Team Member Injuries/Serious Illnesses

Typically, most team member illnesses can be treated by the team. However, if a team member is seriously injured, evacuation may be required. Evacuation may also be required for serious illnesses. Contact information for the in-country U.S. embassy can be obtained at http:// travel.state.gov. The emergency number for the U.S. embassy is (888) 403-4747. Trip insurance is highly recommended because evacuation can cost more than $50,000 and in-country treatment can also be very expensive. Most U.S. medical insurances and Medicare/Medicaid do not provide coverage outside the United States. Trip health insurance can be obtained at http://travel.state.gov/travel/tips/brouchures/ brochures_1215.html.

The online brochure from the Smart Traveler Enrollment Program (STEP) contains excellent information on safety and preparedness. The link is http://travel.state.gov/tips_1232.html.

In-Country Debriefing

Ideally, debriefing should occur each evening in an informal setting. Discussion includes listing what activities went well and what activities should be improved. A list of needed medicines/supplies that are to be purchased while in the country should be compiled and then shared with the host in case the host is able to facilitate the purchase at a discount. A running list of recommendations for the next trip is another task for the team leader. Should team conflicts occur, the team leader and the host deal with the issues.

Post trip Debriefing

Team members need to be given the opportunity to process life-changing experiences, air feelings and reactions, and discuss what worked and what needs to be changed for the future medical brigades. The team leader may need to talk to individuals who had traumatic experiences in caring for patients. Team members may need to receive parasite medications. View Table 6.15 for recommendations on parasite treatments.

ROLE OF THE APRN IN GLOBAL RESEARCH

From a global perspective, the role of the APRN researcher is dynamic and vital to informing and articulating the APN role, shedding light on

TABLE 6.15 Parasitic Treatments

Parasite	Treatment (not recommended during pregnancy or lactation)
Worm (roundworm, hookworm, pinworm, whipworm, etc.) Common local beliefs about symptoms: excess salivation, itchy nose/throat, grinding teeth, craves sweets Roundworm: asymptomatic, but while in lungs produces a nonproductive cough Hookworm: mainly asymptomatic, but early manifestations may be epigastric pain or diarrhea, chronic iron-deficiency anemia Whipworm: chronic abdominal pain, anorexia, bloody or mucoid diarrhea, rectal prolapse Pinworm: chronic anal itching (worse at night), rarely abdominal discomfort, weight loss	**Adults and children 2 and up:** Mebendazole 100 mg twice daily × 3 days or Albendazole 400 mg × 1 dose **Children younger than 2 years:** For ascaris, piperazine 50–75 mg/kg daily × 2 days or For pinworms, piperazine 40 mg/kg daily × 7 days
Giardia Often asymptomatic, early: diarrhea, abdominal pain, bloating, belching, flatus, nausea and vomiting; diarrhea is common, but upper abdominal discomfort predominant Chronic: occasionally diarrhea, most common flatus, loose stools, and sulfurous burping; can cause weight loss	**Adult:** Albendazole 400 mg once daily × 5 days or Metronidazole 250 mg three time daily × 5 days or Metronidazole 2 g daily × 3 days or Tinidazole 2 g × 1 dose **Children:** Albendazole 400 mg once daily × 5 days or Tinidazole 50 mg/kg once daily × 5 days or Metronidazole 5 mg/kg three times daily × 5–7 days
Amebiasis Lower abdominal pain, little diarrhea, malaise, weight loss, abdominal or back pain; can mimic acute appendicitis; small amount of stool but lots of mucus or blood; few have fever	**Adult:** Metronidazole 500–700 mg three times daily × 10 days or Tinidazole 2 g × 2 days (liver abscess × 3 days) **Children:** Metronidazole 15 mg/kg three times daily × 10 days or Tinidazole 50–60 mg/kg/day × 3 days (liver abscess × 5 days)

the health care needs of disadvantaged populations internationally, and establishing a body of evidence of advanced practice nursing knowledge. The scope and perspectives of APRN research are broad ranging and may encompass epistemology; ethnography; role definition, justification, and expansion; exploration of the notion of competence and role-specific competencies; scope of practice and role potential; and disease- and intervention-specific research within APRN roles from an evidence-based practice perspective.

This research reflects both the APRN's own practice perspectives and also those of the national and international health care environments and jurisdictions in which APRNs work. APRN-related research is not confined to APRNs themselves, and the APRN role may be the subject of international research. For example, taking an international perspective and supported by the WHO, Lassi, Cometto, Huicho, and Bhutta (2013) published a systematic review and meta-analysis of 53 studies from the scientific literature comparing the quality of care provided by providers such as APRNs and that by what are considered higher level providers within developed and developing countries, such as the Africa region. The review concluded that there was no difference between the quality, effectiveness, and outcomes of care provided by the two groups of practitioners.

State of APRN Research in the World

Although the APRN role is well established in North America, the role continues to evolve internationally in both developed and developing countries, giving rise to a body of research literature with an evidential and exploratory focus. Researchers use the traditional available resources but also enjoy the use of Google Scholar or access to the Joanna Briggs Institute (JBI) and the JBI Library of Systematic Reviews, available at http://connect.jbiconnectplus.org/JBIReviewsLibrary.aspx. The following journals are also resources and publish international APRN research:

- *American Association of Nurse Practitioners*
- *International Journal of Evidence-Based Healthcare*
- *International Journal of Nursing Practice*
- *International Journal of Nursing Studies*
- *Journal of Advanced Nursing*
- *Journal of Nursing & Care*
- *International Nursing Review*

The following brief review considers APRN research emerging from Australia, Ireland, Japan, Jordan, the Netherlands, and Scandinavia.

Australia

In Australia, where some APRN roles role have been recognized for well over a decade, the research focus tends toward qualitative reviews of the evidence of the effectiveness of the role and discipline-specific interventional research. The focus of the Australian studies presented in this section reflects the scope of practice and the emerging trends in APRN research worldwide. In a systematic review Ramis, Wu, and Pearson (2013), explored the experience of being an APRN within Australian acute care settings. The findings from the study's meta-syntheses reinforced the complexity of the identity, education, and scope of practice of the APRN role.

Kucera, Higgins, and McMillan (2010) explored Australian APRNs' lived experiences and proposed an APRN futures model derived from their narrative analysis of nurses' stories. Earlier Australian studies focused on APRN role definition, role confusion, decision making, and practice autonomy within changing health care environments. In 2006 Gardner, Chang, and Duffield proposed an APRN framework and a "research-informed model of service incorporating operational structures and role parameters" (p. 382).

The Australian Nurse Practitioner Study (AUSPRAC), funded by the Australian Research Council (ARC), undertook a 3-year study of the work, processes, and outcomes of Australian nurse practitioners. An important outcome of the AUSPRAC study was publication of *The Nurse Practitioner Research Toolkit* to guide APRNs in practice, service, and outcome-related research (Gardner, Gardner, Middleton, & Della, 2009).

Ireland

A University of Ireland study by Dowling, Beauchesne, and Murphy (2013) used concept analysis to clarify the meaning of advanced practice nursing from an international perspective and concluded further research and international collaboration are required to establish internationally consistent terminology.

Japan

Kondo (2013), in a review article published in the *Journal of Nursing & Care*, explored the role and contribution of nurse practitioners internationally and the potential for, and barriers to, implementation of the advanced practice role in Japan. In a 2014 article published in *International Nursing Review*, Fukuda et al. reviewed the first nurse practitioner graduate program in Japan and provided an overview of the research and project planning phases preceding implementation of the NP program.

Jordan

Zahran, Curtis, Lloyd-Jones, and Blackett (2012) presented an ethnographic approach to a study of the perceived concept of the introduction of the advanced nurse practitioner and APRN training programs in Jordon. The authors related their findings from the broader APRN literature to the context-specific Jordanian nursing educational and practice environments.

The Netherlands

Noordman, van der Wijden, and van Dulmen (2014) employed a pretest/posttest design to examine the effects of video feedback on the communication skills of APRNs.

Scandinavia

A study by Slatten, Hatlevik, and Fagerstrom (2014), *Validation of a New Instrument for Self-Assessment of Nurses' Core Competences in Palliative Care*, explored the concept of competence as a core prerequisite for APRN quality of care within Scandinavia. The instrument—Nurses' Core Competence in Palliative Care (NCPC)—was developed in Norway in 2007. Findings from this study identified five domains of competence within the palliative care APRN role: knowledge of symptom management, systematic use of the Edmonton symptom assessment system, teamwork skills, interpersonal skills, and life-closure skills.

CONDUCTING GLOBAL RESEARCH

Conducting international nursing research requires an overarching commitment to caring in the context of the local culture. Globally, respect for persons, beneficence, and justice are the foundation for responsible community engagement in the research process. This aligns with the ICN's *Code of Ethics for Nurses*, which states that the universal mandates for nursing practice, and therefore, nursing research, are respect for human rights—the right to life and choice, to dignity, and to be treated with respect. Practically, this requires that APRNs follow the ethical mandates of the professional practice of nursing as they plan and conduct research. Furthermore, all nurse researchers are expected to know the rules and regulations governing human subjects research where the study will be conducted. Yearly, the U.S. Department of Health and Human Services' (DHHS's) Office for Human Research Protections provides an updated international compilation of human research standards (www.hhs.gov/ohrp/international/index.html) and the DHHS's Office of Research Integrity provides a primer on the responsible conduct of research (http://ori.hhs.gov/ori-introduction-responsible-conduct-research). In short, all researchers should know international as well as local professional codes, government regulations, and institutional polices.

All research codes and policies address the issue of informed consent. However, specific cultural factors, such as decision-making processes and issues of literacy, need to be addressed in the research process (Krogstad et al., 2010). In areas where there is a tradition of communal decision making, community leaders may need to be engaged before potential participants are asked to consent. Also, where there is low literacy and consent is obtained verbally, the researcher must recognize the risk of inconsistent information being shared. To minimize the risk of uninformed consent, an adaptation of *teach back* can be employed whereby the participant's level of understanding is evaluated before consent is confirmed (Krogstad et al., 2010).

Often, APRNs may be planning to conduct research as they are providing clinical care. This sets up special concerns. Four particular issues have been identified (Laman, Pomat, Siba, & Betuela, 2013). They include the risk of putting a priority on accomplishing the research activity over patient care, confusing the patient's expectation for clinical care with his or her participation consent, setting up inappropriate inducements, and providing *one-time* clinical services that are not sustainable by the host area. According to international nursing ethical standards, patient care must always take precedence over research. As well, local ethics committees can provide important perspectives to minimize patient confusion, counterproposals for what may be considered *inappropriate inducements*, and partnership with the researcher to work toward creating sustainable clinical services. Overall, nurses engaged in conducting international research must think globally about gaining new scientific knowledge but act wisely at the local level, always moving in accordance with nursing's consistent commitment to ethical practice.

ROLE OF THE APRN IN EDUCATION DELIVERY AND CONSULTATION

The global nursing shortage of both professional nurses providing care and of nursing faculty creates an environment where the pooling of professional resources is critical (Appiagyei et al., 2014; Bell, Rominski, Bam, Donkor, & Lori, 2013; Nardi & Gyurko, 2013). Nursing providers and faculty are increasingly able to come together to increase the capacity and quality of professional nurses through educational consultation. Technology use, communication that makes the world *small,* various iterations of distance education, and the ease and improvement of global transportation may profoundly change the landscape of APRN education globally. Currently, most examples of U.S. participation in APRN or other health care education and consultation has involved face-to-face work, with students coming to the United States or U.S. faculty going to the host country. The selection of clinical sites for APRNs requires particular vigilance—some distance programs expect students to come to the United States for this part of the program, work out experiences at U.S. facilities outside the United States (e.g., military bases, embassies), or scrupulously review the preceptor. One APRN involved in a long-term educational commitment is described in the sidebar.

Box 6.1 Kiwi Conversion: One NP's Educational Experience

In 2008, a good friend contacted me regarding an opportunity to teach with her at the Center for Postgraduate Nursing Studies for the University of Otago. They were looking for a senior lecturer for adult health and pharmacology. I was teaching these courses for Clemson University's graduate nursing program for several years along with working full time

(continued)

Box 6.1 Kiwi Conversion: One NP's Educational Experience—*(continued)*

as a family nurse practitioner. It had been my dream to work and teach internationally. To my surprise, in November 2008, I arrived in Christchurch, New Zealand to begin a career adventure.

Transfer of Registered Nurse licensure was accomplished prior to leaving for New Zealand. However, my nurse practitioner certification did not transfer as ANCC or AANP certification exams are not recognized by the Nursing Council of New Zealand. You must have a minimum of four years of experience and a clinical master's degree, create a portfolio, and pass a panel assessment for nurse practitioner competency (Nursing Council of New Zealand, 2014).

A learning curve both in spelling, health care systems, and nursing ensued. I came from private practice to a public and private health system where health care is a basic human right, not a privilege. A baccalaureate is required for registered nurses with opportunity for specialty certification. Nurse practitioners are expert nurses in specific areas with advanced knowledge and skills, who work independently and in collaboration with other health care professionals (Nursing Council of New Zealand, 2014). To obtain the qualifications for application for nurse practitioner status, I needed an advanced nursing practice position. In the United States, nurse practitioner positions are everywhere—in the newspapers, employment agencies, private practice, and health care institutions. I needed an advanced practice position that would enable me to gain the necessary experience. The director of University of Otago Center for Post Graduate Nursing Studies, Dr. Beverley Burrell, interceded, and I started working for Canterbury University's Student Health Center as a provider once a week. I am grateful and thankful for the support and guidance provided by the staff. In addition, I worked with a nurse practitioner in private practice and a family physician, both of whom provided letters of support. Portfolio development is both an aggravation and enriching experience. It requires you to fully evaluate your practice and qualifications for advanced practice nursing. In February 2011, I successfully passed panel assessment achieving primary care nurse practitioner certification.

The students were bright, creative, highly motivated, and involved with their community. It was a pleasure to teach and mentor such individuals. On September 4, 2010, a 7.1 earthquake struck Christchurch, New Zealand, followed by multiple aftershocks. In February 2011, a more devastating earthquake occurred, killing 185 people. Many of the institutions and individuals I loved were no longer standing or left for safer venues. Although I was safe, after much soul searching, I returned in 2012 and currently work with an Arizona Native American tribal community as a primary care nurse practitioner. Last week, I received an e-mail from two students who recently achieved primary care nurse practitioner certification, making me very happy. I remain active with the Advanced Practice Nursing Network of the International Council of Nurses and plan to work abroad again at the first opportunity.

—Patricia Maybee

Educational consultation can fall into roughly three categories of professional focus.

- **Individuals:** At this level, education consultation occurs within the context of medical brigades.
- **Communities:** Education consultation at this level can occur within the context of medical brigades but also within broader regional or national population health consultation similar to train-the-trainer scenarios (Lasater, Upvall, Nielsen, Prak, & Ptachcinski, 2012).
- **Professional:** Consultation regarding education at this level provides professional infrastructure enrichment, support, or capacity building. Areas for consultation include academic preparation and professional development (Kemp & Tindiweegi, 2001).

This professional consultation can occur in a country where a small group of visiting providers come to receive specialized training/experiences or can occur when a visiting professional can come into a country to provide training or program development. Both areas hold great promise for expanding capacity and quality, yet both raise concerns. Visiting consulters who leave their home for individualized or small group training may not use the training or may not return to their home country at all (Sherwood & Liu, 2005). Visiting single consultants may provide *train-the-trainer* types of experiences within the host country, but they may do so through a cultural lens that is not the same as the host consulter (Palmer & Heaston, 2009).

Process

A similar process undergirds the three categories of educational consultation. At its core, consultation is a process by which people or systems problem solve. This process involves two-way problem solving and is a dynamic method of seeking, giving, and receiving help. Sometimes those receiving the consultation have most of the answers and just need help reaching the goal or solution. The process has three phases: initiation, progression, and culmination.

Initiation

In starting an international education consultation, there are several questions that need to be answered clearly for all parties involved:

- What are the purpose and outcomes of the consultation?
- What questions/topics need to be addressed?
- What resources are available?
- What resources need to be developed?

Clear answers to these questions provide the basis for the interactions and focus of the consultation.

The first point upon which to seek agreement is in regard to the purpose and desired outcome(s). All parties should be specific as to the joint purpose: developing curriculum or programs, addressing specific organizational issues, and/or building infrastructure. That specific purpose will then define the objectives, and they should be concrete and defined and should reflect the consulter's culture, values, state of science, and resources. Each of the parties may have additional purposes that may be served by the consultation, but the primary purpose to be served and goals to be met should be those agreed on by the consultant and consulter (Memmott et al., 2010). For example, building the consultation within the framework of a service learning program emphases the centrality of the agreed-on purpose of the partnership while acknowledging the benefits of the partnership for all involved (McKinnon & Fealy, 2011).

In defining that purpose, the expected role of the consultant should also be clearly expressed. That definition should include expectations of performance (e.g., conducting classes, designing curricula, delivering continuing education) and time (in preparation, while on site, and upon departure) along with workspace (formal academic or in the field) and payment. Forms and amount of communication expected throughout the consultation should also be clarified. Finally, the shared nature of any intellectual property produced as a result of the consultation should be negotiated up front (George & Meadows-Oliver, 2013).

Building on that shared and defined purpose, the next point of agreement is that of the specific questions and topics to be addressed. Does the consulter desire specific subject matter expertise? Who is the intended audience/target learner? Are there programs for professional growth and development to be built or adapted locally or regionally? Are there national, regional, or local implications for practice, licensure, and credentialing that need to be considered and addressed? Awareness of cultural mores and expectations alongside the current practice ecology of the host country is critical for designing and refining content (Scanlan & Abdul Hernandéz, 2014).

Finally, both consultant and consulter need to discuss the resources available. Will translation of materials be needed? What (and in some cases if any) is the access to Internet and library resources? What are the resources necessary for sustaining achievement or reproduction of the final goal? Pioneering work in Somalia and China demonstrates that building capacity with no or minimal indigenous resources can begin by identifying community or governmentally directed needs (Doyle & Morris, 2014; Sherwood & Liu, 2005).

Resources for the consultant (office and living space, fees, and communication assistance overseas and within country through translators if necessary) should all be discussed before the onset of the consultation.

Progression

Once the consultation has begun and the traveler is in country, supports discussed in planning should be identified. Those supports may include translators, teaching and research assistants, evaluators, and collaborators.

Having a cultural *touchstone* or mentor within the host country who can translate expectations and social constructs will prove to be invaluable (Kim, Woith, Otten, & McElmurry, 2006).

Progression throughout the consultation is marked by timeline, benchmarks, and deliverables. All of these should be clearly delineated in the planning stages but may need to be shifted once the consultation is under way. Keeping in mind the scope, purpose, and deliverables of the consultation will keep the project on track. Doing so while attuned to the cultural climate will make the project successful. Clearly identifying the end of the consultation before beginning will help to bound expectations.

Culmination

As the consultation draws to a close, all involved should evaluate the effectiveness of the project. Scheduling for formative and summative evaluations should be set up before beginning the consultation. Several points to consider during evaluation are:

- Were there any secondary responsibilities for program planning, development, or delivery that needed to be met that were not discussed initially?
- Are any return trips needed?
- What follow-on work is needed to foster the consulter's success?
- Does the team that was assembled have plans for other work?
- Are there plans to gauge how the project is doing 3, 6, and 12 months out?
- Did the consultation meet its benchmarks?
- Did the consultation meet the consulter's expectations?
- What were the strengths and weaknesses of the project?
- Can any lessons learned be generalized?

Additional Considerations

Several points should be considered when preparing for international education consultation. The first is to be on guard against cultural tone deafness. The WHO has passed a resolution to set global standards for professional preparation of nurses (Nursing & Midwifery Human Resources for Health, 2009). However, all nurses practice in a local setting. Each setting has different boundaries on and expectations of nursing care. In addition, each setting has specific resources. Those resources determine not only care provision but also the sustainability of education and training for the care providers. Sustainability of projects that come out of the consultation process should be a key consideration in design (Mullan & Kerry, 2014).

Along the lines of sustainability, a point to consider within the consultation planning or delivery is what method or program has the sustainable potential for a *ripple effect*, that is, a far-reaching capacity for change and professional development (Memmott et al., 2010).

Finally, both the consultant and consulter should enter into their relationship with a clear understanding of the ground rules governing their partnership and an appreciation of potential power sharing that may need to occur within the team (Hunter et al., 2013). As international cooperation and collaboration are critical items necessary to expand both the supply of nurses and nursing faculty, educational consultation has the potential to expand and flourish for the advancement of all involved (Haq et al., 2008).

CONCLUSION

The world is opening up to APRNs who want to practice, teach, or conduct research in international settings. Pressing global health care needs and proven APRN track records in health care delivery, education, and research demonstrate this is a time for APRNs to collaborate with colleagues and other medical professionals to improve health for individuals and communities everywhere. Certainly the challenges and obstacles are great, but few professions are as flexible, dynamic, and urgently needed as that of the APRN.

REFERENCES

American Association of Nurse Practitioners. (2014). *ICNNP/APNN aims and objectives.* Retrieved from http://international.aanp.org/About/Aims

Anjana, R.M., Ali, M. K., Pradeepa, R., Deepa, M., Datta, M., Unnikrishnan, R., . . . Mohan, V. (2011). The need for obtaining accurate nationwide estimates of diabetes prevalence in India: Rationale for a national study on diabetes. *Indian Journal of Medical Research, 133*(4), 369–380. Retrieved from http://www.ijmr.org.in/article.asp?issn=0971-5916;year=2011;volume=133;issue=4;spage=369;epage=380;aulast=Anjana

Appiagyei, A. A., Kiriinya, R. N., Gross, J. M., Wambua, D. N., Oywer, E. O., Kamenju, A. K., ... Rogers, M. F. (2014). Informing the scale-up of Kenya's nursing workforce: A mixed methods study of factors affecting pre-service training capacity and production. *Human Resources for Health, 12*(1), 47.

APRN Consensus Work Group & National Council of State Boards of Nursing APRN Advisory Committee. (2008). *Consensus model for APRN regulation: Licensure, accreditation, certification & education.* Retrieved from https://www.ncsbn.org/7_23_08_Consensue_APRN_Final.pdf

Bass, C. (2011). *Megatrends and looking to the future.* Retrieved from http://www.enterprisecioforum.com/en/blogs/cebess/megatrends-and-looking-future

Batancourt, J. R., Green, A. R., Carrillo, J. E., & Owusu, A. (2003). Defining cultural competence: A practical framework for addressing racial/ethnic disparities in health and health care. *Public Health Reports, 118,* 292–302.

Bell, S. A., Rominski, S., Bam, V., Donkor, E., & Lori, J. (2013). Analysis of nursing education in Ghana: Priorities for scaling-up the nursing workforce. *Nursing & Health Sciences, 15*(2), 244–249.

Chase, S., & Hunter, A. (2002). Cultural and spiritual competencies: Curricular guidelines [Monograph]. *National Organization of Nurse Practitioner Faculties,* 19–28.

Dillon, K., & Prokesch, S. (2014). Megatrends in global healthcare. Retrieved from http://hbr.org/web/extras/insight-center/health-care/globaltrends/1-slide

Dowling, M., Beauchesne, M., & Murphy, K. (2013). Advanced practice nursing: A concept analysis. *International Journal of Nursing Practice, 19*(2), 131–140. doi:10.1111/ijn.12050

Doyle, M.-J., & Morris, C. (2014). Development of mental health nursing education and practice in Somaliland. *Nurse Education in Practice, 14*(1), 1–3.

Fukuda, H., Miyauchi, C., Tonai, M., Ono, M., Magilvy, J., & Murashima, S. (2014, August 29). The first nurse practitioner graduate programme in Japan. *International Nursing Review.* Advance online publication. doi:10.111/inr.12126

Gardner, G., Chang, A., & Duffield, C. (2006). Making nursing work: Breaking through the role confusion of advanced practice nursing. *Journal of Advanced Nursing, 57*(4), 382–391.

Gardner, G., Gardner, A., Middleton, S., & Della, P. (2009). *The Australian nurse practitioner study: Nurse practitioner research toolkit.* Retrieved from http://www.nursing.health.wa.gov.au/docs/reports/AUSPRAC_NURSE_PRACTITIONER_RESEARCH_TOOLKIT.pdf

George, E. K., & Meadows-Oliver, M. (2013). Searching for collaboration in international nursing partnerships: A literature review. *International Nursing Review, 60*(1), 31–36.

Hansen-Turton, T. (2014). 2014 International advanced practice nursing symposium. Retrieved from http://www.nncc.us/site/images/pdf/Global-APNSymposiumFINAL.pdf

Haq, C., Baumann, L., Olsen, C. W., Brown, L. D., Kraus, C., Bousquet, G., … Easterday, B. C. (2008). Creating a center for global health at the University of Wisconsin-Madison. *Academic Medicine: Journal of the Association of American Medical Colleges, 83*(2), 148–153.

Hunter, A., & Crabtree, K (2010). Global health and international opportunities. In J. Stanley (Ed.), *Advanced practice nursing: Emphasizing common roles* (pp. 327–348). Philadelphia: F.A. Davis.

Hunter, A., Wilson, L., Stanhope, M., Hatcher, B., Hattar, M., Hilfinger Messias, D. K., & Powell, D. (2013). Global health diplomacy: An integrative review of the literature and implications for nursing. *Nursing Outlook, 61*(2), 85–92.

International Council of Nurses. (2002a). *Definition and characteristics for nurse practitioners/advanced practice nursing roles* [official position paper]. Retrieved from https://acnp.org.au/sites/default /files/33/definition_of_apn-np.pdf

International Council of Nurses (ICN). (2002b). *Guidebook for nurse futurists: A guidebook for future-oriented planning in your national nursing association.* Geneva: Author.

International Council of Nurses. (2014). *Our mission, strategic intent, core values and priorities.* Retrieved from http://www.icn.ch/about-icn/icns-mission/

Kai, Z. (2011, March 20). *Five deadliest effects of global warming.* Retrieved from http://zkmedia.workpress.com/2011/03/20/a-5-infographic/

Kemp, J., & Tindiweegi, J. (2001). Nurse education in Mbarara, Uganda. *Journal of Advanced Nursing, 33*(1), 8–12.

Kim, M. J., Woith, W., Otten, K., & McElmurry, B. J. (2006). Global nurse leaders: Lessons from the sages. *ANS. Advances in Nursing Science, 29*(1), 27–42.

Kondo, A. (2013). Advanced practice nurses in Japan: Education and related roles. *Journal of Nursing and Care,* S5:004. doi:10.4172/2167-1168.S5-004

Krogstad, D. J., Diop, S., Dialto, A., Mzayek, F., Keating, J., Koita, O. A., & Toure, Y. T. (2010). Informed consent in international research: The rationale for different approaches. *American Journal of Tropical Medicine, 83*(4), 743–747.

Kucera, K., Higgins, I., & McMillan, M. (2010). Advanced nursing practice: A futures model derived from narrative analysis of nurses' stories. *Australian Journal of Advanced Practice Nursing, 27*(4), 43–53.

Laman, M., Pomat, W., Siba, P., & Betuela, I. (2013, July 26). Ethical challenges in integrating patient-care with clinical research in a resource-limited setting: Perspectives from Papua New Guinea. *BMC Medical Ethics, 14*(29). Retrieved from Retrieved from http://www.biomedcentral.com/1472-6939/14/29. doi:10.1186/1472-6939-14-29

Lasater, K., Upvall, M., Nielsen, A., Prak, M., & Ptachcinski, R. (2012). Global partnerships for professional development: A Cambodian exemplar. *Journal of Professional Nursing: Official Journal of the American Association of Colleges of Nursing, 28*(1), 62–68.

Lassi, Z. S., Cometto, G., Huicho, L., & Bhutta, Z. A. (2013). Quality of care provided by mid-level health workers: Systemic review and meta-analysis. *Bulletin of the World Health Organization, 3*(91), 824-833. doi:10.2471/BLT.13.118786

Martiniuk, A. L. C., Manouchehrian, M., Negin, J. A., & Zwi, A. B. (2012). Brain gains: A literature of medical missions to low and middle-income countries. *BMC Health Services Research, 12*(134). Retrieved from http://www.biomedcentral.com/content/pdf/1472-6963-12-134.pdf

Massachusetts Institute of Technology. (2014). *Disruptive demographics.* Retrieved from http://agelab.mit.edu/disruptive-demographics

McKinnon, T. H., & Fealy, G. (2011). Core principles for developing global service-learning programs in nursing. *Nursing Education Perspectives, 32*(2), 95–101.

Memmott, R. J., Coverston, C. R., Heise, B. A., Williams, M., Maughan, E. D., Kohl, J., & Palmer, S. (2010). Practical considerations in establishing sustainable international nursing experiences. *Nursing Education Perspectives, 31*(5), 298–302.

Mullan, F., & Kerry, V. B. (2014). The global health service partnership: Teaching for the world. *Academic Medicine: Journal of the Association of American Medical Colleges, 89*(8), 1146–1148.

National Center for Cultural Competence. (2015). *Welcome.* Retrieved from http://nccc.georgetown.edu/index.html

National Nursing Centers Consortium. (2014). *International advanced practice nursing symposium executive summary.* Retrieved from http://www.nncc.us/site/images/pdf/ GlobalAPNSymposiumFINAL.pdf

Nardi, D. A., & Gyurko, C. C. (2013). The global nursing faculty shortage: Status and solutions for change. *Journal of Nursing Scholarship: An Official Publication of Sigma Theta Tau International Honor Society of Nursing / Sigma Theta Tau, 45*(3), 317–326.

Nichols, B. L., Davis, C. R., & Richardson, D. R. (2011). International models of nursing. In the Institute of Medicine's (Eds.), *The future of nursing: Leading change, advancing health* (pp. 565-642). Washington, DC: National Academies Press.

Noordman, J., van der Weijden, T., & van Dulmen, S. (2014). Effects of video-feedback on the communication, clinical competence and motivational interviewing skills of practice nurses: A pretest posttest control group study. *Journal of Advanced Nursing, 70*(10), 2272–2283.

Nursing & Midwifery Human Resources for Health. (2009). *Global standards for the initial education of professional nurses and midwives* (No. WHO/HRH/HPN/08.6). World Health Organization. Retrieved from www.who.int/hrh/nursing_midwifery/hrh_global_ standards_education.pdf

O'Brien, P., & Gostin, L. O. (2011). The global health worker crisis—executive summary. *Health worker shortages and global justice.* New York, NY: Milbank Memorial Fund.

Palmer, S. P., & Heaston, S. (2009). Teaching the teacher program to assist nurse managers to educate nursing staff in Ecuadorian hospitals. *Nurse Education in Practice, 9*(2), 127–133.

Pulcini, J., Jelic, M., Gul, R., & Loke, Y. (2009). An international survey on advanced practice nursing education, practice, and regulation. *Journal of Nursing Scholarship, 42*(1), 31–39.

Ramis, M., Wu, C., & Pearson, A. (2013). Experience of being an advanced practice nurse within Australian acute care settings: A systematic review of qualitative evidence. *International Journal of Evidence Based Healthcare, 11*(3), 161–180.

Samaritans Now. (2014). *Healthcare mission trips: A manual for healthcare mission leaders.* Retrieved from http://www.missiongoal.org/files/resources/Organizing_A_Med_Mission.pdf

Scanlan, J. M., & Abdul Hernandéz, C. (2014). Challenges of implementing a doctoral program in an international exchange in Cuba through the lens of Kanter's empowerment theory. *Nurse Education in Practice, 14*(4), 357–362.

Schober, M. (2011). International report to AANP board of directors. Washington, DC: AANP.

Sherwood, G., & Liu, H. (2005). International collaboration for developing graduate education in China. *Nursing Outlook, 53*(1), 15–20.

Sigma Theta Tau International. (2014). *Sigma Theta Tau International organizational fact sheet.* Retrieved from http://www.nursingsociety.org/aboutus/mission/Pages/factsheet.aspx

Slatten, K., Hatlevik, O., & Fagerstrom, L. (2014). Validation of a new instrument for self-assessment of nurses' core competencies in palliative care. *Nursing Research and Practice, 2014,* article ID 615498. doi:10.1155/2014/615498

United Nations. (2013, June 13). *World population projected to reach 9.6 billion by 2050—UN Report.* Retrieved from http://www.un.org/apps/news/story.asp?NewsID=45165#.VBMUzqOdJ8E

United Nations. (2014). *The millennium development goals report 2014.* Retrieved from http://www.un.org/millenniumgoals/2014%20MDG%20report/MDG%202014%20English%20web.pdf

Sherwood, G., & Liu, H. (2005). International collaboration for developing graduate education in China. *Nursing Outlook, 53*(1), 15–20.

World Health Organization. (2006). *The world health report 2006—Working together for health.* Retrieved from http://www.who.int/whr/2006/en/

World Health Organization. (2008). *The world health report 2008—Primary health care, now more than ever.* Retrieved from http://www.who.int/whr/2008/en/

Zackowitz, M. G. (2014, March). *Medical migration.* Retrieved from http://ngm.nationalgeographic.com/2008/12/community-doctors/follow-up-text

Zahran, S., Curtis, P., Lloyd-Jones, M., & Blackett, T. (2012). Jordanian perspectives on advanced nursing practice: An ethnography. *International Nursing Review, 59*(2), 222–229.

Janet Wessel Krejci and Shelly Malin 7

LEADERSHIP SKILLS AND EXPERTISE: KEYS TO APRN SUCCESS IN HEALTH CARE SYSTEMS

Since the last edition of this book, much has occurred related to advanced practice nursing and the need for leadership skills and expertise. The Institute of Medicine's *The Future of Nursing* report (IOM, 2010) has begun to move the needle on educational progression, leadership, interprofessional collaboration, and expansion of the scope of practice; we now have almost 300 doctorate of nursing practice (DNP) programs across the nation, and the percentage of nurses with bachelor of science in nursing (BSN) degrees is slowly increasing. The Patient Protection and Affordable Care Act (ACA) has been rolled out with many challenges and opportunities. Accountable care organizations, as a result of the ACA, have evolved with some successes and some very hard lessons about the risk and complexity of keeping communities healthy. The term *population health* is no longer a concept; it is shifting the way we need to educate, practice, and lead. More than 80% of nurse practitioners, one segment of advanced practice registered nurses (APRNs), are prepared in primary care, whereas less than 15% of physicians entered a primary care residency and less than 4% of senior medical school students identified interest in primary care. Currently more than two thirds of all Americans have seen an APRN for their primary health care needs, with more than 916 million visits to APRNs each year (American Association of Nurse Practitioners [AANP], 2014). The Federal Trade Commission (2014) has provided an analysis of barriers to fair trade health care practices and identified recommendations concerning state scope of practice legislation.

APRNs can make the difference between chaos and quality in today's complex health care system if and only if they develop leadership competencies needed for the current environment. The changes identified here, as well as revolutionary advances in technology, pharmaceutical research, and surgical innovations, coupled with the organizational complexities and fierce competition for resources, have created unprecedented challenges as well as opportunities for the APRN. In the midst of these awe-inspiring advances, it is clear that the sobering unintended consequences of a complex, highly regulated, and yet fragmented system, first identified by the IOM more than 15 years ago (IOM, 1999, 2001, 2004), have not yet been solved. At a time when the cloning of a human is possible, ensuring the basics, such as hand washing for all providers and preventing falls, remains, at times, elusive. In addition, the incentive structure of the reimbursement system is finally holding providers accountable to keep communities healthy by preventing illness and supporting wellness, creating both intended and unintended consequences. APRNs have incredible opportunities but still face obstacles related to the hierarchy of the health care system that have plagued nurses for decades. O'Neil, Morjickian, Cherner, Hirschkorn, and West (2008) postulated that without a deep commitment to an investment in leadership development for those instrumental in health care outcomes, the future of health care is at risk.

This chapter highlights the opportunity APRNs have in this new world if they embrace this moment with strong leadership competencies and skills to shape the future. We emphasize the importance of leadership competencies for APRNs who have major responsibilities for delivery of quality care, evidence-based practice, patient safety, innovations in nursing practice, and leadership in systems. Different leadership development models and curricula related to leadership in DNP programs are explored. Application of leadership competencies to specific scenarios common to APRNs are presented.

EDUCATIONAL AND PRACTICE CHANGES

Those practicing in APRN roles are aware of major changes both in the practice arena and in the educational requirements for the role. The American Association of Colleges of Nursing (AACN, 2006) identified that the preparation for APRN roles should be the DNP, which, in turn, is influencing educational preparation already and may influence credentialing in the near future. The role of the APRN in the practice setting is also changing. In the past decade, the impact of the APRN has expanded exponentially as the evidence related to APRNs' influence on positive patient outcomes builds (Brooten, Youngblut, Kutcher, & Bobo, 2004; Brooten et al., 2005; Burns & Earven, 2003; Cunningham, 2004; Gawlinski, McCloy, & Jesurum, 2001; Kelly, Kutney-Lee, Lake, & Aiken, 2013; Kleinpell, 2007; Larkin, 2003; Lenz, Mundinger, Kane, Hopkins, & Lin, 2004; Russell, VorderBruegge, & Burns, 2002). More APRNs are responsible for outcomes and providing care at academic health centers, acute care facilities, primary care, specialty clinics, and rural areas. At a time when more than 40 million people are uninsured in the United States and clear disparities exist for minority populations, costs are skyrocketing, reimbursement is changing, and health care providers are scrambling to protect their compensation (Evans, 2014; IOM, 2004).

What does this all mean for APRNs working in a variety of settings with increasing responsibilities, whether working as a clinical nurse specialist (CNS) or as a direct care provider? To be successful in today's complex and political health care system, APRNs cannot rely solely on expertise in practice or naïve optimism about collaboration and cooperation. As the AACN (2004) in its Position Statement on the Practice Doctorate in Nursing indicated, one of the reasons for recommending the DNP as entry into advanced practice was to prepare APRNs with a blend of clinical, organizational, economic and leadership skills because of the complexity they face in trying to influence patient outcomes. Although great strides have been made in licensure, recognition, and reimbursement (Pearson, 2004), patients are at risk for losing the best of what APRNs offer unless they develop skills, knowledge, and competencies not only in clinical practice but in leadership as well.

Senge (1990) and Senge, Kleiner, Roberts, Ross, and Smith (1994) have articulated that the systematic structure of any organization (e.g., the incentives, interdependencies, policies, group norms) provides the context in which all behavior, relationships, and outcomes result. It is the premise of the authors that understanding and mastering this context and developing the competencies to lead in complex health environments is as important, or more so, for APRNs than any other clinical competency they might develop. It is also the premise of the authors that at present, this competency is, at best, not effectively nurtured in either education or practice settings and, at worst, undermined. Historical influences are presented, leadership development models are explored, the DNP curriculum related to leadership in a sample of programs related to leadership is identified, and recommendations for obtaining leadership competencies for APRNs are made here.

INFLUENCE OF HISTORY

To progress successfully into the future, it is imperative to understand the historical context, which has influenced the present state of nursing as well as the role of the APRN as a leader. Nursing's history has resulted in both a light and shadow side of nursing (Ashley, 1979; Nightingale, 1946; Roberts, 1983, 2006). There are two powerful influences of the profession that are highlighted here. The first is the position of power (or lack thereof) nurses held in the hierarchy of health care systems; the second is the way the profession articulated and lived its philosophy and values, specifically as contrasted with the philosophy and values of medicine.

Historically, the predominant thinking and design within other industries influenced the design of hospitals and health care. In the 20th century, the assembly line design was prominent. Most of these industries resembled what Mintzberg (1983) would call a machine bureaucracy, where roles were clearly delineated with the strategic apex (e.g., the thinkers) of the organization, creating the decisions and standardized processes that those in the operating core (e.g., the doers) carried out. The place of nursing was clearly in the operating core, whereas physicians straddled both spheres, enacting their practice in the operating core but influencing decisions in the strategic apex (Mintzberg, 1983). It is important to recognize that the historical differences in gender in these two professions, nursing being predominately female and medicine male, also influenced the alignment within the hospital structure. As Weber (1939/1987) poignantly pointed out, once a hierarchical system is in place, it is easier to annihilate it completely than to make any incremental changes in its structure that are long lasting, as those holding the power have no incentive to relinquish it and those without the power do not have the leverage to obtain it easily.

In addition, nurses have always been steadfast in grounding their values, philosophy, and vision in a framework of care (Gordon, Benner, & Noddings, 1996; Reverby, 1987, 2001). Reverby, a philosopher who studied the nursing profession, articulated that, contrasted with medicine, nurses focused on the *duty to care* rather than the *right to care*, whereas medicine understood that in order to fulfill the *duty to care*, they needed to focus on the *right to care*, which necessitated placing a priority on protecting economic viability and their place in the hierarchy where they could influence decisions. It is important to note that the hierarchical positions were influenced not by differences in inherent contributions to patient care but by philosophical and political positioning. It is interesting to note that the title "doctor" is still almost universally and exclusively believed to belong to MDs. In fact, as identified earlier, almost two thirds of those in the United States have visited an APRN for primary care, but if one listens closely, people continue to talk about "going to the doctor" for health care. It is surprising that even APRNs will use the term *doctor* versus *provider* when talking about seeking health care.

APRNs and the Concept of Power

Given nurses' history, philosophy, and values, the concept of power today holds ambivalence for many nurses, including APRNs. In a graduate course on systems taught by one of the authors, an imagery exercise is conducted on the concept of power (Krejci, 1997). Over the years, images of power experienced in this exercise continue to include negative militaristic, violent, and/or hierarchical images. APRNs are sometimes ambivalent about the concept of power, given how they may have experienced or witnessed power throughout their nursing career. The imagery exercise mentioned also includes a question: "Who wants to be powerful?" Many are tentative about raising their hands, and those that do admit hesitancy, as the desire for power seemed to be in conflict with the prototype of an expert nurse committed to patient care. That being said, in response to the next question, "Who wants to be powerless?" no one raises his or her hand. This is a dilemma; APRNs resent powerlessness and yet are ambivalent about wanting to be powerful.

Although many arguments could be made related to the word *power* and its meaning, it is not coincidental that this ambivalence exists, given our history and our values, contrasted with a health care system that is clearly traditional and hierarchical. In contrast, when this imagery exercise is held with a predominantly male audience, almost all participants raise their hand in response to the question, "Who wants to be powerful?"

For many APRNs, the focus on clinical competence and holistic care is paramount, as it should be. Unfortunately, without development of leadership competencies and influence at decision-making tables, clinical competence will not be enough to affect care. Although APRNs usually clearly believe in and align with Benner's transformational "power with" (1984/2001), they may be uncomfortable making a concerted effort at enhancing the traditional bases of power as articulated in the classic work by French and Raven (1959) and still used today. Nurses tend to rely heavily on their expert power base. Although expert power is crucial, APRNs will do well to develop other bases of power in order to advocate more successfully for their patients.

Nurses by nature strive toward collaboration, often using accommodation as a primary approach to negotiation. Accommodation as a hopeful conduit to collaboration is often a learned approach for women; nurses use it often believing it may be the only way to ensure high-quality care for patients, at least in the short term (Morrison, 2008; Valentine, 2001). Unwittingly, they may be creating the very thing they are wishing to avoid: a continual experience of being at what Kritek (2002) calls the *uneven table*. The systematic structure in most health care settings does not, unfortunately, reward the essence of nursing (Fagin, 1994, 2000; Fagin & Schwarz, 1993) or the unique contribution of APRNs but rather actions and outcomes that facilitate the traditional medical model. This can create a fine line between collaboration and competition, especially for APRNs and physicians (Stewart-Amidei, 2003). Consequently, nurses must develop the leadership, negotiation, and system skills needed to influence systems that may not be designed to naturally highlight their unique contribution. The ACA's goals of preventive health are aligned with the APRN's desired skill set, especially those at the DNP preparation level who are prepared to lead, serve on boards, and advocate for policy initiatives that are aligned with the Community-Based Collaborative Care Network (Lathrop & Hodnicki, 2014). In fact, in the IOM's *The Future of Nursing* report, two of the main recommendations relate to leadership. Recommendation 2 reads, "Expand opportunities for nurses to lead and diffuse collaborative improvement efforts" (p. 2), and recommendation 7 reads "Prepare and enable nurses to lead change to advance health" (p. 5). Unfortunately, calling for leadership and actually enhancing leadership skills are two different things. It will be imperative that both educational and practice settings take these recommendations very seriously by taking focused aim at increasing competencies of APRNs. Curriculum related to leadership in DNP programs is discussed later in the chapter.

Leadership Development in Educational programs

Formal Nursing Education (BSN and MSN)

Leadership development in nursing became more formally recognized and integrated into education with the advent of BSN programs in nursing. The inclusion of leadership content in the curriculum was indeed one of the hallmarks that distinguished a BSN education. *The Essentials for Baccalaureate Education* (AACN, 2008) emphasizes the importance of leadership and identifies "Basic Organizational and Systems Leadership for Quality and Patient Safety" as the second essential for baccalaureate education. Subsequently, BSN programs all have some type of leadership and management course that students take before graduating. However, most of these courses are traditional leadership courses that focus more on content related to delegation, nurse practice acts, magnet hospital designation, evidence-based practice, quality improvement endeavors, and some management content on staffing, productivity, and budgeting. These courses are content driven rather than developing individuals as leaders.

All these concepts are important but insufficient for true leadership development. For nurses, the one senior leadership course may be the only course they get on leadership before being responsible for advocating for clients in a system that renders most clients confused about their bills, their disease, the many providers they encounter, and the technology that they may be dependent on upon discharge.

Traditionally in MSN programs, except for those pursuing the nursing leadership or administrative tracks, graduate students may take only one course addressing health care systems and some leadership content. Given necessities and the knowledge explosion, a majority of the curricula for those pursuing clinical degrees focused on nursing theory, pathophysiology, pharmacology, technology, research, education, professional issues, and management of conditions. In reality however, once practicing, APRNs are expected to be exquisite agents of change, skilled negotiators, astute group leaders, incisive systems thinkers, innovators of practice, and flexible collaborators with a variety of other leaders. Adding complexity to their role, APRNs operate from a basis of expert power, usually in staff roles, while many of the administrative and physician leaders APRNs negotiate with on a day-to-day basis are often those who hold line positions of authority within the organization. In 2011, the AACN published *The Essentials of Master's Education in Nursing*, which explicitly focuses on leadership competencies for all MSN prepared nurses. Essential II, titled "Organizational and Systems Leadership," identifies that any MSN program "recognizes that organizational and systems leadership are critical to the promotion of high quality and safe patient care. Leadership skills are needed that emphasize ethical and critical decision making, effective working relationships, and a systems-perspective" (p. 4). It will be interesting to identify how leadership competencies change as programs begin to realign with the essentials. Although this development will certainly advance the focus on leadership, reading about, writing about, and discussing leadership often fall short of developing new competencies. Given the findings from Burgess and Curry (2014) that lack of leadership was an instrumental influence in sentinel events, we can no longer avoid this.

Outside of Nursing

Industries outside of health care have long understood that leadership development, not just cognitive understanding, is crucial to productivity, satisfaction, profitability, and retention (Buckingham & Coffman, 1999). There have been prestigious fellowships such as the Kellogg Fellowship and in-depth training of business leaders through centers such as the Center for Creative Leadership (CCL, 2008). Interestingly enough, 65% of the leaders trained in the CCL, one of the top-ranked executive education providers worldwide, were men. Many industries have also invested in consultants to provide leadership development for leaders throughout the organization.

However, it is not common for nurse leaders to participate in these leadership fellowships in the same numbers that other leaders do, including leaders of health care systems. As a case in point, the American Council on Education (ACE) has a very well regarded leadership fellowship for leaders in academic settings (www.acenet.edu/leadership/programs/Pages/ACE-Fellows-Program.aspx). This fellowship has launched many presidents and provosts in their careers, but from reviewing credentials from ACE fellows in the past 40 years, fewer than 20 academic nurse leaders have participated in this fellowship, a very small percentage.

Physician leadership development is also alive and well. An Internet search using the words *physician leadership development* turned up leadership development and leadership fellowship programs focused exclusively on physicians at Harvard, Stanford, Johns Hopkins, Duke, and others. The American Association of Medical Colleges (AAMC) created a standard set of competencies called the Physician Competency Reference Set (PCRS) and is tracking competencies across accredited medical schools (www.aamc.org). The PCRS delineates the difference between objectives and competencies and has comprehensive and very specific competencies relevant to effective leadership. For example, under the category of Personal and Professional Development, the competencies include the following: self-awareness, healthy coping, managing conflict, trustworthiness, leadership skills that enhance team functioning, and self-confidence that puts patients, families, and members of health care teams at ease.

The AAMC offers a host of leadership seminars, courses, and institutes and in 2012 reported that the number of medical schools creating "leadership academies" within their schools has grown significantly over a 10-year period.

It is clear to the AAMC and many academic health centers that it is crucial to provide in-depth leadership development for physicians to gain leverage in today's health care system. Crites, Ebert, and Schuster (2008) have recommended a curriculum revision to incorporate in-depth leadership competencies throughout every year of medical school; they believe these skills are crucial to the future success of the profession. They also believe it is imperative to develop physicians as leaders early in their careers to make the biggest difference. They agree with Goleman (2001) that leadership competencies are easier to develop and longer lasting when professionals are just beginning their careers rather than as midcareer development.

Within Nursing

Although nursing leadership development programs are not as extensive or as numerous as the physician and traditional chief executive officer (CEO) programs, several significant and influential programs exist. These programs elucidate the competencies needed for nurses who are agents of change and leaders in the health care system today. One of the most prestigious leadership development programs in nursing has been the Robert Wood Johnson Foundation, Executive Nurse Fellowship (RWJFENF) program (Bellack & Morjikian, 2005). This program developed nurse leaders from practice, public health, and educational environments to have an effect on health policy and patient outcomes. The RWJFENF program identified five main competencies needed for nurses to make a difference in today's health care environment. These competencies include self-awareness, interpersonal and communication effectiveness, risk taking and creativity, strategic visioning, and inspiring and leading change. Since the publication of the last edition, the Robert Wood Johnson Foundation has redirected funds for the Nurse Executive Fellowship and beginning in 2015 will begin to support interprofessional leadership development to align with the IOM *The Future of Nursing* report, which encourages interdisciplinary collaboration.

The University of South Carolina created a Center for Nursing Leadership in 1994. The center focuses on the competencies of organizational communication, self-awareness, resolution and negotiation of conflict, impact of globalization and complexity of organizations (or "circles of influence"), leadership and management of complex systems, and strategic thinking. The center offers the Amy C. Cockcroft fellowship program, developing nurses in all roles in many different settings to become stronger leaders and affect health care throughout the southeastern United States (University of South Carolina, College of Nursing, Center for Nursing Leadership, n.d.).

Recently O'Neil et al. (2008) canvassed the leadership development programs available to nurse leaders. They found that most of the activity for leadership development has occurred since 2000, although leadership development in other industries began strong development in the 1970s (CLC, 2008). They surveyed nursing and nonnursing leaders to ascertain the competencies needed in nursing leaders. They found that both nursing and nonnursing leaders valued building effective teams first and foremost, followed by communicating vision, managing conflict, translating vision into strategy, and maintaining focus on patient and consumer. The authors reported that leaders of health care had a clear preference for developing leadership competencies in nurses but that leadership development of nurses was undercapitalized compared with other industries.

Although these leadership development programs are a great resource for nurses in all roles, it is incumbent upon both nursing practice and education to ensure that APRNs have the sufficient leadership competencies to leverage their clinical contributions and influence health care as we move forward with a new political and economic climate. Although the AACN highlights leadership as one of the main essentials of the DNP curriculum, many programs have yet to integrate leadership development to the depth of the efforts occurring in medical schools.

Within DNP Curriculum

The current explosion of DNP programs provides good evidence of the belief within the nursing community that the health care system, the profession, and the public need nurses who are prepared to be practice leaders. In 2013 almost 15,000 students were enrolled in DNP programs across the country (AACN, 2014a).

The AACN developed the *Essentials for Doctoral Education for Advanced Nursing Practice* in 2006 (AACN, 2006), identifying eight main essentials for curriculum in any DNP program. The DNP essentials document delineates the importance of leadership knowledge and skills throughout the document and specifically addresses leadership in Essentials II, VI, and VIII. Essential II is focused on organizational and systems leadership for quality improvement and systems thinking. Graduates must have advanced communication skills to lead quality improvement and patient safety initiatives. Essential VI is focused on interprofessional collaboration for improving patient and population health outcomes. To be successful, graduates must demonstrate the ability to employ effective communication and collaborative skills, lead interprofessional teams, and employ consultative and leadership skills with intraprofessional and interprofessional teams to create change in health care and complex health care delivery systems. Essential VIII is focused on advanced practice nursing. Among other requirements, DNP graduates must be able to develop and sustain therapeutic relationships and partnerships with patients and other professionals; demonstrate advanced levels of systems thinking; and guide, mentor, and support other nurses to achieve excellence in nursing practice (AACN, 2006).

A review of the AACN website reveals 243 schools currently offer DNP degrees, an increase of almost 300% since the last edition of this book was published. A 2014 study conducted by the RAND Corporation for AACN describes the current state of DNP programs in the United States (AACN, 2014b). Findings suggest almost universal agreement among those surveyed that the content added with DNP programs is highly valuable. While the masters degree continues to be the primary pathway for APRN entry into practice education, the number of DNP degree programs continue to expand steadily. The report provides a detailed analysis of facilitators and barriers to transitioning master's level APRN programs to the DNP and recommends AACN continue with efforts to assist schools facing challenges in offering a BSN to DNP program, particularly programs existing within larger universities.

A search of APRN professional organization's websites resulted in finding readily available resource materials on the website for the National Organization of Nurse Practitioner Faculties (www.nonpf.org) related to leadership core competencies. The website provides access to the "DNP NP Toolkit: Process and Approach to DNP Competency Based Evaluation," as well as sample curriculum "Templates for Doctorate of Nursing Practice (DNP) NP Education." The organization states these are made available to promote quality education for nurse practitioners at the doctoral level and in an effort to ensure national standards are incorporated into DNP programs nationally.

The website of the National Association of Clinical Nurse Specialists (www.nacns.org) includes a statement of neutrality with regard to DNP preparation and a comprehensive set of CNS core competencies (National Association of Clinical Nurse Specialists [NACNS], 2012). Neiminen, Mannevaara, and Fagerstrom (2011) identified five major themes for APRN competencies with leadership in a caring culture as one.

These two APRN roles and relevant competencies, along with the AACN *Essentials for DNP Education* competencies, were compared with the model and framework the authors developed for their leadership development and research work (Krejci & Malin, 2001, 2006). The model is based on more than 20 years of teaching and consulting in the area of leadership development with nurses in a variety of roles (Krejci & Malin, 1997). The model encompasses leadership development for all nurses, not just those in formal leadership positions. The foundation of the model is self-awareness, which the literature on leadership has consistently identified as being a prerequisite for successful leadership (Covey, 2004; Goleman & Boyatzis, 2008; Guthrie & Kelly-Radford, 1998; O'Neil et al., 2008; Senge, 1990). The components in this model are congruent with the essentials document (AACN, 2006) (Figure 7.1). Self-awareness, self-efficacy, and mission occupy the center of the model, surrounded by supporting competencies of systems thinking, circle of influence (personal power), interpersonal communication, building teams, negotiating conflict, moving vision to action, coaching and developing others, and implementing change.

KNOWLEDGE, SKILL, AND COMPETENCIES

The results of this comparison are included in Table 7.1. The lack of consistent language makes it difficult to compare. Without delving into course-level information within individual programs, one can hardly know which competencies students attain in the program. For example, although one might assume that self-awareness is essential for effective interpersonal communication and change implementation, it is not on the list of required competencies. This is despite thought leaders and researchers in organizational development, business, and nursing having consistently and strongly stated the importance of self-awareness for effective leaders (Ancona, Malone, Orlikowski & Senge, 2007; Drucker 1999; Goleman, 1996; Goleman, Boyatzis, & McKee, 2002; McBride 2010).

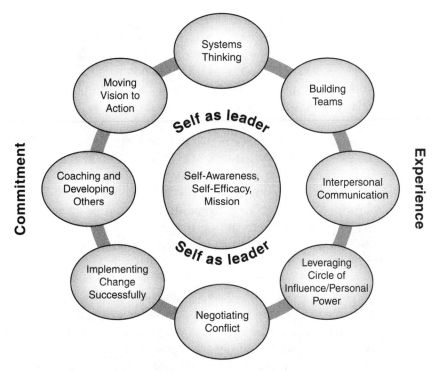

FIGURE 7.1 Krejci and Malin's Leadership Model of Competencies.

TABLE 7.1 Comparison of Nurse Practitioner, Clinical Nurse Specialist, and AACN *Essentials for DNP Education* with Krejci and Malin's Leadership Framework

	NATIONAL ORGANIZATION OF NURSE PRACTITIONER FACULTIES (NONPF) NURSE PRACTITIONER CORE COMPETENCIES	CLINICAL NURSE SPECIALIST CORE COMPETENCIES	AACN ESSENTIALS FOR DNP EDUCATION
Systems thinking	X	X	X
Self-awareness and mission			
Circle of influence (personal power)			X
Interpersonal communication	X	X	X
Negotiating conflict	X	X	X
Building teams		X	X
Moving vision to action	X		X
Coaching and developing others		X	X
Implementing change	X	X	X

Efforts to standardize how we define and evaluate leadership competencies across curricula and advanced practice roles is a crucial step toward ensuring DNP-prepared nurses are ready to be the leaders the U.S. health care system so desperately needs (Fynes, Martin, Hoy, & Cousely, 2014). The goal is for nurses to be as competent in sitting at system-level decision-making tables and advocating for changes necessary to meet the goals of population health as they are in providing care to patients.

Although there seems to be much agreement that leadership competencies are a prerequisite for successful APRNs, at this point nursing education has not overtly delineated this content in its curricula compared with the recommendations to medical school curricula or other industries. As more DNP programs are being created, nursing education has a stunning opportunity to create stronger leaders.

In addition, the authors believe there continues to be a need for leadership development that augments what is learned in formal graduate education programs. Although the numbers of nondegree leadership development programs have grown exponentially, many are created for and offered to those in formal administrative roles, with few focusing on practice leaders. Interestingly, this is not the case in medicine, where practice leadership development programs flourish (Hall, 2005).

A review of websites for relevant national nursing organizations identified very few leadership development opportunities. Although many offer leadership academies or leadership sessions at annual meetings, it was harder to locate leadership development opportunities on most APRN sites (www.nacns.org; www.midwife.org; www.NapNap.org; www.aana.com). One exception was noted; the American Association of Nurse Practitioners (www.aanp.org) has a 12-month Future Leaders Program designed for early career nurse practitioners showing interest and promise in becoming more effective leaders within their practices, within their schools, and nationally.

It is clear that nursing professional organizations for APRNs are engaged in utilizing the IOM *Future of Nursing* report in a variety of ways, often focused on asking relevant entities, such as the Centers for Medicare & Medicaid Services, to allow nurses to practice to the full extent of their education. Sigma Theta Tau International, the nursing honor society, provides many leadership development opportunities, including leadership fellowships aligned with clinical specialties (www.nursingsociety.org). The authors strongly recommend all DNP programs evaluate the DNP curriculum with the goal of ensuring overt, in-depth leadership development throughout the curriculum. Those in APRN roles are strongly encouraged to seek out the leadership development and fellowship opportunities that exist locally, regionally, and nationally.

Application of Competencies to the APRN Role

To demonstrate the importance of leadership competencies, four scenarios are presented. Common issues occurring in many practice settings provide context for examining the critical need for leadership development for APRNs. Both authors have been working with APRNs and other nurses over the past 20 years within leadership development sessions. One of the authors led a department of advanced practice for several years. The scenarios that follow are typical examples of common problems.

Implementing Change, Moving Vision to Action

Jeanne is a seasoned nurse practitioner who has what she believes is an exciting, excellent idea for creating a new clinic that could be staffed solely by the APRNs in the practice, allowing their physician colleagues more time in the operating room and providing a role that would be satisfying to the nurse practitioners. She presents a detailed proposal for the new clinic to the provider group only to have it dismissed by her physician colleagues as cost prohibitive. Her APRN colleagues who agreed to support the proposal before the meeting did not speak in support of the proposal during the meeting. When she asks them why, they shrug and walk away. Jeanne is left confused, disappointed, angry, and unsure of what to do next. Leadership competencies of implementing change successfully and moving vision to action may have helped Jeanne to strategize by partnering with early adopters, proposing a low-cost pilot, and presenting a compelling vision aligned with physician goals. Even if her proposal was not accepted, Jeanne would have been able to reframe the conclusion from "defeat" to "new information" that can be incorporated into her next proposal.

Systems Thinking, Building Teams, Developing and Coaching Others, and Interpersonal Communication

Bruce, an experienced APRN, is approached by a staff nurse working in the practice who is fuming about the encounter she just had with an APRN in the practice. She found the APRN discounting and believes this APRN holds herself above others and devalues nurses as "mere staff nurses." Bruce believes everyone should be responsible for their own "stuff," and although he enjoys the nurse and values her role in the practice, he is not sure how to be helpful. He tells the nurse to shake it off and assures her the APRN does not really mean it. The staff nurse leaves feeling discounted again and begins to question whether she wants to stay. She avoids the other APRN and Bruce by not seeking their consultation. Many leadership skills for either APRN may have produced better results for the APRNs, the patients they serve, and the system. Systems thinking competencies would have allowed both to see this situation from a larger perspective, understanding that individual tensions, events, and relationships are influenced by systematic structure and inherent system patterns. Unfortunately, in this situation, accidental adversaries, a common system archetype (Senge, 1990), has now been created. Competencies in building teams, interpersonal communication, and developing and coaching others might also have helped this situation from escalating into powerlessness and frustration.

Self-Awareness

An effective APRN is one who is self-aware and spends time learning through practice. Betty is a highly productive APRN who consistently works 12 hours a day. She finds herself dreading getting up and going to work these days. Over the past 6 months, she has had a number of formal patient complaints and is mortified about this, hoping no one will mention it, and is very concerned about what has happened; she prided herself in the fact that patients always enjoyed having her work with them. Many APRNs practice in busy practices with little time for colleagueship, mentoring, development, or reflection. Leadership development in the area of self-awareness could have helped Betty understand her particular strengths and challenges and helped her manage her boundaries more effectively. Understanding the importance of self-awareness and exploring growth through strengths is likely to lead to more effective, congruent professionals. The habit of learning through practice is key to excellence in practice.

Negotiating Conflict, Understanding Systems, and Expanding Circle of Influence (Power)

The issue of credentialing and privileging APRNs was under discussion by the Medical Executive Committee at a large academic medical center. Donna, a certified nurse-midwife, tried unsuccessfully to be privileged at the hospital 5 years ago. Her rationale for applying for privileges was to allow her to work with women under her own license versus practicing under supervision. This time she was ready. Shortly after the defeat, Donna had the opportunity to enroll in a leadership development program and gained access to a coach to assist her in understanding the system, politics, and strategic use of power. She learned the structure of decision making around credentialing and privileging at the medical center, including the names of members of the Medical Credentialing and Privileging Committee. She set up one-on-one meetings with committee members to discuss the rationale for privileging APRNs after working closely with her collaborating physicians to ensure their support as well. When the issue came to a vote, it passed, with the majority of members supporting this significant change.

CONCLUSION

Understanding the historical context and the areas of leverage for APRNs is necessary but not sufficient in ensuring that humans have access to the best that APRNs have to offer. To advocate for patient care and affect outcomes for individuals and populations, APRNs need strong and ongoing development of their leadership competencies. The responsibility to enhance the evidence-based leadership skills of the APRN lies with graduate education, professional organizations, and the individual APRN. All three entities need to identify as a priority the development of the APRN as a leader.

These leadership and system skills are as crucial to the success of APRNs in health care organizations as their clinical prowess. Just as APRNs seek ongoing clinical education, they need to seek mentors to help identify how they need to advance their leadership competencies.

Although the ability to operationalize leadership in a measurable way remains elusive, there is now a growing body of literature that has correlated outcomes with leadership, even when measured or articulated in different ways (Bennis, Benne, & Chin, 1969; Buckingham & Coffman, 1999; Burgess & Curry, 2014; Farkas & Wetlaufer, 1996; Goleman, Boyatzis, & McKee, 2002; Kelly, Kutney-Lee, Lake, & Aiken, 2013: Kouzes & Posner, 1995; Kritek, 2002; Porter-O'Grady & Malloch, 2003; Senge et al., 1994). Buckingham and Coffman (1999), leaders in the research conducted by Gallup on managers and outcomes, have identified that strong leadership is correlated with retention, productivity, profitability, and satisfaction. Kelly et al. (2013) found that better work environments, including leadership, were correlated with critical care units that reported fewer hospital-acquired infections. The research on magnet hospitals has supported a need for strong leadership. AACN has now identified a need for stronger leadership presence in the health care system in order to enhance quality care by mandating preparation at the DNP level for advanced practice after 2015 (AACN, 2006). The IOM reports clearly indicate that mastering and coordinating the context of care is an important variable for quality (1999, 2001, 2004, 2010). APRNs need to practice evidence-based practice not only for clinical phenomena but also for system phenomena, of which there is a growing body of supportive evidence (Pfeffer & Sutton, 2006). The National Association for Clinical Nurse Specialist (NACNS) clearly identifies that one dimension of the scope of practice for APRNs is leadership in the organization or system (NACNS, 2004).

APRNs may gain skills in a variety of ways, by reading, attending workshops and training, taking courses, and/or working with a mentor. How they get acquire them is not nearly as important as a focused, systematic effort to enhance their competencies. Hopefully future DNP programs will include a more intense focus on systems and leadership, focusing on individual leadership development with assessment and coaching. Today, most organizations are investing heavily in leadership development for those in administrative positions because they know the impact strong leaders can have on an organization. APRNs need to inquire about participating in these development opportunities.

Second, APRNs need to understand the system and the system politics. APRNs need to be socialized in their graduate education as well as in their professional organizations to study the systems where they are or will be employed. All APRNs should understand the organizational chart, formal and informal (Mintzberg, 1983, 1987), to examine where they are placed within the hierarchy and the place and role of the person to whom they report. APRNs should carefully review their job descriptions and ascertain how words such as *supervision* and *collaboration* are defined.

In essence, how APRNs are described, where they sit in the organization, and over what decisions they have influence are just as important as their clinical expertise in terms of affecting outcomes of care.

Finally, and quite simply, APRNs need to *show up* at the table. APRNs are often so immersed in practice that they may make the mistake of being unintentionally absent at, or even intentionally avoiding, important system decision-making bodies (formal and informal) because they do not want to engage in "politics." APRNs need to network with their colleagues to ensure adequate representation through themselves or other strong nursing leaders, when discussions or decisions are being carried out that affect their role. APRNs must take every opportunity to be present, particularly when invited to the table. Missing these opportunities unfortunately signals disinterest and lack of professional involvement.

In summary, demonstrating and advancing leadership competencies is critically important to ensuring effective, high-quality APRN practice in systems. Being knowledgeable about the current state and understanding when and how to choose high-leverage targets for change is essential for APRNs to evolve practice to the level of respect in the system where they are universally accessible, receive appropriate compensation for services rendered, and sit at the appropriate decision-making tables. Other health professionals clearly understand the importance of in-depth leadership development. It is imperative that APRNs not be left behind; patient care outcomes and the future of nursing depend on their leadership.

REFERENCES

American Association of Colleges of Nursing (2004). Position statement on the practice doctorate in nursing. http://www.aacn.nche.edu/dnp/dnp-position-statement

American Association of Colleges of Nursing. (2006). *Essentials of doctoral education for advanced practice nurses.* Washington, DC: American Association of Colleges of Nursing. Retrieved from http://www.aacn.nche.edu/DNP/pdf/Essentials.pdf

American Association of Colleges of Nursing. (2008). *Essentials of baccalaureate education for professional nursing practice.* Washington, DC: American Association of Colleges of Nursing. Retrieved from http://www.aacn.nche.edu/education-resources/baccessentials08.pdf

American Association of Colleges of Nursing. (2011). *Essentials of master's education.* Retrieved from http://www.aacn.nche.edu/education-resources/MastersEssentials11.pdf

American Association of Colleges of Nursing. (2014a). *DNP fact sheet: The doctor of nursing practice (DNP).* Retrieved from http://www.aacn.nche.edu/media-relations/fact-sheets/dnp

American Association of Colleges of Nursing. (2014b). *The DNP by 2015: A study of the institutional, political, and professional issues that facilitate or impede establishing a post-baccalaureate doctor of nursing practice program.* Retrieved from http://www.aacn.nche.edu/dnp/DNP-Study.pdf

American Association of Nurse Practitioners. (2014). NP Infographic. http://www.aanp.org/images/about-nps/npgraphic.pdf

Ancona, D., Malone, T. W., Orlikowski, W. J., & Senge, P. M. (2007). In praise of the incomplete leader. *Harvard Business Review, 85*(2), 92–100.

Ashley, J. (1979*). Hospitals, paternalism, and the nurse.* New York, NY: Teachers College.

Association of Medical Colleges. (2012). *Leadership development academies help shape the future of medicine.* Retrieved from https://www.aamc.org/ members/gip/strategicplanning/352092/leadershipdevelopmentacademieshelpshapethefutureofmedicine.html

Bellack, J. P., & Morjikian, R. L. (2005). The RWJ executive nurse fellows program, Part 2. *Journal of Nursing Administration, 35*(12), 533–540.

Benner, P. (2001/1984). *From novice to expert: Excellence and power in clinical nursing practice.* Upper Saddle River, NJ: Prentice Hall.

Bennis, W. G., Benne, D., & Chin, R. (Eds.). (1969). *The planning of change.* New York, NY: Holt, Rinehard & Winston.

Brooten, D., Youngblut, J. M., Kutcher, J., & Bobo, C. (2004). Quality and the nursing workforce: APRNs, patient outcomes and health care costs. *Nursing Outlook, 52*(1),45–52.

Brooten, D., Youngblut, J., Blais, K., Donahue, D., Cruz, I., & Lightbourne, M. (2005). APRN-physician collaboration in caring for women with high-risk pregnancies. *Journal of Nursing Scholarship, 37*(2), 178–184.

Buckingham, M., & Coffman, M. (1999). *First, break all the rules: What the world's greatest managers do differently.* New York, NY: Simon & Schuster.

Burgess, C., & Curry, M. (2014). Patient safety first: Transforming the health care environment collaborative. *Association of periOperative Registered Nurses Journal, 99*(4), 529–539.

Burns, S. M., & Earven S. (2003). Improving outcomes for mechanically ventilated medical intensive care unit patients using advanced practice nurses: A 6-year experience. *Critical Care Nursing Clinics of North America, 14*(3), 231–243.

Center for Creative Leadership. (2008). Retrieved from http://www.ccl.org/ leadership/pdf/community/harvardbusinesswhitepaper.pdf

Covey, S. (2004). *The 8th habit.* New York, NY: Free Press.

Crites, G., Ebert, J., & Schuster, R. (2008). Beyond the dual degree: Development of a five-year program in leadership for medical undergraduates. *Academic Medicine, 83*(1), 52–58.

Cunningham, R. S. (2004). Advanced practice nursing outcomes: A review of selected empirical literature. *Oncology Nursing Forum, 31*(2), 219–232.

Drucker, P. F. (1999). Managing oneself. *Harvard Business Review, 77*(2), 64–74.

Evans, M. (2014). Not-for-profit hospitals: Pressure for revenue growth . . . more patients expected . . . smaller DSH payments . . . value based reimbursement. *Modern Healthcare, 44*(1), 16.

Fagin, C. (1994). Cost effectiveness of nursing care revisited: 1981-1990. In C. Harrington & C. Estes (Eds.), *Health policy and nursing.* Boston, MA: Jones & Bartlett.

Fagin, C., & Schwarz, M. R. (1993). Can APRNs be independent gatekeepers? *Hospitals & Health Networks, 7*(11), 8–9.

Fagin, C. M. (2000). *Essays on nursing leadership.* New York, NY: Springer.

Farkas, C. M., & Wetlaufer, S. (1996). The ways chief executive officers lead. *Harvard Business Review, 74*(3), 110–122

Federal Trade Commission. (2014). *Policy perspectives: Competition and the regulation of advanced practice nurses.* Retrieved from http://www.ftc.gov/policy/ policy-actions/advocacy-filings/2014/03/policy-perspectives-competition-regulation-advanced

French, J.R., & Raven, B. (1959). The base of social power. In D. Cartwright (Ed.), *Studies in social power* (pp. 150–167). Ann Arbor, MI: Institute for Social Research. University of Michigan.

Fynes, E., Martin, D., Hoy, L., & Cousely, A. (2014). Anesthetic nurse specialist role: Leading and facilitating in clinical practice. *Journal of Perioperative Practice, 24*(5), 97–102.

Gawlinski, A., McCloy, K., & Jesurum, J. (2001). Measuring outcomes in cardiovascular APRN practice. In R. Kleinpell (Ed.), *Outcome assessment in advanced practice nursing* (pp. 131–188). New York, NY: Springer.

Goleman, D. (1996). *Emotional intelligence: Why it can matter more than IQ.* New York, NY: Random House.

Goleman, D. (2001). What makes a leader? In *Harvard Business Review: On What Makes a Leader.* Boston, MA: Harvard Business School Publishing.

Goleman, D., & Boyatzis, R. (2008). Social intelligence and the biology of leadership. *Harvard Business Review, 8*(9), 74–81.

Goleman, D., Boyatzis, R., & McKee, A. (2002). *Primal leadership: Realizing the power of emotional* intelligence. Boston: Harvard Business Review.

Gordon, S., Benner, P., & Noddings, N. (1996). *Caregiving: Readings in knowledge, practice, ethics, and politics.* Philadelphia, PA: University of Pennsylvania.

Guthrie, V., & Kelly-Radford, L. (1998). Feedback-intensive programs. In C. McCauley, R. Moxley, & E. VanVelor (Eds.), *The center for creative leadership: Handbook of leadership development* (pp. 66–105). San Francisco, CA: Jossey-Bass.

Hall, L. (2005). *National leadership development programs.* Washington, DC: American Association of Medical Colleges.

Institute of Medicine. (1999). *To err is human: Building a safer health system.* Washington, DC: National Academies of Science.

Institute of Medicine. (2001). *Crossing the quality chasm: A new health system for the 21st century.* Washington, DC: National Academies of Science.

Institute of Medicine. (2004). *Insuring American's Health: Principles and Recommendations.* Washington, DC: National Academies of Science.

Institute of Medicine. (2010). *The future of nursing: Leading change, advancing health.* Washington, DC: National Academies of Science.

Kelly, D., Kutney-Lee, A., Lake, E., & Aiken, L. H. (2013). The critical care work environment and nurse reported health care associated infections. *American Journal of Critical Care, 22*(6), 482–489.

Kleinpell, R. M. (2007). APRNs: Invisible champions? *Nursing Management, 38*(5), 18–22.

Kouzes, J., & Posner, B. Z. (1995). *The leadership challenge.* San Francisco, CA: Jossey-Bass.

Krejci, J. W. (1997). Imagery: Stimulating critical thinking by unearthing mental models. *Journal of Nursing Education, 36*(10), 482–484.

Krejci, J. W., & Malin, S. (1997). Impact of leadership development on leadership competencies. *Nursing Economics, 15*(5), 235–241.

Krejci, J., & Malin, S. (2001, October). *Leadership critical incidents, before and after leadership development.* National Nursing Administration research conference. Cincinnati, OH.

Krejci, J.W., & Malin, S. (2006) Leadership skills and expertise: Keys to APN success in health care systems. In M. P. Mirr Jansen and M. Zwygart-Stauffacher (Eds.). *Advanced Practice Nursing: Core concepts for professional role development* (3rd ed., pp. 61–78). New York, NY: Springer Publishing.

Kritek, P. (2002). *Negotiating at an uneven table: Developing moral courage in resolving our conflicts.* San Francisco, CA: Jossey-Bass.

Larkin, H. (2003). The case for nurse practitioners. *Hospitals & Health Networks, 77*(8), 54.

Lathrop, B., & Hodnicki, D. (2014). The Affordable Care Act: Primary care and the doctor of nursing practice nurse. *Online Journal of Issues in Nursing, 19*(20). Retrieved from http://www.nursingworld.org/MainMenuCategories/ANAMarketplace/ANAPeriodicals/OJIN/TableofContents/Vol-19-2014/No2-May-2014/Articles-Previous-Topics/Affordable-Care-Act-Doctor-of-Nursing-Practice.html.

Lenz, E. R., Mundinger, M. O., Kane, R. L., Hopkins, S. C., & Lin, S. X. (2004). Primary care outcomes in patients treated by nurse practitioners or physicians: Two-year follow-up. *Medical Care Research Review, 61*(3), 332–351.

McBride, A. B. (2010). *The growth and development of nurse leaders.* New York, NY: Springer Publishing.

Mintzberg, H. (1983). *Structure in fives: Designing effective organizations.* Englewood Cliffs, NJ: Prentice-Hall.

Mintzberg, H. (1987). The five basic parts of the organization. In J. M. Shafritz & J. S. Ott (Eds.), *Classics of organization theory* (2nd ed.). Pacific Grove, CA: Grove. (Originally published 1979.)

Morrison, J. (2008). The relationship between emotional intelligence competencies and preferred conflict-handling styles. *Journal of Nursing Management, 16*(8), 974–983.

National Association of Clinical Nurse Specialists. (2004). *Statement on clinical nurse specialist: Practice and education.* Harrisburg, PA: National Association of Clinical Nurse Specialists.

National Association of Clinical Nurse Specialists. (2012). *Clinical nurse specialist core competencies.* Retrieved from http://www.nacns.org/docs/CNSCore CompetenciesBroch.pdf

Neiminen, A., Mannevaara, B., & Fagerstrom, L. (2011). Advanced practice nurses' scope of practice: A qualitative study of advanced clinical competencies. *Scandinavian Journal of Caring Sciences,* Volume 25, 661–670.

Nightingale, F. (1946). *Notes on nursing: What it is and what it is not.* Philadelphia, PA: Lippincott.

O'Neil, E., Morjickian, R. L., Cherner, D., Hirschkorn, C., & West, T. (2008). Developing nursing leaders: An overview of trends and programs. *Journal of Nursing Administration, 38*(4), 178–181.

Pearson, L. (2004). Sixteenth annual legislative update. *Nurse Practitioner, 29*(1), 26.

Pfeffer, J., & Sutton, R. I. (2006). *Hard facts, dangerous half-truths and total nonsense: Profiting from evidence-based management.* Boston, MA: Harvard Business Publishing.

Porter-O'Grady, T., & Malloch, K. (2003). *Quantum leadership.* Boston, MA: Jones & Bartlett.

Raven, B. H. (2008). The bases of power and the power/interaction model of interpersonal influence. *Analyses of social issues and public policy, 8*(1), 1–22.

Reverby, S. (1987). *Ordered to care: The dilemma of American nursing, 1850-1945.* New York, NY: Cambridge University.

Reverby, S. (2001). A caring dilemma: Womanhood and nursing in historical perspective. In E. C. Hein (Ed.), *Nursing issues in the 21st century: Perspectives from the literature.* Philadelphia, PA: Lippincott.

Roberts, S. (1983). Oppressed group behavior: Implications for nursing. *Advances in Nursing Science, 5*(4), 21–30.

Roberts, S. (2006). Oppressed group behavior in nursing. In K. Wolf & P. Nicholas, *A History of Nursing Ideas.* London, UK: Jones & Bartlett Publishers.

Russell, D., VorderBruegge, M., & Burns, S. (2002). Effect of an outcomes-managed approach to care of neuroscience patients by acute care nurse practitioners. *American Journal of Critical Care, 11*(4), 353–364.

Senge, P. (1990). *The fifth discipline: The art and practice of the learning organization.* New York, NY: Doubleday.

Senge, P. M., Kleiner, A., Roberts, C., Ross, R. B., & Smith, B. J. (1994). *The fifth discipline fieldbook: Strategies and tools for building a learning organization.* New York, NY: Currency, Doubleday.

Stewart-Amidei, C. (2003). Collaboration or competition. *Journal of Neuroscience Nursing, 35*(4), 183.

University of South Carolina, College of Nursing, Center for Nursing Leadership (n.d.). The Amy V. Cockroft Leadership Development Program. Retrieved from http://www.sc.edu/study/colleges_schools/nursing/centers_institutes/center_nursing_leadership/cockcroft_program/index.php

Valentine, P. B. (2001). A gender perspective on conflict management strategies for nurses. *Journal of Nursing Scholarship, 33*(1), 69–74.

Weber, M. (1987). Bureaucracy. In J. M. Shafritz & J. S. Ott (Eds.), *Classics of organization theory* (2nd ed.). Pacific Grove, CA: Grove. (Originally published 1946.)

PART II: IMPLEMENTATION OF THE APRN ROLE

Rhonda D. Squires

8

ADVANCED CLINICAL
DECISION MAKING

Clinical decision making in advanced practice nursing occurs as a continuous, purposeful, theory- and knowledge-based process of assessment, analysis, strategic planning, and intentional follow-up. It is both a cognitive and affective problem-solving activity for defining patient problems and selecting appropriate management approaches (Buckingham & Adams, 2000). Lunney (2009) states, "The personal strengths of tolerance for ambiguity and reflective practice need to be developed because decisions are so complex in nursing and the use of clinical judgment needs to be an ongoing learning process. Each decision is relative to context of situation and specific nature of the individual, family, or community" (p. 7).

The role of the advanced practice registered nurse (APRN) is multifaceted, and the scope of decision making is similarly complex. It incorporates health promotion, disease prevention, risk reduction, management of functional health needs, subjective concerns, program planning, biomedical diagnostics, and disease management. Large amounts of data are elicited, sorted, and organized into meaningful patterns. Conducted within the context of nurse–patient relationships, APRN clinical decision making is frequently characterized by changing health circumstances and complex social variables. The nursing and biomedical decision making involved may be straightforward or of low, moderate, or high complexity. The level of patient health risk may range from very low to very high. These parameters are used to direct allowable and appropriate billing charges in clinical practice. Reimbursement is higher for increased decision making complexity and increased patient health care risk.

PROCESSES, FOCUS, AND FRAMEWORKS

To understand clinical decision making at the APRN level, it is necessary to examine at least three interrelated aspects of practice: decision-making processes, the focus of APRN practice, and APRN frameworks for practice. Each of these components contributes essential elements to the process of clinical decision making in advanced practice nursing, resulting in a unique and valuable clinical practice role.

Decision-Making Processes: Research in Clinical Reasoning

Research in clinical judgment and decision making has been an important area of study for more than 50 years. Much of the decision-making and problem-solving research began in the cognitive sciences (Newell & Simon, 1972; Tversky & Kahneman, 1974), with early application to diagnostic reasoning and clinical problem solving in nursing and medicine (Elstein, 1976; Elstein, Shulman, & Sprafka, 1978; Hammond, 1964; Hammond, Kelly, & Castellan, 1966). Strong interest in this field of study has continued with distinctions more clearly discerned between clinical problem solving in nursing and medicine. Nursing problem solving frequently focuses on expert judgment about changes in a patient's overall status; anticipating and preventing potential problems; ensuring safe passage through uncertain health–illness trajectories; addressing the functional needs and capacities and quality-of-life issues for the whole person; understanding and responding to complex human responses; and protecting individuals and groups in their health–illness vulnerabilities (Benner, Hooper-Kyriakidis, & Stannard, 1999; Carnevali & Thomas, 1993; Tanner, Benner, Chesla, & Gordon, 1993). Medical reasoning, in contrast, focuses more specifically on the management of illness, pathology and disease, biomedical hypothesis generation with probability determination, and medical treatment decisions (Schwartz & Elstein, 2008). In medicine, a very different set of problem-solving skills and knowledge bases are required: pathophysiologic causal reasoning, use and interpretation of diagnostic tests, prognostic determination, and disease-oriented therapeutic decision making (Kassirer & Kopelman, 1991). Advanced practice nursing involves a complex blending of both nursing and medical decision making. It is important to be able to synthesize decision-making skills from both fields.

Commonalities in Clinical Reasoning Across Health Disciplines

Several common or core features of clinical reasoning across health disciplines have been identified in the research (Higgs & Jones, 2008). First, clinical reasoning and clinical knowledge are now accepted as being strongly interdependent. At one time, particularly in medicine, it was hypothesized that clinical reasoning and clinical knowledge could be learned independently (Patel & Kaufman, 2000). Many educational programs attempted to deal with the rapidly escalating volume of biomedical information by emphasizing the development of problem-solving skills and devoting less time to content. Research has shown, however, that the development of expertise in clinical reasoning requires considerable depth and organization of domain-specific clinical knowledge (Boshuizen & Schmidt, 1992). Growth in clinical expertise is accompanied by increasing depth and complexity of knowledge structures (Higgs & Jones, 2008). Thus, in addition to clinical reasoning skills, expert clinicians need to demonstrate clinical knowledge for care delivery, not just the ability to access knowledge such as clinical decision-making tools.

Another core feature of clinical reasoning across health disciplines is that an array of higher-order cognitive skills and processes is necessary for effective clinical reasoning. Various theorists identify these higher-order cognitive skills differently, but some that have been emphasized in the literature are clinical appraisal (Brookfield, 2008), categorization (Loftus & Higgs, 2008), and propositional knowledge (Titchen & Higgs, 2000). Clinical appraisal consists of critically evaluating the totality of presenting information for the most relevant clinical features and accurately defining what those features represent, such as assessing a patient to determine the pertinent positives or negatives. Categorization is a way of both learning complex content and using relevant features and pattern recognition to relate novel instances to known categories. For instance, categorization would be used to judge the level of severity or acuity of patient presentation. Risk stratification is an important current application of categorization, selecting management approaches based on the level of severity or risk and statistically predicted patient care outcomes. Propositional knowledge incorporates hypothesis generation and the development of plausible and probabilistic relationships between events. For example, the APRN uses propositional knowledge to hypothesize the most probable diagnosis given a certain patient presentation. When clinicians make prospective predictions about the likely course of a condition based on clinical signs and symptoms, they are engaging in a combination of categorization and probabilistic reasoning.

The third feature associated with clinical reasoning is that it is highly context dependent. The context within which clinical reasoning occurs is determined by the patient's health concern(s), the specific health setting, the care provider's disciplinary background and level of experience, the patient's unique personal context, the stage of case management (e.g., initial diagnosis versus long-term stabilization versus exacerbation management), and elements of the wider health care environment (Higgs & Jones, 2008). Research attending to context-specific factors (e.g., Benner et al., 1999) demonstrates that expert clinical reasoning is complex, interpretive, and personalized. Other clinicians have likened this to good clinical jazz (Flynn & Becker, 2004). Good jazz needs structure and improvisation. Structure in health care is the clinical evidence, and improvisation is the patient's personal situation. A good clinician blends these two components uniquely for each patient as a part of clinical reasoning and decision making.

Clinical reasoning depends on the clinician's language tools and skills. Knowledge and ability to use appropriate "terminology, categories and category systems, metaphors, heuristics and mnemonics, ritual, narrative, rhetoric and hermeneutics" (Loftus & Higgs, 2008, p. 340) is critical to construct a diagnosis and plan and to communicate those recommendations in a way that conveys a need for action.

Clinical Reasoning in Nursing

Multiple approaches have been used to study clinical reasoning in nursing, including information processing theory (Corcoran, 1986a), decision analysis (Corcoran, 1986b), skill acquisition or hermeneutic processes (Benner, 1984), cognitive continuum theory (Lauri & Salantera, 2002), and use of heuristics (Cioffi & Markham, 1997). Information processing derives primarily from the cognitive sciences. It focuses on memory capacity, the chunking or clustering of complex information into recognizable patterns, weighing alternative options, and searching for pathways to solutions (Elstein, 1976; Newell & Simon, 1972).

Information is accessed from long-term memory and cue assessment, then transformed into units that can be cognitively manipulated in short-term memory. This theoretical approach assumes that there are limits to the amount of information a person can process at any specific time and effective problem solving is an adaptation to those limits. In nursing, information processing has been used with verbal, or thinking-aloud, protocols to study cognitive processes used in clinical decision making (Corcoran, 1986a; Simmons, 2002). The tendency of information-processing models to be overly linear and mechanistic has been addressed through the addition of heuristics, contextual variables, varying degrees of task complexity, and varying levels of uncertainty (Higgs & Jones, 1995; Narayan & Corcoran-Perry, 1997; Tanner, Padrick, Westfall, & Putzier, 1987). Information processing provides a better theoretical match for the dynamic environments and ambiguity of decisions in clinical practice.

Analytical decision making relies on a more structured process of identifying options and possible outcomes, assigning values to the outcomes, and determining probability relationships between the options and anticipated outcomes. Formal (mathematically based) or informal (conceptually based) models are used to systematize decision making using decision trees, grids, or decision flow diagrams (Corcoran, 1986b; Narayan, Corcoran-Perry, Drew, Hoyman, & Lewis, 2003). Decision analysis has been reported as being useful for evaluation of medical treatment options, cost analysis, sensitivity analysis, quality improvement decisions, and policy decisions (Narayan et al., 2003).

Skill acquisition theory, also referred to as the hermeneutic model, has been used by Benner and colleagues (Benner, 1984; Benner & Wrubel, 1989; Benner, Tanner, & Chesla, 2009) to study expertise in clinical nursing practice. Benner and colleagues argue that experienced nurses often use the nurse–patient relationship and their intimate knowledge of a patient's response patterns to make clinical judgments about patient care. From their contributions, definitions of clinical judgment, particularly at the level of expert practice, have been expanded to include both deliberate analytic thinking and unconscious holistic discrimination of a patient's clinical status. In the hermeneutic model, expert judgment includes ethical decision making on what is good and right, a repertoire of extensive knowledge from practice, emotional engagement with patients and with one's practice, and a deep understanding of specific contexts for care (Benner et al., 2009). Components of the hermeneutic model have been identified as pattern recognition, similarity recognition, common sense understanding, skilled know-how, sense of salience, and deliberative rationality (Dreyfus & Dreyfus, 1986). Ultimately, data have to be selected and synthesized into an understandable narrative through the clinician's interpretative process.

As language has evolved in nursing to name and examine the cognitive processes and activities of expert clinical decision making, reference is often made to "intuition" in expert nursing practice (Benner et al., 2009; Pyles & Stern, 1983; Rew, 1988; Smith, 1987). *Intuition* refers to the capacity of the expert clinician to process quickly large amounts of complex data, simultaneously discern patterns, and act on hypotheses without consciously naming all the factors involved in his or her decision making. It is the highly expert application of rational processes and cue analysis, occurring at a pace too rapid for each step to be discretely named or recognized.

Cognitive continuum theory (Hamm, 1988; Lauri & Salantera, 2002) suggests a range of analytical thinking approaches with varying combinations of intuitive and analytical thinking. In this theory, the task to be accomplished exhibits features that determine the degree of intuition and/or analysis used by the decision maker. Particularly salient here are these three features: the complexity of task structure (number and redundancy of cues, form of an accurate organizing principle), the ambiguity of task content (availability of organizing principles, familiarity with the task, and possibility of high accuracy), and the form of task presentation (task decomposition, cue definition, and response time). In this model, greater analytical thinking is assumed to be related to fewer cues, less redundancy of cues, and more complex procedures for combining evidence to result in correct answers. The availability of organizing principles, greater task familiarity, and the possibility for high accuracy also contribute to greater use of formal reasoning.

The use of heuristics, as proposed by Tversky and Kahneman (1974), is a method for reducing the complexity of judgment tasks by cognitively estimating probabilities, typically based on prior experience via these three categories: representativeness, availability, and anchoring-adjustment. *Representativeness* can be used to compare signs and symptoms in a new clinical situation to previously encountered clinical conditions. *Availability* is the ease with which particular instances or cases of a condition can be brought to mind. *Anchoring-adjustment* is used to determine a baseline set of indicators for a condition and then shifting that baseline to account for the clinical factors present in a specific situation. For their part, Cioffi and Markham (1997) examined relationships between the use of heuristics and task complexity in midwifery. In simulated clinical decision-making situations, heuristic processes were used more frequently in situations of greater clinical risk and complexity, in situations with less predictability, and when less clinical information was available. Heuristic techniques were used effectively (with a high rate of accurate diagnoses) and more frequently as task complexity increased. Cioffi (1997) has proposed that heuristic strategies are an important component of advanced practice nurses' decision making in ambiguous clinical situations and in deriving intuitive judgments.

Moving from data collection to diagnosis is difficult for novice APRNs. A small number of studies have focused specifically on the clinical reasoning of APRNs. Using an information-processing model to study diagnostic reasoning among nurse practitioners, White, Nativio, Kobert, and Engberg (1992) concluded that study participants made decisions reflective of hypothetic–deductive models proposed in the information-processing literature. Experienced nurse practitioners demonstrated greater expertise in making hypothesis-driven choices about what data were necessary for making accurate diagnoses. Nurse practitioners with less expertise in a clinical area used data widely rather than focusing assessments on the basis of diagnostic hypotheses. Not all participants had the content expertise needed to correctly interpret the significance of findings or to make correct management decisions. Findings from this study demonstrate that both the process of clinical decision making and the nurse practitioner's content expertise were necessary for effective patient care.

In a study of 70 entry-level nurse practitioners, Sands (2001) found that 76% of the participants were able to develop differential diagnoses, acquire relevant data, refine their hypotheses, and make an accurate diagnosis with a common health concern (pregnancy). Characteristics of novice practice were demonstrated in the tendency of participants to acquire a great deal of data, "seemingly in an effort 'not to miss something'" (p. 137). Entry-level nurse practitioners with at least 5 years of registered nurse (RN) experience demonstrated stronger scores on the test of diagnostic reasoning. Participants with less than 2 years of RN experience were at increased risk for inadequate reasoning through the clinical problem.

Ritter (2003) examined the diagnostic reasoning of 10 expert nurse practitioners using both information-processing and hermeneutic models. Specific steps of either information processing or hermeneutics accounted for 99% of participants' think-aloud responses. Within information processing, gathering information accounted for 32% of the responses. Within hermeneutics, skilled know-how accounted for 25% of the responses. Information processing was found to begin the process. Hermeneutics were then used for cue acquisition, thereby bringing structure to the clinical problem and determining what information was salient.

APRN Practice Focus

One factor that can be used to distinguish clinical decision making in advanced practice nursing from other autonomous health care providers is the focus of APRN practice. Smith (1995) identified the core of advanced practice nursing as lying within nursing's disciplinary perspectives on health, healing, person–environment interactions, and nurse–patient relationships. Huch (1995) echoes this in identifying the need to use nursing theory as the basis for advanced nursing practice.

APRNs focus their clinical decision making on health promotion, health protection, disease prevention, and management of health concerns (National Association of Clinical Nurse Specialists [NACNS], 2008; National Organization of Nurse Practitioner Faculties [NONPF], 2012). As outlined by nurse practitioner and clinical nurse specialist organizations, health promotion activities include lifestyle concerns, principles of lifestyle change, and behavioral change. Health protection includes knowledge of health risks, use of epidemiologic principles, and community/population-level measures to protect health. Disease prevention includes primary and secondary prevention measures addressing major chronic illness, disability, and communicable disease. Management of health concerns focuses on assessing, diagnosing, monitoring, and coordinating the care of individuals and populations (NACNS, 2008; NONPF, 2012). Depending on the APRN's role and specialty preparation, the practice focuses include both disease- and non disease-based etiologies that affect health, wellness, and quality of life. For nurse practitioners, the focus is generally on providing direct patient care. For clinical nurse specialists, the focus tends to be on influencing the outcomes of care more widely within an area of population focus, at individual patient, population, and health system levels. With the advent of the doctorate of nursing practice (DNP), practice doctorate APRNs are educated to practice with increased emphasis on the health care system and population health care outcomes (American Association of Colleges of Nursing [AACN], 2004; NONPF, 2006, 2012).

APRN Practice Frameworks

Advanced practice nursing has been consistently characterized as based in holistic perspectives, the formation of partnerships with patients or populations, the use of research and theory to guide practice, and the use of diverse approaches in health and illness management (Davies & Hughes, 2002). These characteristics are now built into nationally recommended educational guidelines for advanced practice educational programs (AACN, 2006; NACNS, 2008; NONPF, 2012). For example, the NONPF (2012) core competencies for nurse practitioner clinical decision making incorporate the following expectations for practice: "Critically analyzes data and evidence for improving nursing practice" (p. 2). The core competencies and associated domains of practice were developed based on studies by Benner (1984), Brykcyznski (1989), and Fenton (1983). As advanced practice education moves to the practice doctorate level, AACN's (2006) *The Essentials of*

Exhibit 8.1 APPROACHES FOR INCORPORATING CORE NURSING PERSPECTIVES INTO APRN CARE

- Make an effort to understand meanings that patients attribute to their health situation.
- Learn about patients' lived social world, support systems, and role responsibilities.
- Work with patients to identify personal and social health obstacles or facilitators.
- Determine patients' preferences for and abilities to participate in health care decision making and self-health management.
- Jointly determine appropriate health care goals and priorities.
- Work with patients as they struggle through personal crises, losses, or transitions.
- Learn about patients' spiritual point of view and how they view the relationship between their health status and spirituality.

Doctoral Education for Advanced Practice Nursing outlines advanced clinical decision making as part of the core of APRN work: "Demonstrate sound critical thinking and clinical decision making" (p. 23).

An important feature of clinical decision making in advanced practice nursing is that the nursing focus continues to be evident in daily practice. This can be done, for example, by making an effort to understand the meanings that patients attribute to their health situation; by learning about the patients' lived social world, support systems, and role responsibilities; and by working with patients to identify personal and social health obstacles or facilitators. Several additional approaches for incorporating basic nursing perspectives into APRN care are listed in Exhibit 8.1.

In addition to the specialty knowledge required for health and illness management, these patient-centered, holistic dimensions of clinical decision making are necessary to maintain the quality of APRN care and the ability to distinguish advanced practice nursing from other forms of autonomous health practice.

CLINICAL DECISION MAKING AS UNDERSTOOD FROM PRACTICE

In addition to influences from nursing research, theory, and professional organizations, much has been learned about APRN clinical decision making directly from clinical practice as well as research and practice experiences from other disciplines.

Skilled communication and interaction are essential components of clinical decision making at all levels, whether the APRN is posing wide-field or focused inquiries, clarifying diverse perspectives, providing guidance for lifestyle health behaviors, or evaluating a patient's responses to treatment. As Chase (2011) points out, clinical decision making is not a process that occurs with the APRN in isolation. It occurs as dialogue and interaction between the patient and provider, with experiences of satisfaction significantly influenced by the quality of communication and engagement with the clinical situation (Benner, Stannard, & Hooper, 1996).

Most descriptions of APRN clinical decision making begin with an expanded nursing process model that integrates elements of hypothetic–deductive reasoning. Carnevali and Thomas (1993) describe the diagnostic reasoning process in nursing as reviewing pre-encounter data, entering into the assessment situation, collecting the database, coalescing cues into working clusters, selecting pivotal cues or cue clusters, determining possible diagnostic explanations, further comparing the clinical situation with diagnostic categories, and assigning the diagnosis.

White et al. (1992) outlined a clinical decision-making framework for APRNs that adds elements from hypothetic–deductive reasoning. Hypotheses formed are used to guide the process of inquiry (i.e., decisions about how to focus the history, examination, and diagnostic testing). The process outlined by White et al. adds many of these elements to nursing clinical decision making: reviewing pre-encounter data, generating early hypotheses, engaging in clinical inquiry, determining working hypotheses, conducting diagnostic testing, testing the final hypothesis, specifying the diagnosis, determining patient management, and evaluating the total clinical situation.

Chase (2004) configures this process specifically for nurse practitioner practice. She lists the phases of clinical judgment as follows: conducting an early wide-field search for the primary concerns; generating an early hypothesis on probable causes of the concerns; engaging in focused data acquisition related to supporting the active hypotheses and ruling out other serious conditions; evaluating various hypotheses by clustering and analyzing the data for the appropriate fit with diagnostic categories; naming the priority problems; determining appropriate therapeutic goals; determining an appropriate management plan; evaluating the effectiveness of the clinical process; and confirming or revising the diagnoses and plans. Table 8.1 provides a comparison of these three approaches.

In advanced practice nursing, each of these approaches might be appropriate for differing clinical scenarios or problems and stages. The decision-making processes can be used with both disease- and non-disease-based concerns, as well as with medical or nursing diagnoses. Hypothetic–deductive models are perceived generally to be more useful during data collection and implementation. Intuitive–interpretive models are reported in use more during data processing, whereas during planning both models are perceived to be equally in use (Bjork & Hamilton, 2011). Clinical nurse specialists might place less relative emphasis on the biomedical diagnostic content, tending more often to work collaboratively with medical care providers for these decision-making components. Nurse practitioners emphasize greater autonomy in medical diagnostic and treatment elements but place less overall emphasis on specialty nursing care and system-level thinking. With either role, however, keys to the process are clinician characteristics of perception and engagement, discipline-specific knowledge, commitment to quality

TABLE 8.1 Comparison of Nursing and APRN Clinical Decision-Making Frameworks

CARNEVALI AND THOMAS (1993), DIAGNOSTIC REASONING IN NURSING	WHITE, NATIVIO, KOBERT, AND ENGBERG (1992), APRN CLINICAL DECISION MAKING	CHASE (2004), PROCESS OF CLINICAL JUDGMENT FOR NURSE PRACTITIONERS
Collecting pre-encounter data	Reviewing pre-encounter data	Conducting wide-field data search
Entering into the assessment situation	Generating an early hypothesis	Generating a hypothesis
Collecting the database	Clinical inquiry	Acquiring data
Coalescing cues	Determining working hypotheses	Evaluating the hypothesis
Selecting pivotal cues	Performing diagnostic testing	Naming priority problems
Determining diagnostic explanations	Testing final hypothesis	Determining therapeutic goals
Comparing with diagnostic categories	Specifying the diagnosis	Determining management plan
Assigning the diagnosis	Determining patient management	Evaluating effectiveness
	Evaluating	Confirming or revising

practice, and know-how related to "think clinically" under differing clinical role expectations. Skilled clinical decision making occurs as an intentional process of problem solving, critical thinking, and reflection in action (Benner et al., 1996). It is guided by content expertise and deliberate decisions about how to proceed through the current clinical encounter as well as reasoning through the anticipated trajectory of the health concern.

Relationship Between Critical Thinking and Clinical Decision Making

Critical thinking skills can assist with sorting out the aforementioned complexities. In a 1990 consensus statement on critical thinking, Facione (1990) defines *critical thinking* as a tool of inquiry characterized by "purposeful, self-regulatory judgment" resulting in "interpretation, analysis, evaluation, and inference" (p. 3). It is not "rote, mechanical, unreflective" (p. 8) or disconnected from other thought activities. Critical thinkers are able to examine and evaluate their own reasoning processes and apply critical thinking skills in a variety of contexts. The consensus components of critical thinking are provided in Table 8.2.

Scheffer and Rubenfeld (2000) used a Delphi method to develop a consensus statement on critical thinking in nursing, describing both

TABLE 8.2 Consensus Components of Critical Thinking

CRITICAL THINKING SKILL	IDENTIFIED COMPONENTS OF THE SKILL
Interpretation	Categorizing
Evaluation	Clarifying meanings
	Assessing claims and arguments
Inference	Examining evidence
	Drawing conclusions
	Proposing alternatives
Explanation	Stating results
	Presenting arguments
	Justifying procedures
Self-regulation	Self-examination
	Self-correction
Dispositional skills	Inquisitiveness
	Eagerness for reliable information

its affective and cognitive components. In addition to the components described by Facione (1990), the nursing study identified creativity and intuition as two additional affective components.

Although *critical thinking* is defined by educators as a broad set of cognitive skills and habits of mind, applying these skills in clinical practice requires large amounts of discipline-specific knowledge. Research-based understandings of relationships between critical thinking and clinical decision making are not yet well developed. Clearly, however, the skills of interpretation, analysis, evaluation, and inference are highly necessary in advanced clinical practice, where both nursing and medical knowledge must be distinguished and applied. Well-developed critical thinking skills and habits of mind are an important foundation for the discipline-specific processes of clinical thinking required in advanced practice nursing.

Thinking Clinically

As suggested earlier, the meaning of *thinking clinically* will vary widely from one advanced practice nursing clinical setting and role to another. General elements can be described, however. From these elements it becomes incumbent upon nurses in advanced practice who are pursuing future research agendas to discern the particulars for their practice areas.

Organizing Clinical Knowledge for Practice

Ultimately, cognitively organizing diagnostic and treatment concepts for clinical practice is hard work that individual practitioners must do for themselves (Carnevali & Thomas, 1993). A systematic approach is recommended, based on building a repertoire of specific diagnostic/prognostic/treatment concepts and exemplars from practice. For knowledge from nursing, such cognitive categories could be built around human response categories, broad nursing diagnostic categories, functional health patterns, or population health needs. As the depth of knowledge increases with various phenomena, increasing expertise is developed relating to manifestations, underlying mechanisms, risk factors and complications, prognostic variables and anticipated trajectories, and efficacy of treatment options. Increasing depth of medical knowledge, on the other hand, relates to the complexity of pathophysiologic explanations and relationships, variations in disease attributes and manifestations, use and interpretation of diagnostic tests, increasingly precise probabilistic and prognostic thinking, and increasingly sophisticated risk–benefit analyses. Building interprofessional and nursing knowledge for advanced clinical practice is an ongoing process of study and practice.

Clinical Decision Making in Health–Illness Management

In the realm of biomedical knowledge, diagnosis and management of health–illness places greater emphasis on probabilistic thinking and inferential or inductive reasoning, with greater attention to the specificity of the data and the precision of decisions. Rational justification, confirmation and elimination strategies, and judgment of value are critical reasoning skills within this domain. As outlined by Kassirer and Kopelman (1991), the first step in the diagnostic process is hypothesis activation or the identification of diagnostic possibilities. Hypothesis activation is based on preliminary information such as the patient's age, medical history, clinical appearance, and presenting concerns. The next step is information gathering and interpretation. This step is strongly influenced by probabilistic thinking and inductive reasoning. The likelihood of various diagnostic hypotheses is carefully considered, with new data used to assist with confirming, eliminating, or discriminating between diagnoses. The working diagnosis is then selected based on causal attribution (i.e., whether all physiologic features are consistent with the favored diagnosis and underlying cause).

This hypotheses generation and revision occur in both novices and experienced clinicians, although the experienced clinicians' hypotheses are of higher quality. It is also noted that some of diagnostic reasoning variation between novices and experts does not appear to be problem-solving variations but instead dependent on the experts' increasing use of pattern recognition based on their knowledge organization and experiences. Retrieval of those patterns can be based on previous experienced exemplars or more abstract prototypes. Thus, expert–novice differences can be somewhat explained in terms of the volume of experts' experienced exemplars available for pattern recognition (Schwartz & Elstein, 2008).

The working diagnosis becomes the basis for therapeutic action, prognostic assessment, or further diagnostic testing. Final verification of the diagnostic hypothesis is determined through tests of adequacy and coherence. Adequacy ascertains whether the suspected disease process encompasses all of the patient's findings. Coherence determines whether all the patient's illness manifestations are appropriate for the suspected health concern. The final diagnostic hypothesis then becomes the basis for treatment decisions, in combination with evidence-based analysis of treatment options and patient-specific cost–benefit analyses for each of the treatment options.

Probability decision making is used to narrow the hypotheses. As new data are obtained, each diagnostic probability is recalculated. The posttest probability is then used to guide additional data collection and to generate the pretest probability of the usefulness of that data. The formal mathematical rule for this process is Bayes' theorem. Inaccurate application of Bayes' theorem explains some of the errors that occur in the diagnostic reasoning process, such as overestimation of pretest probability. The clinician tends to overemphasize rare conditions with inflation of pretest probabilities because those are the cases most memorable. In general, small probabilities are overestimated and large probabilities are underestimated by clinicians. Experience and mentoring are clearly necessary to learn biomedical decision making. Kassirer and Kopelman (1991) also advise parsimony in medical reasoning (i.e., seeking a simple, direct, and clear explanation for the patient's health–illness findings whenever possible). As commonly stated, if you hear hoof beats, look for horses, not zebras.

Heuristics in Advanced Practice Nursing

Heuristics are specific cognitive techniques used by skilled clinicians to make reasoning more efficient by reducing complex tasks to simpler and more automatic processes (Tversky & Kahneman, 1974). They can be thought of as mental rules of thumb acquired over time through experience that promote reasoning. Heuristics are domain specific (e.g., medical–surgical nursing, critical care nursing, mental health nursing) and are thought to operate strongly in what has been understood as the "intuitive" knowing of clinical experts.

Simmons (2002) identified 11 heuristics used by experienced nurses to reason about assessment findings: recognizing patterns, enumerating lists, forming relationships, searching for information, setting priorities, providing explanations, judging value, stating practice rules, stating propositions, drawing conclusions, and summing up.

Other heuristics used by expert nurses have been identified by Benner and colleagues. These include clinical grasp (making qualitative distinctions, engaging in clinical puzzle solving, recognizing changing clinical relevance, and developing population-specific clinical knowledge) and clinical forethought (future think, clinical forethought about specific diagnoses or conditions, anticipation of crises, assessment of risks and vulnerabilities, and seeing the unexpected; Benner et al., 1999).

Central to clinical grasp are understanding and recognizing clinical patterns and attending very closely to the clinical situation. It is essential to get an accurate story and then observe carefully for patient responses and trends. Clinical forethought involves thinking ahead to common eventualities and using this knowledge to be prepared for, or, when possible, to prevent the unfolding of detrimental scenarios. Expertise in clinical forethought requires not only expert textbook knowledge but an array of personal case experiences, providing firsthand experience from which to generate understandings of the clinical terrain, timing issues, and practical knowledge on how to read and interpret clinical cues. Chase (2004) and Dains, Baumann, and Scheibel (2011) describe multiple heuristics specific to nurse practitioner judgment and decision making. The heuristics described are too numerous to elaborate here, but these and other clinical reasoning texts provide very valuable compendia of practice knowledge central to nurse practitioner decision making.

Errors in Clinical Reasoning

Several types of clinical practice errors are described in the literature, broadly grouped as skill-based errors, knowledge-based errors, and errors caused by psychoemotional factors. Skill- and knowledge-based errors in this context are not the same as not possessing the necessary skills or knowledge. Rather, the assumption is made that the necessary skills and knowledge are present, but errors are made in their application. Skill-based failures include lack of attention at crucial moments, distraction or preoccupation resulting in missed crucial events, failure to carry out specific activities or intentions, and errors resulting from mixing up behaviors or activities.

Knowledge-based failures include errors resulting from the use of heuristics. Despite the value of heuristics, overuse has the potential to increase errors in clinical judgment. Care must be taken to maintain a reflective balance between formal reasoning and the use of knowledge from practice. Being overconfident about the correctness of one's knowledge (overconfidence bias), using personal case experience alone as the basis for a decision (hindsight bias), and neglecting the underlying base rate of a health condition when diagnosing or treating (base rate neglect) are three common types of errors in the application of practice knowledge (Thompson, 2002). Conservatism is the failure to revise diagnostic probabilities as new data are presented. Confirmation bias is the tendency to seek information that confirms a diagnosis but failing to efficiently test competing hypotheses (Schwartz & Elstein, 2008). Psychological commitment takes place early in the hypothesis generation process, and clinicians find it difficult to restructure the problem. A psychoemotional error occurs (value-induced bias) when the clinician exaggerates the probability of a diagnosis when one possible outcome is perceived as exceedingly unfavorable compared with others (Buckingham, 2002; Kassirer & Kopelman, 1991).

Errors in the information-processing components of practice are also categorized using terminology from hypothesis testing. Type I errors, claiming a significant difference when there is none (analogous to rejecting a true null hypothesis), occur in clinical decision making through naming a clinical problem when there is none. In this situation the disease model used by the clinician may be too broad, perhaps causing the clinician to overestimate the allowable range of variation for findings in a given diagnosis and not recognizing that the actual findings are at odds with the favored diagnosis.

Type II errors, claiming no significant difference when there is one (analogous to accepting a false null hypothesis), occur with failing to name a clinical problem when there is one. This may occur through missing significant clinical indicators of a health problem or failing to realize the significance of specific signs or symptoms. A correct diagnosis may have been eliminated even though the findings are consistent with the diagnosis.

Type III errors, solving the wrong problem, phrasing the problem incorrectly, setting the boundaries or scope of the problem too narrowly, or failing to think systematically (Kassirer & Kopelman, 1991). Based on this information, habits of practice that promote sound clinical reasoning can be cultivated by the APRN. These are summarized in Table 8.3.

Tools to Support and Enhance Clinical Decision Making in Advanced Practice Nursing

A final aspect of APRN decision making is the increasingly important role of a variety of tools that can be used to support and enhance clinical decision making. A listing of these tools is provided in Exhibit 8.2.

Multiple nursing standards of practice have been developed by the American Nurses Association and by specialty nursing organizations. These are organized both by specialty practice areas and by practice-related frameworks, such as the nursing code of ethics and the nursing social policy statement. They continue to serve as basic frameworks for nursing practice and are especially important documents for clinical nurse specialists. The North American Nursing Diagnosis Association (NANDA)/Nursing Intervention Classification (NIC)/Nursing Outcomes Classification (NOC) taxonomies, although not necessarily complete and not universally used, help organize ways of naming nursing diagnoses and begin the process of building common expectancies for nursing interventions and outcomes. Midlevel theories help guide practice by addressing the needs or experiences of specific populations, typically relative to one or more human responses or areas of concern. Incorporating information or concepts from midlevel theories is an excellent way to begin addressing the holistic care considerations of health care populations and build depth at an advanced practice level.

Evidence-based practice has been described as basing clinical decisions and practice on the best available evidence (Melnyk & Fineout-Overholt, 2011). Not all elements of practice are based on empirical evidence, however. Many areas of practice do not have adequate bodies of evidence. In addition, context-specific problems sometimes warrant decisions not addressed by the research literature. Thus, it is imperative that critical

TABLE 8.3 Habits That Promote Sound Clinical Reasoning in Advanced Practice Nursing

PHASE OF CLINICAL REASONING	HABITS THAT PROMOTE SOUND REASONING
Data acquisition	Use a systematic and comprehensive approach.
	Use nursing and medical hypotheses in combination with a systems approach to focus the data collection.
	Integrate new findings into the emerging model.
	Search for and attend to both confirming and disconfirming data.
	Critically evaluate the significance and reliability of findings.
	Attend to variations in clinical attributes and manifestations.
Hypothesis generation	Formulate preliminary hypotheses early in the encounter.
	Develop reasonable competing hypotheses.
	Remain vigilant for serious or life-threatening conditions.
	Use the hypotheses as models against which to seek and compare findings.
	Adjust the hypotheses as new data emerge.
	Carefully compare the hypotheses to reliable information on manifestations, prevalence, and probability.
	Eliminate hypotheses that fail to remain tenable.
Diagnostic testing	Consider test results as further probability information.
	Decide whether a test result could alter the probability of disease enough to alter management.
	Use highly sensitive tests (low rate of false-negative results) to exclude serious disease.
	Use highly specific tests (low rate of false-positive results) to confirm a diagnosis.
Hypothesis evaluation	Determine the "working hypothesis."
	If competing hypotheses remain, determine a strategy for discriminating between them.
	Test the hypothesis for coherence, adequacy, and parsimony.
	Avoid premature closure.
	Continue testing the working hypothesis against test results, clinical course, and response to therapy.
Comprehensive care	Identify the most fundamental problems and concerns.
	Incorporate risk stratification.
	Include disease- and non disease-based perspectives.
	Incorporate nursing theory, human responses, and personhood.

(continued)

TABLE 8.3 Habits That Promote Sound Clinical Reasoning in
Advanced Practice Nursing *(continued)*

PHASE OF CLINICAL REASONING	HABITS THAT PROMOTE SOUND REASONING
	Include health promotion, disease prevention, and risk reduction.
	Engage the patient as a partner in care.
Goal setting	Include the patient in establishing goals.
	Determine management priorities and plan care accordingly.
	Identify specific and realistic goals for treatment.
	Incorporate clinical standards in goal setting.
Determination of management plans	Employ intervention modalities from both nursing and medical perspectives.
	Initiate effective care for emergency or life-threatening conditions.
	Consult with appropriate colleagues in complex care situations.
	Consider patient's social context, preferences, abilities, lifestyle, and individual needs.
	Anticipate and discuss possible conflicts in values, priorities, and beliefs.
	Use evidence-based therapies appropriately.
	Consider treatment efficacy as compared to risks, costs, and desired outcomes.
	Think ahead to probabilistic disease progression needs.
	Incorporate evidence-based approaches, accepted treatment guidelines, and current standards of care.
	Provide effective and appropriate management for comorbidities.

Adapted from Chase (2004).

Exhibit 8.2 TOOLS TO SUPPORT AND ENHANCE CLINICAL DECISION MAKING IN
ADVANCED CLINICAL PRACTICE

Nursing Standards of Practice
North American Nursing Diagnosis Association (NANDA)/Nursing Intervention Classification (NIC)/Nursing Outcomes Classification (NOC)
Midlevel theories
Evidence-based practice guidelines
Web-based information systems
Smartphone applications (apps)
Electronic health record systems

thinking, research appraisal, and clinical decision making skills be used in combination with one another. Typically, evidence-based practice is assumed to refer to external, population-based evidence derived through systematic research. There is the expectation that APRNs will seek the available evidence and use this evidence to inform their decision making in the context of a patient's unique situation.

Evidence-based practice guidelines can be formalized by specific managed care organizations with the expectation that the guidelines are used to direct practice, or they may simply refer to concise informational outlines and algorithms intended to assist clinicians with the massive amounts of diagnostic and management information available. Utilization of practice guidelines do assist in minimizing cognitive and systemic sources of clinician error such as the bias that occurs from over-emphasizing risk for rare conditions and the potential for the clinician to overreact to that perceived risk. They can also constrain and over-simplify practice by focusing on more common problems (Tracy, 2009). If they are overly relied on, practice guidelines can result in failing to attend to the individual needs and nuanced presentations of a patient's condition. Many web-based information systems have been developed that are now viewed as part of the standard support tools for practice. These include intranet and Internet systems, as well as online journals and texts, databases, and governmental and organizational websites. The advent of smartphone and associated apps have provided the opportunity to have support tools in all clinical settings at the point of care. One entry-level advanced practice competency is the ability to access, search, and critically evaluate the appropriateness of practice guidelines and electronic resources for practice (AACN, 2006).

CONCLUSIONS

Expertise in clinical decision making is vital for clinical competency. At the advanced practice level, this is a complex undertaking for both the individual provider and the profession. Keeping the core of nursing theory and perspectives central and visible while gaining competency in the knowledge base and probabilistic thinking of advanced practice requires continual attention to practice-based cognitive skills and processes. It is recommended that advanced practice clinical decision making be approached as a continual and deliberate process of knowledge expansion and reflective practice, maintaining the personhood and holistic needs of the patient and the importance of the nurse–patient relationship central to practice.

Acknowledgment

The author acknowledges the contributions of Sheila Smith to this chapter in the previous edition.

REFERENCES

American Association of Colleges of Nursing (AACN). (2004). *AACN position statement on the practice doctorate in nursing.* Washington, DC: Author.

American Association of Colleges of Nursing (AACN). (2006). *The essentials of doctoral education for advanced practice nursing.* Washington, DC: Author.

Benner, P. (1984). *From novice to expert: Excellence and power in clinical nursing practice.* Upper Saddle River, NJ: Prentice-Hall.

Benner, P., Hooper-Kyriakidis, P., & Stannard, D. (1999). *Clinical wisdom and interventions in critical care: A thinking in action approach.* Philadelphia, PA: W.B. Saunders Company.

Benner, P., Stannard, D., & Hooper, P. L. (1996). A "thinking-in-action" approach to teaching clinical judgment: A classroom innovation for acute care advanced practice nurses. *Advanced Practice Nursing Quarterly, 1*(4), 70–77.

Benner, P., Tanner, C. A., & Chesla, C. A. (2009). *Expertise in nursing practice: Caring, clinical judgment, and ethics.* New York, NY: Springer Publishing.

Benner, P., & Wrubel, J. (1989). *The primacy of caring.* Menlo Park, CA: Addison-Wesley.

Boshuizen, H. P. A., & Schmidt, H. G. (1992). On the role of biomedical knowledge in clinical reasoning by experts, intermediates, and novices. *Cognitive Science, 16,* 153–184.

Bjork, I. T., & Hamilton, G. A. (2011). Clinical decision making of nurses working in hospital settings. *Nursing Research and Practice, 2011* (524918), pp. 1–8. doi:10.1155/2011/524918

Brookfield, S. (2008). Clinical reasoning and generic thinking skills. In J. Higgs, M. A. Jones, S. Loftus, & N. Christensen (Eds.), *Clinical reasoning in the health professions* (pp. 65–75). Philadelphia, PA: Butterworth-Heinemann Elsevier.

Brykczynski, K. (1989). An interpretive study describing the clinical judgment of nurse practitioners. *Scholarly Inquiry for Nursing Practice: An International Journal, 3*(2), 75–111.

Buckingham, C. D. (2002). Psychological cue use and implications for a clinical decision support system. *Medical Informatics and the Internet in Medicine, 27*(4), 237–251.

Buckingham, C. D., & Adams, A. (2000). Classifying clinical decision making: A unifying approach. *Journal of Advanced Nursing, 32,* 981–989.

Carnevali, D. L., & Thomas, M. D. (1993). *Diagnostic reasoning and treatment decision making in nursing.* Philadelphia, PA: J.B. Lippincott.

Chase, S. K. (2004). Clinical judgment and communication in nurse practitioner practice. Philadelphia, PA: F.A. Davis.

Chase, S. K. (2011). The art of diagnosis and treatment. In L. M. Dunphy, J. E. Winland-Brown, & D. Thomas (Eds.), *Primary care: The art and science of advanced practice nursing* (pp. 43–61). Philadelphia, PA: F.A. Davis.

Cioffi, J. (1997). Heuristics, servants to intuition in clinical decision making. *Journal of Advanced Nursing, 26,* 203–208.

Cioffi, J., & Markham, R. (1997). Clinical decision making by midwives: Managing case complexity. *Journal of Advanced Nursing, 25,* 265–272.

Corcoran, S. A. (1986a). Task complexity and nursing expertise as factors in decision making. *Nursing Research, 35*(2), 107–112.

Corcoran, S. A. (1986b). Planning by expert and novice nurses in cases of varying complexity. *Research in Nursing & Health, 9,* 155–162.

Dains, J. E., Baumann, L. C., & Scheibel, P. (2011). *Advanced health assessment and clinical diagnosis in primary care*. St. Louis, MO: Mosby.

Davies, B., & Hughes, A. M. (2002). Clarification of advanced nursing practice: Characteristics and competencies. *Clinical Nurse Specialist, 16*(3), 147–152.

Dreyfus, H. L., & Dreyfus, S. E. (1986). *Mind over machine: The power of intuition and expertise in the era of the computer*. New York, NY: Free Press.

Elstein, A. S. (1976). Clinical judgment: Psychological research and medical practice. *Science, 194*, 696–700.

Elstein, A. S., Shulman, L. S., & Sprafka, S. A. (1978). *Medical problem solving: An analysis of clinical reasoning*. Cambridge, MA: Harvard University Press.

Facione, P. (1990). *Critical thinking: A statement of consensus for purposes of educational assessment and instruction*. Fullerton, CA: American Philosophical Association, California State University.

Fenton, M. V. (1983). Identification of the skilled performance of master's prepared nurses as a method of curriculum planning and evaluation. In P. Benner (Ed.), *From novice to expert: Excellence and power in clinical nursing practice* (pp. 262–274). Upper Saddle River, NJ: Prentice-Hall.

Flynn, C. A., & Becker, L. (2004). Clinical jazz: Harmonizing clinical experience with evidence-based medicine. In W. Rosser, D. Slawson, & A. Shaughnessy (Eds.), *Information mastery: Evidence based family medicine* (pp. 61–65). Hamilton, Ontario: BC Decker.

Hamm, R. M. (1988). Clinical intuition and clinical analysis: Expertise and the cognitive continuum. In J. Dowie & A. Elstein (Eds.), *Professional judgment: A reader in clinical decision making* (pp. 78–105). New York, NY: Cambridge University Press.

Hammond, K. R. (1964). An approach to the study of clinical inference in nursing: Part II. *Nursing Research, 13*(4), 315–319.

Hammond, K., Kelly, K., & Castellan, E. A. (1966). Clinical inference in nursing: Use of information seeking strategies by nurses. *Nursing Research, 15*(4), 330–336.

Higgs, J., & Jones, M. (1995). Clinical reasoning. In J. Higgs & M. Jones (Eds.), *Clinical reasoning in the health professions* (pp. 3–10). Oxford: Butterworth-Heinemann.

Higgs, J., & Jones, M. (2008). Clinical reasoning in the health professions. In J. Higgs, M.A. Jones, S. Loftus, & N. Christensen (Eds.), *Clinical reasoning in the health professions* (pp. 3–17). Philadelphia, PA: Butterworth-Heinemann Elsevier.

Huch, M. H. (1995). Nursing science as a basis for advanced practice. *Nursing Science Quarterly, 8*(1), 6–7.

Kassirer, J. P., & Kopelman, R. I. (1991). *Learning clinical reasoning*. Baltimore, MD: William & Wilkins.

Lauri, S., & Salantera, S. (2002). Developing an instrument to measure and describe clinical decision making in different nursing fields. *Journal of Professional Nursing, 18*(2), 93–100.

Loftus, S., & Higgs, J. (2008). Learning the language of clinical reasoning. In J. Higgs, M.A. Jones, S. Loftus, & N. Christensen (Eds.), *Clinical reasoning in the health professions* (pp. 339—348). Philadelphia, PA: Butterworth-Heinemann Elsevier.

Lunney, M. (2009). Assessment, clinical judgment and nursing diagnosis: How to determine an accurate diagnosis. In North American Nursing

Diagnosis Association, *Nursing diagnoses: Definitions and classification 2009–2011* (pp. 1–17). Ames, IA: Wiley-Blackwell.

Melnyk, B. M., & Fineout-Overholt, E. F. (2011). Making the case for evidence-based practice and cultivating a spirit of inquiry. In B. M. Melnyk & E. F. Fineout-Overholt (Eds.), *Evidence-based practice in nursing and healthcare: A guide to best practice* (pp. 3–24). Philadelphia, PA: Lippincott, Williams & Wilkins.

Narayan, S. M., & Corcoran-Perry, S. (1997). Line of reasoning as a representation of nurses' clinical decision making. *Research in Nursing & Health, 20,* 353–364.

Narayan, S. M., Corcoran-Perry, S., Drew, D., Hoyman, K., & Lewis, M. (2003). Decision analysis as a tool to support an analytical pattern-of-reasoning. *Nursing and Health Sciences, 5,* 229–243.

National Association of Clinical Nurse Specialists (NACNS). (2008). *Clinical nurse specialist core competencies executive summary.* Philadelphia, PA: Author.

National Organization of Nurse Practitioner Faculties (NONPF). (2006). *Practice doctorate nurse practitioner entry-level competencies.* Washington, DC: Author

National Organization of Nurse Practitioner Faculties (NONPF). (2012). *Nurse practitioner core competencies.* Washington, DC: Author.

Newell, A., & Simon, H. A. (1972). *Human problem solving.* Englewood Cliffs, NJ: Prentice-Hall.

Patel, V. L., & Kaufman, D. R. (2000). Clinical reasoning and biomedical knowledge: Implications for teaching. In J. Higgs & M. Jones (Eds.), *Clinical reasoning in the health professions* (pp. 33–44). Oxford: Butterworth-Heinemann.

Pyles, S., & Stern, P. (1983). Discovery of nursing gestalt in critical care nursing: The importance of the gray gorilla syndrome. *Image: The Journal of Nursing Scholarship, 15,* 51–57.

Rew, L. (1988). Intuition in decision making. *Image: The Journal of Nursing Scholarship, 20,* 150–155.

Ritter, B. J. (2003). An analysis of expert nurse practitioners' diagnostic reasoning. *Journal of the American Academy of Nurse Practitioners, 15*(3), 137–141.

Sands, H. M. (2001). *Making the diagnosis: Factors shaping diagnostic reasoning among entry level nurse practitioners* (Unpublished doctoral dissertation). University of California, Los Angeles.

Scheffer, B. K., & Rubenfeld, M. G. (2000). A consensus statement on critical thinking in nursing. *Journal of Nursing Education, 39*(8), 352–359.

Schwartz, A., & Elstein, A. S. (2008). Clinical reasoning in medicine. In J. Higgs, M. A. Jones, S. Loftus, & N. Christensen (Eds.), *Clinical reasoning in the health professions* (pp. 223–234). Philadelphia, PA: Butterworth-Heinemann Elsevier.

Simmons, B. (2002). *Clinical reasoning in experienced nurses.* (Unpublished doctoral dissertation). Loyola University, Chicago.

Smith, M. C. (1995). The core of advanced practice nursing. *Nursing Science Quarterly, 8,* 2–3.

Smith, S. K. (1987). An analysis of the phenomenon of deterioration in the critically ill. *Image: The Journal of Nursing Scholarship, 20*(1), 12–15.

Tanner, C. A., Padrick, K. P., Westfall, U. E., & Putzier, D. J. (1987). Diagnostic reasoning strategies of nurses and nursing students. *Nursing Research, 36,* 358–362.

Tanner, C. A., Benner, P., Chesla, C., & Gordon, D. (1993). The phenomenology of knowing the patient. *Image: The Journal of Nursing Scholarship, 25,* 273–280.

Thompson, C. (2002). Human error, bias, decision making and judgment in nursing: The need for a systematic approach. In C. Thompson & D. Dowding (Eds.), *Clinical decision making and judgment in nursing* (pp. 21–45). Edinburgh: Churchill Livingstone.

Titchen, A., & Higgs, J. (2000). Facilitating the acquisition of knowledge and reasoning. In J. Higgs & M. Jones (Eds.), *Clinical reasoning in the health professions* (pp. 222–229). Oxford: Butterworth-Heinemann.

Tracy, M. F. (2009). Direct clinical practice. In A. B. Hamric, J. A. Spross, & C. M. Hanson (Eds.), *Advanced practice nursing: An integrative Approach* (pp. 123–158). St. Louis, MO: Saunders Elsevier.

Tversky, A., & Kahneman, D. (1974). Judgment under uncertainty: Heuristics and biases. *Science, 185,* 1124–1131.

White, J. E., Nativio, D. G., Kobert, S. N., & Engberg, S. J. (1992). Content and process in clinical decision making by nurse practitioners. *Image: The Journal of Nursing Scholarship, 24,* 153–158.

Evelyn G. Duffy

9

HEALTH CARE POLICY: IMPLICATIONS FOR ADVANCED NURSING PRACTICE

Since the Patient Protection and Affordable Care Act (ACA) was passed in 2010, the opportunities for advanced practice nurses (APRNs) have increased tremendously. This has been referred to as the "golden age" for APRNs. The release of the Institute of Medicine (IOM) report that same year, *The Future of Nursing: Leading Change, Advancing Health,* has been another factor in adding opportunities for APRNs. These events were preceded by the publication in 2008 of the *Consensus Model for APRN Regulation: Licensure, Accreditation, Certification & Education*, completed through the work of the APRN Consensus Work Group and the National Council of State Boards of Nursing APRN Advisory Committee. While state laws that govern APRN practice will need to be updated to fully realize all the changes proposed by the *Consensus Model*, changes have already occurred in educational programs, certification examinations, and the accreditation processes. The effect of these factors combined to advance the opportunities for APRNs and helped unify their voice and purpose.

As the public has become better informed of the full capacity of APRNs to provide health care, groups outside of health care have advocated for the removal of boundaries that prevent APRNs from practicing to the full extent of their education and training. The *Center to Champion Nursing in America* is a joint initiative of the Robert Wood Johnson Foundation (RWJF) and AARP. The *Campaign for Action* (accessible at www.campaignforaction. org), coordinated by the RWJF through the Center to Champion Nursing in America, is a national campaign that works to implement the recommendations of the IOM report on the *Future of Nursing: Leading Change, Advancing Health* (2010). The Center helps form coalitions of professionals, the public, and businesses to remove barriers to practice and care. Another key contribution to removing barriers came from the Federal Trade Commission (FTC) in 2014 as it addressed the threat to competition in the marketplace that results from the requirement for physician supervision of APRNs. *Policy Perspectives: Competition and the Regulation of Advanced Practice Nurses* added support for allowing APRNs to practice to the full extent of their preparation and licensure (FTC, 2014).

An important development for nurse practitioners (NPs) was consolidation in 2012 of the two largest NP organizations, the American College of Nurse Practitioners and the American Academy of Nurse Practitioners, into one organization: the American Association of Nurse Practitioners (AANP). NPs now have one voice addressing issues that affect practice and a coordinated front to address policy issues. The AANP has the potential to achieve results that neither organization had been able to accomplish alone. The consolidation of these two major NP organizations addresses the observation by O'Grady (2011) that APRN organizations were fragmented and that unification would be a key to increasing APRNs influence in health policy. In 2014, the new AANP celebrated reaching the 50,000-member milestone.

APRNs today more than ever before need to be informed health professionals who are aware of the current health policy issues, the process necessary to make change happen, and the advocacy groups for nursing and advanced practice nursing that are working to remove barriers and support policy that will allow them to provide the best care to their patients. Patient-centered care is the hallmark of nursing and has become the focus of health care nationally and the motivation for the formulation of coalitions to support the advancement of APRN practice.

No matter the scale of the health policy issue or the size of the community it affects, the process of creating health policy is basically the same on the local, state, and national levels. Knowing how that process works and ways to influence it empowers the APRN to stand up for health policies on any level. The purpose of this chapter is to help the APRN understand and engage in that process.

LEADERSHIP AND HEALTH POLICY

APRNs provide excellent patient care; this is supported by multiple studies (Stanik-Hutt, 2013). They are comfortable advocating for their patients, but they may not see the connection between advocating for health policy and providing quality care. Without development of leadership competencies and influence at decision-making tables, clinical competence will not be enough to affect care. Leadership skills that are especially important in advocacy for health policy include vision, timing, risk taking, communication, and relationship building. Others have cited the legacy of Florence Nightingale and her response to the "moral imperative" as a model for leadership in health policy development today (Falk-Rafael, 2005, p. 213). Florence Nightingale's vision for change was informed by her practice on the battlefields in Crimea. APRNs also bring that practice experience to the policy tables. It is their stories that personalize for decision makers the impact of the policies they create.

The National Organization of Nurse Practitioner Faculties (NONPF) published updated *Nurse Practitioner Core Competencies* in 2012. At least four leadership competencies directly relate to leadership in health policy:

> (1) Assumes complex and advanced leadership roles to initiate and guide change
> (2) Provides leadership to foster collaboration with multiple stake-holders (e.g., patients, community, integrated health care teams, and policy makers) to improve health care
> (4) Advocates for improved access, quality and cost-effective health care
> (7) Participates in professional organizations and activities that influence advanced practice nursing and/or health outcomes of a population focus (p. 2)

These competencies reflect NONPF's endorsement of the doctorate of nursing practice (DNP) as entry level for nurse practitioner practice. *The Essentials of Doctoral Education for Advanced Nursing Practice* (American Association of Colleges of Nursing [AACN], 2006) Essential II addresses leadership and includes the expectation that DNP graduates will engage in policy development to improve health care quality and access.

Why should APRNs care about becoming leaders in health policy? For many APRNs, moving from leadership in clinical practice to leadership in health policy is not an obvious choice. However, APRNs need to understand how the skills used in motivating patients to improve their health are the same skills that can move legislatures to pass laws and develop rules that will allow APRNs to practice to their full scope and remove the obstacles to providing quality care to their patients. Policy makers at the federal, state, and local levels influence what nursing professionals can do, how they do it, and what they are paid. Public policies dictate who has insurance and what insurance will pay. Public policies and how they are implemented shape the direction of health care delivery. They affect the experience of providers as they practice and the experience of consumers as they attempt to receive care in an increasingly complex and expensive system. APRNs need to have the resources to stay informed and respond to proposed changes to local, state, and national policies that will affect their practice and the care their patients receive.

PUBLIC POLICY: THE PROCESS

The U.S. Constitution was written by men of vision. Their ability to frame a document that not only addressed current issues but allowed for adaptation to challenges faced in the future has been cited as the reason the Constitution has remained relevant. The document set forth broad principles in general terms that allowed future interpretation based on the context at that time (Stone & Marshall, 2011). When laws contain specific language, adaptation to changes in the future environment may be stymied. Medicare Law P.L. 89-97, passed in 1965, specified that authority for many actions was limited to physicians. Lawmakers did not envision future changes to a physician-dominated health care system because most of the advanced practice roles did not exist at that time. This limitation has resulted in a number of barriers to APRN practice and provided strong motivation to include provider-neutral language in laws and rulemaking. Inclusion of provider-neutral language is one of the key priorities of the APRN *Health Affairs* agenda today.

The Constitution describes three branches of government and delineates the responsibilities of each. The *legislative branch,* which includes the Senate and the House of Representatives, creates the laws, confirms presidential appointments, and has the power to declare war. The *executive branch* includes the president, the vice president, and the cabinet and is charged with carrying out and enforcing the laws, including the responsibility for rulemaking. The *judicial branch* includes the Supreme Court and other federal courts; it is responsible for settling conflicts that occur over the law, interpreting the law, and deciding whether a law is constitutional (USA.gov, 2014).

Process Models

Work by Kingdon (1995), Wakefield (2006), and Longest (2010) identify key factors in moving legislation forward and understanding the process. Longest (2010) proposed a "Model for Health Policy Making in the United States" (p. 51; Figure 9.1). Although the model was designed around the federal system, it is also applicable to state, county, and local governments. The process is cyclical, which underscores the fact that laws are subject to change. Laws introduced each year generally are modifications of some existing law.

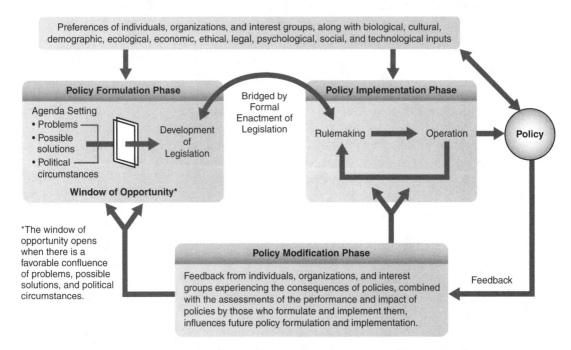

FIGURE 9.1 Model of the public policy-making process.
Source: Longest (2010).

Influential Factors: Lessons for APRNs

The Longest (2010) model also emphasizes the influence that individuals, organizations, and special interest groups have on every aspect of the process. For Kingdon (2010) these are the "actors" that influence the agenda, including elected officials, the public, the media, experts, and interest groups. There is overlap between Kingdon's actors and Wakefield's (2006) nine factors that influence legislation. These factors include constituents (the public), research findings (the experts), special interest groups, the media, crisis, market forces, fiscal pressures, personal experience, and political ideology (Figure 9.2).

For Kingdon (2010) the foremost actors in the policy-making process are the *elected officials*. At the federal level the president and members of Congress set the national agenda. The governor and legislature serve the same role on a state level. Members of Congress decide what proposals or bills will be introduced, which will have public hearings, and which will be debated.

The role of the public (constituents) is not insignificant. Constituents have the ability to influence what policies are discussed and ultimately what policy changes occur when they support candidates who represent their perspectives and values. APRNs need to be engaged citizens so that their voices are heard. They become involved when they communicate with legislators, attend hearings, testify at hearings, visit their legislators, and attend events that legislators hold. The attention that Congress gives to their constituents is illustrated in this comment from the *Christian Science Monitor*, "Members of Congress put their own political needs ahead of the body's institutional effectiveness" (Grant, 2012). It is this situation that has been cited in explaining the lack of action by recent congressional bodies. The fear of displeasing constituents and risking re-election exceeds their responsibility to govern the country.

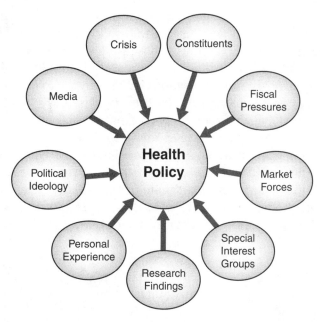

FIGURE 9.2 Nine factors that influence legislation.
Source: Wakefield (2006).

Elected officials may gain awareness about certain issues through their own personal experiences. They may become acutely aware of a problem or develop a unique insight because of personal events. Rob Portman, a Republican senator from Ohio, in March 2013 went against his party and supported same-sex marriage after his son told his parents that he was gay. Senator Portman wanted to think that his son could experience the same supportive relationship that he shared with his wife (Portman, 2013). Portman did not cite any other compelling argument for this shift in his support of this initiative. Without the context of his personal experience, it is not clear whether he would have made that policy shift.

Media are in a powerful position to shape the national discussion of issues and get these onto the policy-making agenda. When Dr. Sam Foote resigned from the Phoenix Veteran's Administration (VA) hospital in December 2013 after 24 years, he used the media to inform the public of the corruption he had observed. Before he resigned, he sent two letters to the VA inspector general requesting an investigation into the secret waiting lists, but his requests fell on deaf ears. After he resigned, he contacted the House Veteran Affairs Committee and a reporter with the *Arizona Republic* to discuss the problems at the Phoenix VA (Foote, 2014). The news stories about the corruption enraged the public, and the investigation that occurred in the wake of this public outcry uncovered a widespread problem involving a number of VA hospitals across the country. In response, multiple actors worked together to create and pass legislation—that is, the Veterans' Access to Care through Choice, Accountability and Transparency Act of 2014, P.L. 113-146, which was signed into law by President Obama on August 7, 2014. The bipartisan support in both the House and the Senate was a highly unusual occurrence for this 113th session of Congress, "the least productive Congress ever" (Cillizza, 2014). APRNs need to learn to use the media to advance their agendas. Education of the public regarding APRN practice and the barriers APRNs face to providing optimal care to their patients may be as effective in accomplishing policy change as contacting their representatives. Social media can also be a useful tool for APRNs. For example, by acquiring Twitter followers APRNs are able to get their messages out, and if they become recognized by their tweets, APRNs may be sought out by the media for their expertise and commentary.

Experts from government agencies, universities, think tanks, congressional committees, and associations provide advice and counsel to the elected officials, and much of this is based on research findings. Experts often disagree, and ultimately, the elected officials who make the laws will choose the expert advice that most closely aligns with their personal agenda. Special interest groups look after their constituents and advocate for preferred policy choices based on the preferences of their members. There were nearly 12,353 lobbyists registered with the government in 2013, and they received $3.24 billion in fees (Center for Responsive Politics, 2014).

Nursing has coordinated their special interest groups; the Nurse Practitioner Roundtable (NPRt), the Extended Roundtable, the APRN Workgroup, and the Nursing Community are of particular interest to

APRNs. When O'Grady (2011) noted the importance of a coordinated front by nursing, she did not recognize the many nursing health advocacy groups that work together to present a unified message to policy makers. The NPRt is one of those advocacy groups and includes the American Association of Nurse Practitioners, Gerontological Advanced Practice Nurses Association, National Association of Pediatric Nurse Practitioners, NONPF, and Nurse Practitioners in Women's Health. Representatives from each of the organizations, as well as their lobbyists, meet weekly by conference call to review current issues and develop a coordinated message to present to policy makers. They advocate not only to legislatures but also to federal agencies such as the Centers for Medicare & Medicaid Services (CMS) and the Health Resources and Services Administration.

The Extended Nurse Practitioner Roundtable expands the NPRt membership to include the American Nurses Association, the AACN, and the American Academy of Nursing. The group meets twice a month by conference call. This provides an opportunity for the agenda agreed on by the NPRt to be shared and discussed with these other influential professional organizations. These conversations help coordinate the messages that are presented and resolve differences when they exist.

The APRN Workgroup was originally formed in 2009; it includes the organizations in the NPRt and the Extended Nurse Practitioner Roundtable, as well as the American Association of Nurse Anesthetists; Association of Women's Health, Obstetric and Neonatal Nurses; American College of Nurse Midwives; and the National Association of Clinical Nurse Specialists. In a personal communication from Frank Purcell, Senior Director, Federal Government Affairs for the American Association of Nurse Anesthetists (September 4, 2014), he describes the group as a "coalition of the willing" that was formed to develop a document that would describe the barriers to APRN full practice authority. The "barriers" document, identified federal regulatory, statutory, and policy barriers to the use of APRNs. This document has been used by the member groups for organizing advocacy efforts on Capitol Hill and in agencies. The group meets face to face in various locations in Washington, DC, and by conference call on a monthly basis. Issues may arise with a very short turnaround time, and the APRN Workgroup drafts letters and documents to send to policy makers expressing the unified voice of the members of the group. This rapid response cycle would be difficult for one organization to track, and again the unified message is important in communicating concerns to policy makers.

The Nursing Community (www.thenursingcommunity.org) expands the reach of the APRN organizations to include the larger nursing community in its membership, a total of 61 nursing organizations. A typical letter from the Nursing Community begins with the words: "On behalf of the undersigned organizations representing the Nursing Community, we write in support of…Collectively, our organizations represent over one million registered nurses, advanced practice registered nurses, nurse faculty, researchers, and students, and we are committed to promoting efforts that advance the health of our nation through nursing care" (see www.thenursingcommunity.org). An individual professional organization, even one with 50,000 members, does not have the impact of a coalition of professional organizations representing more than 1 million members. APRNs need to be familiar with these coalitions and provide their professional organizations with examples of barriers APRNs face that affect patient care to help them illustrate the problems that result from the inability to practice to full the extent of their preparation and licensure.

Kingdon's (1995) actors and Wakefield's (2006) factors do not work in isolation. It is the combination of these influences that ultimately result in setting the agenda. When APRNs understand the multiple forces involved in the development of health policy, they are better equipped to find ways to become involved and to work to accomplish their professional agenda.

Policy Formulation Phase: Agenda Setting

Setting the political agenda prioritizes concerns and guides the policy-making process. Many problems require solutions, and there is a limited amount of time to address those problems. In developing his model of public policy-making process, Longest (2010) drew on the prior work of Kingdon (1995). Kingdon noted that public policy starts with agenda setting, deciding to which issue or problem policy makers and outside interests will pay attention. With so many voices and influences, how does a single idea move to the top of the agenda? Kingdon described three Ps—problems, possible solutions, and political circumstances—that are involved in setting the agenda. For policy change to occur, policy makers must be convinced that a problem is serious. Reaching agreement on what constitutes a serious problem can be a challenging task among policy makers. Crisis, one of Wakefield's (2006) factors, is clearly influential. The rapid bipartisan response from an otherwise underperforming legislature to a crisis in the Middle East in 2014 is an excellent example of the impact of crisis on legislative priority. When Americans were being beheaded by a radical Islam faction in September 2014, within a span of 3 days an amendment went from the House of Representatives to the Senate to the president and became part of the continuing budget resolution, PL 113-164, and signed into law. A crisis can create a sense of urgency or the desire to get something done. As Rahm Emanuel, President Barack Obama's then–chief of staff, said shortly before the president's inauguration, "You never want a serious crisis to go to waste" (Seib, 2008).

Policy Formulation Phase: Development of Legislation

The possible solutions are the policy proposals that are created, debated by committees, and presented to the legislative body. The less conflict there is regarding a possible solution to a serious problem, the more likely it will actually be heard in Congress. There is a strong relationship between the problems and the solutions that are proposed. How a problem is defined influences and limits the solutions that are proposed to address it. Two policy makers can look at the same problem and describe it differently because they are defining the problem based on what *they* think the solution ought to be. As Thomas Birkland (2005) states in his book on the policy process, "the actual act of identifying a problem is as much a normative judgment as it is an objective statement of fact" (p. 15). That is, whether something is really a problem is actually part of the debate itself.

A well-defined problem and reasonable solution are not enough to guarantee that a policy proposal will move forward. A third factor, the political circumstances, is also involved in opening the window of opportunity. When there is a recognized problem, a solution available in the policy community to solve that problem, and a favorable political environment, a policy window is open. Kingdon (1995) writes, "Policy windows open infrequently, and do not stay open long. Despite their rarity, the major changes in public policy result from the appearance of these opportunities" (p. 166). When the ACA was passed in 2010, it was the result of a unique combination of problem, proposal, and political circumstances. Democrats had a majority in the both the House of Representatives and the Senate, and President Obama had identified health care as his top priority. After the midterm elections, the control of the House shifted to the Republican Party, and the window was closed, not only for legislation about health care, but for almost any legislation at all. APRNs need to use the open window when it exists to help remove barriers to their practice and allow them the opportunity to care for their patients as they were prepared to do.

How a Bill Is Created

When a problem has been identified as important and a reasonable solution is proposed, a congressperson introduces a bill. Only a congressperson may introduce a bill, but he or she may receive the language of the bill from interested parties who ask the congressperson to sponsor the legislation. The bill is evaluated by the Office of Legislative Counsel to put it into proper legislative language. There is a separate legislative counsel for the House and the Senate. The counsel consists of groups of lawyers with specific expertise who will aid in the development of the bill and identify what current laws the bill will affect. The law or laws the bill affects will determine to which committee the bill will be assigned. There are 22 committees in the House and 16 in the Senate, plus numerous subcommittees. Health care policies usually involve either Medicare or Medicaid law. In the Senate, bills affecting either of these laws would be sent to the Senate Finance Committee. In the House, bills that affect Medicare law would go to the House Ways and Means Committee, and those that affect Medicaid law go to the House Energy and Commerce Committee.

A committee chair calls the committee together, sets the committee agenda, and prioritizes the bills that will be addressed by the committee. The majority party appoints the committee chairs, so party politics has a strong influence on which bills will be addressed by the committee and the amount of time given to the hearings. Each year thousands of bills are introduced to committee, but only about 11% of them find that "policy window" that allows them to go to the floor for debate (GovTrack.us, 2013). Committees hold hearings to address bills, and during the interaction between committee members and interested parties, it may be obvious that there are issues in common with other bills. When a bill is important but does not have the urgency to bring it to the top of the political agenda, it may be included in a bill that does reach the level of introduction. Bills can also be *packaged* so that less popular bills are combined with bills that are more likely to be passed. They may be included in other legislation as amendments or written into "clean bills."

Bills must pass both the House and the Senate to become law. From January 3, 2011, to January 3, 2013, the 112th Congress passed only 3% of bills that were introduced. Bills that are passed go from the Congress to the president for his signature. When the president signs a bill, it becomes law. If the president doesn't sign the bill, it may still become law after 10 days as long as Congress is still in session. If Congress adjourns before the 10 days pass, the bill is pocket vetoed and does not become law. The president may also actively veto the bill, but the bill may still become law if a two-thirds majority in both the House and the Senate override the presidential veto.

Incrementalism

Laws are imperfect, and the cyclical process allows for modifications over time. The small changes that are made in laws define the concept of incrementalism. Kingdon (1995) describes *incrementalism* as a strategy used to enact policy change a little piece at a time. As legislation is debated and competing proposals are presented, compromise is necessary to make change happen. If one group refuses to accept the compromise, the important problem may not get any solution at all. Through incremental changes some aspect of the problem may be solved now, which will open the window for more complete change in the future. Even though it can succeed, the strategy of incrementalism is controversial. It can achieve results in the long run, but it may seem as if not enough is being done in the short term to solve the big problems of the day. Advocates of all or nothing should understand that compromise is the best method of achieving change and that they should not allow the perfect to become the enemy of the good (Hitt, 2009; Wakefield & Wangsness, 2009).

Incrementalism is the way that APRNs have achieved increasing independence in practice. In 1997 APRNs in the state of Ohio first received license recognition, the Certificate of Authority (COA) for Advanced Practice, but this did not include prescriptive authority. APRNs were allowed to order laboratory tests and could prescribe medications that were available over the counter. In January 2000, Ohio granted prescriptive authority to APRNs who held a COA. This included the ability to prescribe Schedule III through V drugs with limited authority for prescribing Schedule II drugs. In 2011 the Ohio legislature expanded the authority of APRNs to prescribe Schedule II drugs. The goal of independent authority is still not a reality in Ohio, but with each of the incremental steps that have spanned over a decade, soon that may become a reality.

Policy Implementation Phase: Rulemaking

After a bill becomes law, it is assigned to the appropriate federal agency for rulemaking. Rulemaking authority was defined by the Administrative Procedure Act of 1946, which governs the way an agency may propose regulations. An agency may not exceed statutory authority in writing the rules and may not violate the Constitution. All proposed and final rules must be published in the *Federal Register*. The *Federal Register* is published every business day by the Government Printing Office and includes the Federal Agency Regulations, Proposed Rules and Public Notices, Executive Orders, Proclamations, and other presidential documents. It is available online at www.gpo.gov/fdsys/. Important resources for information about rulemaking include the review of federal regulations available on the Office of Information and Regulatory Affairs website (www.Reginfo.gov) and the website for submitting comments regarding the proposed regulations (www.regulations.gov). Regulations.gov provides a venue for the public to submit feedback regarding any proposed rule. APRNs engaged in health policy should be aware of these resources. Typically there is 30- to 60-day window of opportunity for the public to provide feedback regarding the proposed rule.

There is an important distinction between law and regulation. APRNs need to be mindful of this difference when advocating for change locally or nationally. When an issue is specifically addressed in the law or statute, it requires a new law to make a change in the existing statute, as illustrated in Longest's (2010) cyclical model. However, if the issue is specified in regulation, it can be changed by a revision of the regulation using the rulemaking process. The less detail that is included in the statute, the more opportunity there will be for response to changes in the future environment by the use of rulemaking.

One example that directly affects APRNs is the stipulation in the Medicare Law of 1965 that only physicians can certify a patient for home health care. Because it is in the law, it cannot be changed by rulemaking; it requires a new law. Another example is the restriction prohibiting APRNs from ordering portable x-rays, but this resulted from a regulation in the 1969 *Conditions for Coverage* (CMS, 2012). Each year the CMS develops *The Physician Fee Schedule*, which specifies what services under Medicare Part B will be covered and reimbursed. It is a regulation that is published in the *Federal Register* and provides an opportunity to change rules that have been created in the past. In July 2012, the CMS submitted its *Proposed Rule for Revisions to Payment Policies Under the Physician Fee Schedule* with clarification of a restriction regarding who could order portable x-rays. The new regulation stated, "we propose revisions to the Conditions for Coverage at § 486.106(a) and § 486.106(b) to permit portable x-ray services to be ordered by a physician or nonphysician practitioner in accordance with the ordering policies for other diagnostic services under § 410.32(a)." Once a rule is finalized, it is reviewed by the House and the Senate. The House and Senate can pass a resolution of disapproval, which then can be approved or vetoed by the president. This review process began in 1996, and since then, only one rule has been disapproved by Congress (Office of the Federal Register, 2011).

THE APRN AS ENGAGED CITIZEN

Scanning the Environment

How well APRNs use their "golden age" depends on the engagement of each individual (see Table 9.1). Developing leadership skills and increasing the understanding of the political process will support the effectiveness of APRNs as they seek to increase their engagement. Business theory has described the concept of "scanning the environment," the monitoring of the organization's internal and external environment. APRNs can use this concept in the monitoring of the local and national health policy environment. The individual APRN can extend his or her reach at the federal and state levels by participating in professional organizations whose staff scan the environment daily. Scanning the local environment is just as important and provides an opportunity for direct involvement, especially for the fledgling political activist.

Locally, APRNs can scan for opportunities to educate others about their role and respond to barriers when identified. It may be as simple as having the language on the school health form changed from physician to provider. When institutional policies set up barriers to full practice authority, the well-informed APRN is positioned to respond. Institutional policies that are more restrictive than necessary may be a result of a knowledge gap. The administrators who created the policy may lack an understanding of changes in federal and state laws that govern APRN practice. When an informed APRN presents data with a request for a change in policy and emphasizes the effect on improved patient care and the benefit to the organization, that APRN will be presenting a strong argument in support of his or her agenda. The uninformed APRN is at the mercy of policies from others that may not represent the current regulations. For example, a portable x-ray company, unaware of the change that occurred in the regulation in the physician fee schedule, may refuse to accept an order from an APRN. This may negatively affect the patient of an informed APRN who acquiesces to the policy. However, an informed APRN could use the strategy of providing data, emphasizing the effect on the patient and the benefit to the organization, and may successfully accomplish the objective and benefit colleagues as well.

Working Collaboratively

Collaboration not only with other APRNs but also with other health care providers will be a growing requirement in new regulatory models. With the redesign of health care delivery systems, all health professionals find their traditional roles and responsibilities changing. New delivery models include accountable care organizations, medical/health homes, and retail clinics. These models are intended to be patient centered and to help contain costs. The Center for Medicare and Medicaid Innovation at the CMS was an agency created as a result of ACA. The center is charged with testing new health care delivery models. APRNs need to be aware of these initiatives and become active participants in the development of the models.

As the public became more aware of the value of the patient-centered care provided by APRNs, coalitions formed outside of health care to support expansion of advanced practice nursing. It is equally important for APRNs to articulate their expertise and the contribution that advanced practice nursing can make to the success of the new delivery models, working together with other professionals to meet the objectives of improved quality at a cost savings. With increased emphasis on interprofessional collaboration and new graduates who are prepared with interprofessional educational experiences, obstacles that have separated professionals in the past will hopefully be removed. Interprofessional models emphasize collaboration and increase the understanding of the expertise that each profession brings to the care of the patient.

The Policy Process and the Nursing Process

The cyclical nature of Longest's (2010) Health Policy Making Model has similarities with the nursing process: assessment, planning, intervention, and evaluation. As one nursing scholar on policy and politics put it, "Nursing and politics are a good match" (Leavitt, Cohen, & Mason, 2002, p. 71). The policy-making process, moving from a problem to the implementation of a program that aims to fix it, requires the separation of one problem from another. It requires us to understand that many solutions exist, to prioritize our needs, to interact and compromise with many other interests, and to be ready to respond to change, which is certain to come in a highly dynamic environment. With a more in-depth understanding of the legislative process, the rulemaking, and the development of regulation that follows, APRNs are prepared to apply that understanding to address their own concerns. Developing their leadership ability and connecting to their colleagues at the local, state, and national levels is essential to accomplishing policy change.

Resources for Developing the Engaged Citizen

TABLE 9.1 Policy Resources

Legislative Branch	Websites	Description
Federal Legislative Information	www.congress.gov	Is the official website for up-to-date information on legislation presented by the Library of Congress
Library of Congress	www.loc.gov	Serves as an archival resource
House of Representatives	www.house.gov	Provides a directory of Representatives, leadership, committees, and legislation
U.S. Senate	www.senate.gov	Provides a directory of Senators, committees, and legislation
GovTrack.us	www.govtrack.us	Is not a government site but independently tracks the bills that are considered by Congress
Executive Branch		
White House	www.whitehouse.gov	Provides a directory of the executive branch, the executive offices, the White House schedule, and issues
Health and Human Services (HHS) Administration	www.hhs.gov	Cabinet department
Centers for Disease Control and Prevention	www.cdc.gov	A department under HHS resource for many health statistics; publishes the *Morbidity and Mortality Weekly Report*
Centers for Medicare & Medicaid Services	www.cms.hhs.gov	Provides comprehensive information on Medicare, Medicaid, Children's Health Insurance Program (CHIP), and resource for statistics
Food and Drug Administration	www.fda.gov	Provides safety information, regulatory information
Substance Abuse and Mental Health Services Administration	www.samhsa.gov	Is a resource for mental health services and data

(continued)

TABLE 9.1 Policy Resources *(continued)*

Health Resources and Services Administration	www.hrsa.gov	Provides information on National Health Service Corps, loans and scholarships, federally qualified health centers
National Institute of Nursing Research	www.ninr.nih.gov	Provides funding for nursing scientists
Rulemaking and Regulation		
Federal Register	www.gpo.gov/fdsys	Includes all proposed and final rules; is published daily
Office of Information and Regulatory Affairs	www.Reginfo.gov	Publishes the Unified Agenda and Regulatory Plan
Regulations.gov	www.regulations.gov	Provides access to federal regulatory content; submits comments on documents published in the *Federal Register*
State Resources		
National Conference of State Legislatures	www.ncsl.org	Provides information and resources to state legislatures
National Governors Association	www.nga.org	Bipartisan coalition of governors to create a unified response to national issues
Research and Policy Institutes		
Cato Institute	www.cato.org	A public policy research organization focused on a wide variety of topics, including health care and welfare
Center on Budget and Policy Priorities	www.cbpp.org	Works on federal and state fiscal policies and programs that affect low- and moderate-income people
The Commonwealth Fund	www.common wealthfund.org	Private foundation that supports health care systems
The Heritage Foundation	www.heritage.org	Mission is to formulate and support conservative public policies
Kaiser Family Foundation	http://kff.org	Provides policy analysis on national health issues

(continued)

TABLE 9.1 Policy Resources *(continued)*

National Center for Policy Analysis	www.ncpa.org	Policy research with the goal to promote free enterprise including health care initiatives

Coalitions

Future of Nursing Campaign for Action	http://campaignforaction.org/	An initiative of AARP, AARP Foundation, and the Robert Wood Johnson Foundation to implement the recommendations in the Institute of Medicine report on nursing
Robert Wood Johnson Foundation	www.rwjf.org	Shares evidence and promotes change in health care through partnerships and collaboration
The Nursing Community	www.thenursingcommunity.org	A coalition of 61 national nursing organizations that strive to "Speak With One Voice"

TABLE 9.2 National APRN Professional Organizations

ORGANIZATION	WEBSITE
American Academy of Nursing	www.aannet.org
American Association of Colleges of Nursing	www.aacn.nche.edu
American Association of Critical Care Nurses	www.aacn.org
American Association of Nurse Anesthetists	www.aana.com
American Association of Nurse Practitioners	www.aanp.org
American College of Nurse Midwives	www.acnm.org
American Nurses Association	www.nursingworld.org
Association of Women's Health, Obstetric, and Neonatal Nurses	www.awhonn.org
Gerontological Advanced Practice Nurses Association	www.gapna.org
National Association of Clinical Nurse Specialists	www.nacns.org
National Association of Pediatric Nurse Practitioners	www.napnap.org
National Organization of Nurse Practitioner Faculties	www.nonpf.org

(continued)

TABLE 9.2 National APRN Professional Organizations *(continued)*

ORGANIZATION	WEBSITE
National Organization of NPs in Women's Health	www.npwh.org
Oncology Nurses Society	www.ons.org

Acknowledgment

The author acknowledges the contributions of Linda Reivitz to this chapter in the previous edition.

REFERENCES

American Association of Colleges of Nursing. (2006). *The essentials of doctoral education for advanced nursing practice.* Retrieved from http://www.aacn .nche.edu/publications/position/dnpessentials.pdf

APRN Consensus Workgroup and APRN Joint Dialogue Group. (2008). *Consensus model for APRN regulation: Licensure, accreditation, certification & education.* Retrieved from http://www.aacn.nche.edu/Education/pdf/APRNReport .pdf

Birkland, T. (2005). *An introduction to the policy process: Theories, concepts and models of public policy making* (2nd ed.). Armonk, NY: M. E. Sharpe.

Centers for Medicare & Medicaid Services. (2012). Medicare Program; Revisions to payment policies under the physician fee schedule, proposed rules. *Federal Register* (July 30, 2012). Retrieved from https://www.federalregister. gov/articles/2012/07/30/2012-16814/medicare-program-revisions-to-payment-policies-under-the-physician-fee-schedule-dme-face-to-face#h-138

Center for Responsive Politics. (2014). *Lobbying data base.* Retrieved from https:// www.opensecrets.org/lobby/index.php

Cilliza, C. (2014, April 10). Yes, President Obama is right. The 113th Congress will be the least productive in history. *The Washington Post* [blog entry]. Retrieved from http://www.washingtonpost.com/blogs/the-fix/wp/2014/04/10/president-obama-said-the-113th-congress-is-the-least-productive-ever-is-he-right/

Falk-Rafael, A. (2005). Speaking truth to power: Nursing's legacy and moral imperative. *Advances in Nursing Science, 28*(3), 212–223.

Federal Trade Commission. (2014). *Policy perspectives: Competition and the regulation of advanced practice nurses.* Retrieved from http://www.ftc.gov/system/files/documents/reports/policy-perspectives-competition-regulation-advanced-practice-nurses/140307aprnpolicypaper.pdf

Foote, S. (2014, May 23). Why I blew the whistle on the VA. *The New York Times*, p. A 21.

Govtrack.us. (2013). *Bill prognosis analysis.* Retrieved from https://www.govtrack. us/about/analysis#prognosis

Grant, D. (2012, May 14). Top 9 reasons Congress is broken. *Christian Science Monitor.* Retrieved from http://www.csmonitor.com/USA/DC-Decoder/2012/0514/Top-9-reasons-Congress-is-broken/Congress-is-back-to-the-future

Hitt, G. (2009, February 5). GOP wields more influence over the stimulus bill. *The Wall Street Journal.* Retrieved from http://online.wsj.com/article/SB123376269235148125.html

Institute of Medicine. (2010). *The future of nursing: Leading change, advancing health.* Retrieved from http://books.nap.edu/openbook.php?record_id=12956&page=R1

Kingdon, J. W. (2010). *Agendas, alternatives, and public policies* (2nd ed.). New York, NY: Longman

Leavitt, J., Cohen, S., & Mason, D. J. (2002). Political analysis and strategies. In D. J. Mason, J. K. Leavitt, & M. W. Chaffee (Eds.), *Policy & politics in nursing and health care* (pp. 71–91). St Louis, MO: W.B. Saunders.

Longest, B. B. (2010). *Health policy making in the United States* (5th ed.). Chicago, IL: Health Administration Press.

National Organization of Nurse Practitioner Faculties. (2012). *Nurse practitioner core competencies.* Retrieved from http://c.ymcdn.com/sites/www.nonpf.org/resource/resmgr/competencies/npcorecompetenciesfinal2012.pdf

Office of the Federal Register. (2011). *A guide to the rulemaking process.* Retrieved from https://www.federalregister.gov/uploads/2011/01/the_rulemaking_process.pdf

O'Grady, E. T. (2011). Advanced practice nursing and health policy. In J. M. Stanley (Ed.), *Advanced practice nursing: Emphasizing common roles* (pp. 351–377). Philadelphia, PA: F.A. Davis.

Portman, R. (2013, March 15). Gay couples also deserve a chance to get married. *The Plain Dealer.* Retrieved from http://www.dispatch.com/content/stories/editorials/2013/03/15/gay-couples-also-deserve-chance-to-get-married.html

Seib, G. (2008). In crisis, opportunity for Obama. *The Wall Street Journal.* Retrieved January 2, 2009, from http://online.wsj.com/article/SB122721278056345271.html

Stanik-Hutt, J. (2013). The quality and effectiveness of care provided by nurse practitioners. *Journal for Nurse Practitioners, 9*(8), 492–500.

Stone, G. R., & Marshall, W. P. (2011). The framers constitution. *Democracy Journal. org.* Summer 2011, pp. 61–66. Retrieved from http://www.democracyjournal.org/pdf/21/the_framers_constitution.pdf

USA.gov. (2014). U.S. federal government. Retrieved from http://www.usa.gov/Agencies/federal.shtml

Wakefield, M., & Wangsness, L. (2009, February 18). Doctors criticize Massachusetts health law. *The Boston Globe.* Retrieved February 23, 2009, from http://www.boston.com/news/ politics/politicalintelligence/2009/02/doctors_critici.html

Wakefield, M. (2006, February 19). So you want to be an advocate? Strategies for advocacy, knowledge, resources, colleagues and actions (PPT slides). Presented at the American College of Nurse Practitioners Health Policy Conference, Washington, DC.

Michaelene P. Jansen

10

PRACTICE ISSUES: REGULATION, CERTIFICATION, CLINICAL PRIVILEGES, PRESCRIPTIVE AUTHORITY, AND LIABILITY

Advanced practice registered nurses (APRNs) encounter a variety of professional issues in their practices. Most questions focus on what APRNs can or cannot do within the scope of nursing practice. Although APRNs have made progress in terms of removing barriers to practice, many barriers continue to exist. As health care reform evolves in individual states or on a national level, it will be critical for APRNs to be fully cognizant of legislative or regulatory activity that may impede their ability to perform within their full scope of practice. At the same time, APRNs are expanding their educational focus, bringing forth new issues and challenges. In an ideal world, APRNs would have the same privileges and legal and prescriptive authority across all states.

Proposed models for uniform APRN practice and the progress toward full practice authority will be discussed later in this chapter. In the interim, as APRNs seek new or continued employment, they must consider what regulations will allow or limit their practice in their specific states. In doing so, they can choose positions that are congruent with their educational scopes of practice. They should also know what credentials might be needed to practice in a certain state, institution, or organization. For example, if they choose to practice in a selected state, would they be able to prescribe medications, sign death certificates, admit patients to hospitals, sign worker's compensation claims or disabled parking permits? Would they be required to be supervised by a physician, develop a collaborative agreement, or have restrictions placed on their billing? These are all practice issues that surround regulation, certification, scope of practice, and liability.

The terms *regulation, certification,* and *credentialing* as they apply to all APRNs can be very confusing to the public as well as health care providers.

These terms are often used incorrectly, and they can cause misperceptions or confusion among consumers. There are distinct differences in the meaning of each term and the things that APRNs are allowed to do. Understanding these terms will help APRNs carry out their roles while avoiding any barriers that may exist.

REGULATION

A regulation is a law that has been passed by the state or federal legislature and signed by the governor of that state or the president of the United States. Nursing practice is regulated by each state in accordance with state statutes and interpreted through administrative rules. In most states, APRNs are regulated under the authority of a board of nursing. In a review of state APRN regulation in 2014, one state had a separate advanced practice board; advanced practice nurses from three states were controlled by Boards of Nursing and Medicine; one state was regulated by a Nursing Care Quality Assurance Commission and one state regulated APRNs through their state's Education Department (Phillips, 2014). Buppert (2015) provides the state statutes and regulatory rules for each state.

Regulation of APRNs varies from state to state, and changes occur yearly. This variability inhibits APRNs moving from state to state with the same authority and scope of practice. As of 2014, 24 states—with three additional states having pending legislation—have enacted a Nurse Licensure Compact for registered nurses and vocational licensed nurses to increase mobility between states (National Council of State Boards of Nursing, 2014). Only three states—Iowa, Texas, and Utah—have APRN compacts. It is anticipated that Nurse Licensure Compact states will be able to implement the APRN compact in the near future (Nurse Licensure Compact Administrators, 2012).

The road to removing regulatory barriers for APRNs has been bumpy, to say the least. However, thanks to the perseverance and endless efforts of individual and professional advanced practice advocates, APRNs can practice and prescribe medications in every state. That said, however, much more work needs to be done to educate legislators, interprofessional groups, and the public in order to provide access to safe, competent care for all consumers.

A hallmark publication by the committee on the Robert Wood Johnson Foundation Initiative on the Future of Nursing at the Institute of Medicine (IOM) has provided support and foundation for state legislatures to update nurse practice acts to allow APRNs to practice to the full extent of their licenses. The publication, *The Future of Nursing. Leading Change, Advancing Health* (IOM, 2011), makes four recommendations:

1. Nurses should practice to the full extent of their education and training.
2. Nurses should achieve higher levels of education and training through an improved education system that promotes seamless academic progression.

3. Nurses should be full partners, with physicians and other health professionals, in redesigning health care in the United States.
4. Effective workforce planning and policy making require better data collection and an improved information infrastructure. (p. S-3)

The implications of this publication continue to unfold and provide a positive forum for APRNs to remove barriers from practice. It is interesting that the report is not asking or recommending expanding the scope of APRN practice or additional money (American Association of Nurse Practitioners [AANP], 2011). The timing of this publication, along with the Patient Care and Affordable Care Act of 2010 (ACA), has been helpful for nursing and APRNs to promote legislation in their states and encourage provider-neutral terminology. As of 2014, 20 states have full practice authority for nurse practitioners (NPs) (AANP, 2014).

Title Protection

Title protection limits the use of a title unless the user meets the regulations mandated by state regulation. Currently, 39 states have legislation that protects the title *nurse* (American Nurses Association [ANA], 2013). Restriction of the term *nurse* provides reassurance to the public that the individual using that title has met all the requirements mandated for licensure in that state. Eleven states do not provide title protection; however, these states do regulate professional nursing. Without title protection, persons can call themselves nurses without meeting the requirements in those states.

All states have some form of title protection for NPs (Pearson, 2014; Phillips, 2014), but they vary in who has the legal authority to regulate APRN practice. Clinical nurse specialists (CNSs) are advocating among state legislators to promote title protection for their role (National Association of Clinical Nurse Specialists [NACNS], 2004). Title protection for nurse-midwives and nurse anesthetists (NAs) also varies among states. There is variability as to the title for APRN in each state. Currently there are 13 titles associated with recognition of APRNs by state regulatory boards. Table 10.1 provides a list of these titles. The APRN Consensus Workgroup and APRN Joint Dialogue Group (2008) identify NPs as certified nurse practitioners (CNPs), one of the four APRN roles.

Title protection is not synonymous with autonomous or uniform regulation. APRNs must continue to promote legislation to remove statutory restrictions that limit advanced practice nursing. The APRN Consensus Workgroup and APRN Joint Dialogue Group (2008) proposed the title *advanced practice registered nurse* (APRN) as the licensing title for the four advanced practice roles. Since the publication of this model, several states have incorporated the model and titling in their state statutes to be in compliance with the APRN regulatory model, which is one of the driving forces for revising state regulatory statutes.

TABLE 10.1 APRN Titles Recognized by State Regulatory Bodies

APN	Advanced practice nurse
APNP	Advanced practice nurse prescriber
APPN	Advanced practice professional nurse
APRN	Advanced practice registered nurse
ARNP	Advanced registered nurse practitioner
CNM	Certified nurse-midwife
CNP	Certified nurse practitioner
CNS	Clinical nurse specialist
CRNA	Certified registered nurse anesthetist
CRNM	Certified registered nurse-midwife
CRNP	Certified registered nurse practitioner
NA	Nurse anesthetist
RNP	Registered nurse practitioner

Even as advanced practice education moves toward requiring the clinical doctorate for practice at the entry level, several states have statutory restrictions against doctorally prepared NPs being addressed as *doctor* (Pearson, 2009). Several advanced practice nursing organizations developed a unified statement outlining Doctor of Nursing Practice certification, education, and use of the title *doctor* (Nurse Practitioner Roundtable, 2008). The unified statement acknowledges that a medical doctor or doctor of osteopathy may be title protected, but notes that recognition of the title *doctor* for APRNs who are doctorally prepared facilitates parity within health care.

APRN Regulatory Model

Given the variability in scope of practice, recognized advanced practice roles, criteria for entry into advanced practice, and accepted certification examinations, it can be difficult for APRNs to move between states. A model has been developed that includes four essential elements—licensure, accreditation, certification, and education (LACE)—as a means to protect the public and decrease barriers for APRNs who practice in multiple states (APRN Consensus Workgroup & APRN Joint Dialogue Group, 2008).

The APRN regulatory model includes registered NAs, certified nurse-midwives (CNMs), CNSs, and CNPs. The consensus group recognized that there are many nurses with graduate preparation, such as nurse educators, informatics specialists, or administrators; however, their focus is not direct care to individuals. The model provides for APRNs to "be licensed as independent practitioners for practice at the level of one of the four APRN roles within at least one of the six identified population foci. Education, certification, and licensure of an individual must be congruent in terms of role and population foci. APRNs may be specialized but they cannot be licensed solely within a specialty area" (APRN Consensus Workgroup & APRN Joint Dialogue Group, 2008, p. 5).

The APRN regulatory model (Figure 10.1) illustrates the four advanced practice roles educated by an accredited academic program in at least one of six population foci: family/individual across the life span, adult/gerontology, neonatal, pediatrics, women's health/gender related, and psychiatric/mental health. Licensing will occur at the level of role and population focus, and certification will reflect the population focus. APRN specialties are areas of focus beyond the role and population. Implementation of the model will occur incrementally by state boards of nursing. Full implementation is anticipated by 2015, when the entry education level for advanced practice will be the doctor of nursing practice, although that projected deadline seems somewhat optimistic.

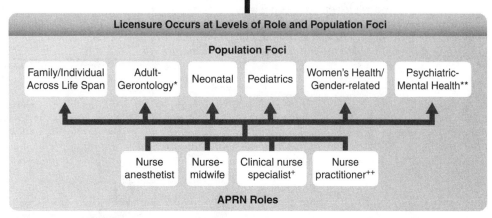

* The population focus, adult-gerontology, encompasses the young adult to the older adult, including the frail elderly. APRNs educated and certified in the adult-gerontology population are educated and certified across both areas of practice and will be titled adult-gerontology CNP or CNS. In addition, all APRNs in any of the four roles providing care to the adult population (e.g., family or gender specific) must be prepared to meet the growing needs of the older adult population. Therefore, the education program should include didactic and clinical education experiences necessary to prepare APRNs with these enhanced skills and knowledge.

** The population focus, psychiatric/mental health, encompasses education and practice across the lifespan.

+ Clinical nurse specialist (CNS) is educated and assessed through national certification process across the continuum from wellness through acute care

++ Acute or primary care certified nurse practitioners (CNPs)

FIGURE 10.1 APRN regulatory model. *Source:* APRN Consensus Workgroup and APRN Joint Dialogue Group (2008, p. 9).

Figure 10.2 illustrates the relationship among educational competencies, licensure, and certification in the role/population foci and education and credentialing in a specialty.

CERTIFICATION

The introduction of the APRN regulatory model has put a greater emphasis on certification. Certification by a national board has been a requirement for regulatory processes and prescriptive authority. Certification differs from licensure in that certification is a process by which a nongovernmental agency or association certifies that an individual licensed to practice a profession has met certain predetermined standards specified by that profession for population or specialty practice. The purpose of certification is to assure various publics that an individual has mastered a body of knowledge and acquired skills for a particular population or specialty.

Historically, certification in nursing has been murky with no uniform standards. Many specialty organizations certified nurses with varying educational backgrounds at one general level. Most certification agencies now require a master's or higher degree to be eligible for certification at an advanced practice level. As the APRN regulatory model is implemented,

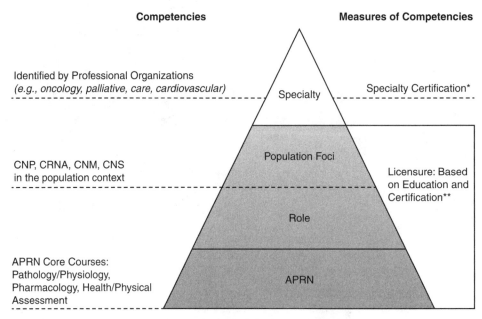

Competencies   **Measures of Competencies**

Identified by Professional Organizations
(e.g., oncology, palliative, care, cardiovascular) - - - - - Specialty - - - - - Specialty Certification*

CNP, CRNA, CNM, CNS
in the population context - - - - - - - - - - Population Foci - - - - - - - - - - Licensure: Based on Education and Certification**

Role

APRN Core Courses:
Pathology/Physiology,
Pharmacology, Health/Physical
Assessment   APRN

* Certification for specialty may include exam, portfolio, peer review, etc.

** Certification for licensure will be a psychometrically sound and legally defensible examination by an accredited certifying program.

FIGURE 10.2 Relationship among educational competencies, licensure and certification in the role/population foci, and education and credentialing in a specialty. *Source:* APRN Consensus Workgroup and APRN Joint Dialogue Group (2008, p. 14).

certification for licensing at an advanced practice level will reflect the six populations identified and entry level will be at the practice doctorate level. Specialty certification will occur by the same or additional certifying bodies. Specialty certification will not suffice alone for licensing as an APRN.

Certifying Bodies

American Association of Critical-Care Nurses Certification Corporation

The certification arm of the American Association of Critical-Care Nurses (AACN), the American Association of Critical-Care Nurses Certification Corporation (AACNCC), began offering certification for clinical nurse specialists in 1999.

The AACN Certification Corporation now has population and specialty certifications for APRNs (AACNCC, 2014). Their advanced practice consensus model–based certifications include Acute Care Nurse Practitioner (Adult-Gerontology) (ACNPC-AG) and Clinical Nurse. AACNCC offers a certification for critical care nurses and APRNs who influence patients, nurses, and/or organizations to have a positive impact on acutely and/or critically ill adult, pediatric, or neonatal patients but do not work at the bedside (CCRN-K).

American Association of Nurse Practitioners —Certification Program

The AANP has an affiliated organization, the AANP—Certification Program (AANPCP), that provides entry-level, competency-based examinations in three areas: adult, family and adult-gerontology primary care. The purpose of this certification is "to provide a valid and reliable program for entry-level NPs to recognize their education, knowledge and professional expertise" (AANPCP, 2014). Medicare, Medicaid, the Veterans Administration, and private insurance companies recognize nurse practitioners in all 50 states, as well as certification by the AANPCP. NPs receiving certification by the AANPCP use NP-C (nurse practitioner-certified) as their credential.

American Nurses Credentialing Center (ANCC)

The ANCC provides certification for the nursing profession, guaranteeing to the public that nurses have a certain level of knowledge or skill. The ANCC is an outgrowth of the ANA certification program, which was established in 1973 to function as an independent center through which the ANA would serve as its own credentialing program. ANCC certification "protects the public by enabling anyone to identify competent people more readily. Simultaneously it aids the profession by encouraging and recognizing professional achievement. Certification also recognizes specialization, enhances professionalism, and, in some cases, serves as a criterion for financial reimbursement. It may also foster an enlarged role within the employment setting" (ANCC, 2014).

The ANCC offers certification for CNSs in two areas: adult/gerontology and pediatric nursing. The ANCC no longer certifies CNSs in adult, gerontology, adult and adolescent psychiatric and mental health, public and community health, or home health but will continue to recertify these individuals. They will continue to recertify CNSs in advanced diabetes management as a specialty certification. In a collaborative effort with the NACNS, the ANCC formerly offered a core clinical nurse specialist (CNS) examination that addressed CNS competencies across the life span regardless of specialty, but that examination has been retired due to a move toward population-based certification.

The ANCC also certifies NPs in five clinical areas: (a) adult/gerontology primary care, (b) adult/gerontology acute care, (c) family, (d) pediatric primary care, and (e) psychiatric and mental health. Certification examinations for adult, gerontology, adult psychiatric and mental health, school, and advanced diabetes management will no longer be offered, but individuals can continue to recertify.

Over the years, the ANCC has granted multiple credentials to designate certification at an advanced practice level. Over the past 15 years, APRNs have seen multiple changes in their credentials. For example, before 1993, NPs certifying with the ANCC were given the title "C" to indicate certification. CNSs were given the credential "CS." From 1993 to 2000, both CNSs and NPs were given "CS" as the certifying credential. After 2000, NPs and CNSs were first given the credential APRN-BC; then APRN, BC, to indicate advanced practice registered nurse, board certified. Currently, NPs and CNSs have their own certification credential that reflects the clinical focus. For example, a family NP would have the following credentials: FNP-BC representing family nurse practitioner–board certified. An adult/gerontology CNS would use the credentials AGCNS-BC to signify board certification for this population.

American Midwifery Certification Board

The American Midwifery Certification Board (AMCB) is the certifying body for CNMs and certified midwives (AMCB, 2014). Students who have completed graduate programs accredited by the Accreditation Commission for Midwifery Education are eligible to take the examination. Certification by the AMCB is the gold standard for CNMs and is recognized in all 50 states. Certified midwives require a graduate degree, but not nursing degree, for certification and are recognized in four states. Certified professional midwives (CPM) are certified by the North American Registry of Midwives. No educational degree is required for the CPM designation, which is regulated in 27 states.

National Board of Certification and Recertification of
Nurse Anesthetists (NBCRNA)

Since 1956, certified registered nurse anesthetists (CRNAs) have been certified by the NBCRNA. There are more than 113 accredited CRNA programs and, of those programs, 16 award the Doctor of Nursing Practice

(DNP). CRNAs take the National Certification Exam (NCE) and are required to take a minimum of 40 hours of approved continuing education every 2 years, maintain state licensure, and document substantial anesthesia practice for a minimum of 850 hours. The NBCRNA recently increased passing standards in 2014 (NBCRNA, 2014).

Other Certification Opportunities

Although most specialty organizations provide certification for professional nursing practice, few offer certification at an advanced practice level. The organizations that offer advanced practice examinations are often at the specialty level of the APRN regulatory model. The American Psychiatric Nurses Association (APNA) considered offering certification for advanced practice psychiatric mental health nurses, but currently the certification as a psychiatric/mental health CNS or NP comes through the ANCC.

Women's Health

The National Certification Corporation (NCC) offers certification for women's health care NPs and neonatal NPs. The NCC also offers a subspecialty certification in gynecologic reproductive health along with the two core certifications (NCC, 2014). The NCC was formerly known as the Nurses' Association of the American College of Obstetricians and Gynecologists (NAACOG) Certification Corporation. The NAACOG was renamed the Association for Women's Health, Obstetrics and Neonatal Nursing and became an independent certification organization in 1991.

Pediatrics

Pediatric NPs can also be certified by the Pediatric Nursing Certification Board (PNCB). The PNCB offers certification for primary care pediatric NPs and acute care pediatric NPs. Certified pediatric NPs, pediatric CNSs, and family NPs are also eligible to take the pediatric primary mental health specialists certification examination offered by PNCB if they meet the eligibility criteria (PNCB, 2014).

Oncology

The Oncology Nursing Society through the Oncology Nursing Certification Corporation (ONCC) offers certification for NPs (Advanced Oncology Certified Nurse Practitioner [AOCNP]) and CNSs (Advanced Oncology Certified Clinical Nurse Specialist [AOCNS]). The ONCC also offers an Advanced Oncology Certification Nurse (AOCN) designation for nurses with master's degrees or higher working in administration, clinical practice, education, or research (ONCC, 2014). Other examples of specialty certification include orthopaedic nurse practitioners (ONP-C) and clinical nurse specialists (OCNS-C) certified by the Orthopaedic Nurses Certification Board (ONCB, 2014).

The Council for the Advancement of Comprehensive Care (CACC), established in 2000, is a consortium of academic and health policy leaders who are committed to ensuring high standards of doctoral nursing practice. In 2008, the CACC collaborated with the Board of Medical Examiners to develop and administer a certification examination for doctorate of nursing practice (DNP). The comprehensive care certification examination is comparable to the performance standards in Step 3 (the final step) in the United States medical licensing exam (USMLE) for medical students. Although the examinations are similar, the comprehensive care certification examination is only for graduates of DNP programs, and the candidate must be certified as an APRN. APRNs who pass this examination are designated diplomats in comprehensive care by the American Board of the CACC (CACC, 2014). The AACN released a statement in March 2009 to clarify that this examination is considered a specialty exam defined by Columbia University and is not a population-based examination (AACN, 2009). The CACC examination is an examination for DNP graduates from comprehensive care programs.

Criteria for Certification

Each certifying body has its own set of eligibility criteria. Certification corporations that certify NPs, CNSs, and CRNAs require a master's degree. Some of the early NPs and CRNAs graduated from nonmaster's certificate programs and have been grandfathered in. In the future, most eligibility criteria will require a practice doctorate to apply for certification.

Each certification area (e.g., family, adult, acute care, women's health) may have different practice or recertification requirements. Given the dynamic nature of certification and professional standards, the reader is referred to the specific certification website for the desired advanced practice role. Exhibit 10.1 provides a list of some websites offering information on eligibility and the application process.

Accreditation of Educational Programs

Accreditation of educational programs for APRNs will become integrated with the APRN Regulation Model. Competencies for NPs and CNSs have been developed by the NACNS and the National Organization of Nurse Practitioner Faculties (NONPF), respectively (NACNS, 2009; NONPF, 2012a). The NONPF has also developed criteria for evaluation of NP programs (NONPF, 2012b). The American Association of Colleges of Nursing (AACN) has developed an *Essentials* document that provides guidance to existing and developing DNP programs (AACN, 2006). CNM and CRNA programs are accredited by the Accreditation Commission for Midwifery Education (ACME) and the Council on Accreditation of Nurse Anesthesia Educational Programs (COA), respectively.

Exhibit 10.1 CERTIFICATION WEBSITES

- American Association of Critical-Care Nurses Certification Corporation: www. aacn.org/DM/MainPages/CertificationHome.aspx
- American Board of Comprehensive Care: http://nursing.columbia.edu/dnpcert/index.shtml
- American Midwifery Certification Board: www.amcbmidwife.org
- American Nurses Credentialing Center: www.nursecredentialing.org
- American Academy of Nurse Practitioners Certification Program: www.aanpcert. org/ptistore/control/index
- Oncology Nursing Certification Corporation: www.oncc.org
- Orthopaedic Nurses Certification Board: http://oncb.org/
- National Board of Certification and Recertification for Nurse Anesthetists: www. nbcrna.com/Pages/default.aspx
- National Certification Corporation: www.nccnet.org
- Pediatric Nursing Certification Board: www.pncb.org/ptistore/control/exams/index

---

Credentials

One of the concerns related to certification is the multiplicity of acronyms that are used to indicate certification and that each certifying body uses its own credentials. The frequent change in credentials, as well as the variety of terms used to indicate advanced practice nursing, is confusing for the consumer as well as other health care professionals. As regulatory bodies become more uniform and as certification corporations align their examinations with the APRN regulatory model, there may be more consistency and understanding of the titles that reflect advanced practice.

In the interim, APRNs can facilitate common terminology within their organizations. For example, having a common format for name badges that is consistent with documentation signatures would be a first step. Smolenski (2005) provides guidance for listing credentials in the following order: degree, licensure, state designation or requirement, national certification, honor or awards, then other certifications. An illustration of this titling is as follows: Jane Doe, DNP, APRN, ANP-BC, FAAN.

Clinical Privileges

Clinical privileges are "authorizations granted by the governing body of a hospital to provide specific patient care services within well-defined limits, based on the qualifications reviewed in the credentialing process" (Cooper, 1998, p. 30). The credentialing process ensures the protection of patients by providing a process for institutions to select competent practitioners (Klein, 2003). The Joint Commission, formerly known as the Joint Commission on Accreditation of Health Care

Organizations (JCAHO), specifies characteristics of a process for the delineation of clinical privileges. The Joint Commission's 2012 accreditation manual for hospitals states that medical staff must credential and privilege all licensed independent practitioners (LIP) (JCAHO, 2012). The process and procedural details must be outlined in medical staff bylaws. Nonlicensed independent practitioners, such as physician assistants (PAs) and APRNs, may be privileged through an established medical staff process that reflects The Joint Commission's credentialing and privileging standards.

Clinical privileges have been successfully obtained for CNMs and CRNAs. Set standards are processes typically established through the appropriate medical departments (i.e., obstetrics or anesthesia). Clinical privileges for CNSs and NPs have been more difficult to obtain. The great diversity in qualifications for APRNs, including CRNAs and CNMs, makes it difficult for agencies to develop uniform clinical privileging guidelines for all APRNs.

Although there is some variability in the credentialing process, The JCAHO recommends a series of steps for medical staff. Credentialing is the first step in the process that leads to privileging. Typically, the credentialing process includes the application, verification of credentials, evaluation of applicant-specific information, and a recommendation to the governing medical board for appointment and privileges. The medical staff has the discretion to use the information provided to make the appropriate decision regarding privileges. The information that is required should include data on qualifications, such as licensure, education, experience, and clinical competence. A period of focused professional practice is implemented for all successful applicants who have requested privileges (JCAHO, 2012).

APRNs must go through a similar process of credentialing to obtain clinical privileges. Each institution has a specific process and form, although they all contain components required by the JCAHO. As a result, an APRN requesting clinical privileges at four different hospitals is likely to undergo four separate application procedures and reviews. The title given to the APRN will also likely vary, depending on each institution. Designations such as *allied health provider, associate allied health provider,* and *nonphysician provider* are often used in granting clinical privileges for APRNs.

Institutions must have not only a credentialing process in place, but also a review process, including peer review every 2 years, for the renewal of clinical privileges. However, temporary privileges may be granted for a limited time. Most institutions use the same application forms and processes for LIPs and non-LIPs. These forms are medically focused and often difficult for providers who are not physicians to use. Some institutions tailor their credentialing process specifically for APRNs with appropriate terminology that reflects current regulations. State laws and hospital policies determine who can practice independently. The JCAHO defines an LIP as "any individual permitted by law and organization to provide care, treatment, and services, without direction or supervision" (JCAHO, 2012). In states that require a collaborating or supervising physician, practice agreements are required as part of the credentialing process. Additional information on practice agreements is presented in Chapter 16.

As APRNs continue to practice within their full scope of practice in acute care facilities, clinical privileges become more important. There continues to be confusion among medical staff as to specific requirements for cosigning clinical documentation for PAs, APRNs, interns, residents, and fellows. Unfortunately, some institutions require physicians to cosign all clinical documentation, whether or not law requires it, to avoid any errors in documentation for billing purposes. There is also ongoing discussion regarding whether CNSs and NPs who are credentialed in acute care facilities should be certified as acute care NPs or CNSs.

The process for obtaining clinical privileges will be facilitated by the use of a common language about advanced nursing practice among institutions and across states. The placement of nurses in high administrative posts in agencies as well as having APRNs on credentialing panels will also make it less difficult for APRNs to obtain clinical privileges. Educating staff, physicians, institutions, and communities regarding advanced nursing practice will be necessary before clinical privileges are granted without question for all APRNs.

PRESCRIPTIVE AUTHORITY

Historically, the issue of prescriptive authority has been a barrier to autonomy in advanced nursing practice. The ability to prescribe medications allows the APRN more flexibility in implementing holistic care for patients. Although great strides have been made legislatively to allow full prescriptive authority in each state, there continues to be inconsistency among states. To review or learn the prescriptive authority for APRNs in individual states, the reader is referred to the annual reviews conducted by the American Association of Nurse Practitioners, Linda Pearson, and/or Susanne Phillips. In addition, Pearson (2014) provides extensive information on regulation, titling, legislation, practice authority, advanced practice programs, and consumer rating for NP regulation.

Prescriptive authority can be granted in several ways. The greatest independence is in those states where APRNs have full practice authority and are allowed to prescribe medications, including controlled substances, independent of any required physician involvement. The first states to provide legislation granting prescriptive authority were Washington, Oregon, and Alaska during the 1970s. All states allow APRNs to prescribe medications, including controlled substances, but require some degree of physician collaboration or delegation or limit controlled substances (Phillips, 2014).

Another issue surrounding prescriptive authority is the language used in regulations and legislation. Some rules and regulations specify "nurse practitioner," excluding CNSs, CNMs, and CRNAs. Increasingly, legislation is written to reflect the expanded advanced nursing practice title. Terms that have been used include midlevel practitioner, midlevel provider, advanced practice nurse, and APRN. Terms such as *midlevel provider/practitioner* often refer to NPs, CNSs, and PAs. Active participation in the political process by professional nursing lobbyists and individuals has resulted in provider-neutral terminology for all APRNs.

Once legislation is passed, most laws go to an administrative rules committee comprised of legislators who develop rules for interpreting the law. Administrative rules committees often seek input from professionals, consumers, and parties affected by the law. It is extremely important for APRNs to be "at the table" during these discussions. Special interest groups can influence whether rules are broadly or literally interpreted. One such example is how states define collaboration or supervision in their administrative rules. With implementation of the APRN regulatory model and the recommendations of the IOM's *The Future of Nursing* report, it is hoped that most states will move toward full practice authority for all APRNs.

Other trends serve to restrict or limit prescriptive practice. These include a movement toward joint regulation (a joint board with representatives from pharmacy, medicine, and nursing); reluctance to grandfather in nurses with existing prescriptive authority; ignoring state boards of nursing actions by other governmental agencies; restricting drug utilization review boards to pharmacists and physicians; and reluctance by insurance companies to fill prescriptions written by APRNs. Inconsistencies among states related to prescriptive authority contribute to the frustration of APRNs whose authority to prescribe medications is called into question.

In 1991, the U.S. Drug Enforcement Administration (DEA) proposed rules for affiliated practitioners (e.g., NPs, PAs) that would have imposed restrictive regulations for APRNs that superseded state laws. The DEA rules did not acknowledge the existing prescriptive regulations in states. Nurses in independent practice would have been affected by the ruling. However, the DEA withdrew these proposed rules subsequent to huge protest from the nursing community. A second ruling entitled Definition and Registration of Mid-Level Practitioners was proposed in 1992 (*Federal Register*, 1992). The 1992 ruling is less restrictive regarding prescriptive authority for APRNs. DEA registration is required to prescribe controlled substances. The national provider identification number (NPI) is required on all noncontrolled substance prescriptions. APNs can apply for DEA registration online at www.deadiversion.usdoj.gov, and NPI numbers can be obtained or accessed online at https://nppes.cms.hhs.gov. A practitioner prescribing manual is also available through the DEA (2014) at www.deadiversion.usdoj.gov/pubs/manuals/pract/pract_manual012508.pdf.

Drug Utilization Review programs mandated by the Omnibus Budget Reconciliation Act of 1990, effective January 1, 1993, were designed to reduce fraud, abuse, overuse, or unnecessary care among physicians, pharmacists, and patients. Currently, no state specifically provides for the inclusion of nurses or other health care members on the review program board. The exclusion of APRNs from these boards is a concern because prescriptive practice by APRNs will be evaluated by individuals lacking a nursing perspective.

Prescriptive authority of medications, including controlled substances, is not only a privilege; it is a responsibility that APRNs cannot take lightly. The provider is fully responsible for understanding the regulatory parameters for prescribing these drugs. Ongoing pharmacotherapeutics education is essential in safe prescribing practices. All prescribers should avoid any prescribing practices that would put their prescriptive privileges at risk.

LIABILITY

As APRNs assume more autonomy and independence, liability issues arise. It is critical that APRNs work within their scope of practice; maintain certification, including continuing education requirements; and maintain adequate liability coverage.

To practice within their scope of practice, APRNs must comply with state regulatory statutes. Laws are interpreted through administrative rules, as discussed previously. The interpretation of each specific law will determine whether APRNs are practicing within their scope of practice.

An example of the importance of administrative rules in interpreting state statutes is illustrated in the following case. A pediatric NP became interested in pain management and was hired by a pain clinic. After working there for some time, it was requested that she obtain prescriptive authority to allow her to prescribe pain medication, including controlled substances for all age groups. Based on the administrative rule that allows prescription orders appropriate to the APRN's area of competence as established by education, training, or experience, the board of nursing deemed the NP eligible to obtain prescriptive privileges because of her experience in the pain clinic. However, the NP believed that it was in her best interest to return to school and obtain post-master's certification as an adult NP to expand her scope of practice to include all the populations to which she provided care.

There has been an increase in malpractice claims filed against APRNs in recent years, because more APRNs are employed than ever before. Some people believe that attorneys often name anyone associated with the case as a way to increase their client's award or recovery costs (Buppert, 2015). Overall, however, APRNs—particularly NPs— have had fewer adverse claims against them compared with doctors of osteopathy (DOs) or physicians (MDs). Pearson (2014) performs an annual analysis to further examine adverse actions taken against NPs. She uses data from the National Practitioner Data Bank (NPDB) and the Healthcare Integrity and Protection Data Bank (HIPDB) to evaluate the number of accumulated malpractice actions, regulatory or civil judgments, and criminal convictions submitted by NPs, DOs, and MDs. Pearson evaluates each state, lists actions against NPs, and calculates the ratio between NPs compared with DOs and MDs. In 2014, Vermont boasted the best ratio, 1:545; and Oklahoma the worst, 1:10 (Pearson, 2014).

Another retrospective study of the NPDB examined anesthesia-related malpractice payments from 2004 to 2010. There were 369 anesthesia-related malpractice payments associated with CRNAs. The most common complaints were related to improper performance, problem with intubation, or failure to monitor (Jordan, Ouraishi, & Liao, 2013).

One question that many APRNs raise is whether they should carry their own malpractice insurance in addition to their employer's liability coverage. Some legal experts recommend that APRNs do so because there may often be a conflict of interest within a given claim. The other side of the argument is that APRNs may be named in a claim specifically because they do carry their own insurance (Wright, 2004). Buppert (2008) advises APRNs who are thinking about how much liability insurance to carry to buy "as much as you can get and afford" (p. 406).

Malpractice occurs when an APRN fails to "exercise that degree of skill and learning commonly applied by the average prudent, reputable member of the profession" whereas negligence is "predominant legal theory of malpractice liability" (Buppert, 2015, p. 272). Most malpractice claims against APRNs are related to missed diagnosis, failure to refer, mishandling of medicine, or failure to provide preventive care or routine screening (Buppert, 2015). Negligence can occur when an APRN fails to follow up with a patient appropriately, refer the patient when necessary, disclose information to a patient, or provide appropriate care. This would include a failure to monitor or observe a patient's health status; a failure to diagnose or a delayed diagnosis; a failure to perform procedures safely and competently; a failure to treat a patient appropriately, including prescribing and minimally administering medications; a failure to communicate patient information in a timely manner; a failure to protect a patient from avoidable injuries; and/or a failure to practice within the scope of the APRN's nursing education and position description. For further in-depth discussion and information related to liability and legal issues, the reader is referred to Buppert's excellent legal reference (2015).

APRNs must become familiar with legal terminology to avoid committing unintentional acts of negligence. Table 10.2 briefly outlines terms that are often unfamiliar. The term *intentional tort*, meaning that an APRN commits an act that brings about an intended result, may be confusing for the APRN. Intentional torts can include assault and battery (forcing an individual to take a medication), invasion of privacy (breaking confidentiality), and defamation (slander or libel), among others (Wright, 2004).

Malpractice is covered under tort law. Klutz (2004) has called for state or federal tort reform to decrease the skyrocketing cost of malpractice insurance premiums. States that have set caps on liability awards have not experienced the insurance crisis. One of the contributing factors to high insurance premiums is that some insurance companies underwrite the cost of malpractice policies in investments, and when the stock market is unstable, insurance companies either fail or increase the cost of their premiums significantly. Once a rare occurrence, providers are increasingly leaving their practices due to the high cost of insurance premiums. Another result of increased malpractice litigation is the tendency to practice defensive medicine rather than use evidence-based practice

TABLE 10.2 Legal Terminology

Tort	An injury or wrongdoing
Tort liability	The right of an injured individual to be made whole again
Intentional tort	An individual (APRN) commits an act with intent to bring about the result in question
Negligence	A failure to fulfill a responsibility that subsequently results in injury to an individual

guidelines. Defensive practices—for example, ordering unnecessary tests to rule out all possible diagnoses—only contribute to increasing health care costs (Klutz, 2004).

APRNs should learn what type of insurance policy best fits their needs. The two most common types of insurance available are "occurrence" and "claims made." An occurrence policy covers an APRN for any incident that occurs during the time insured. For example, an APRN is covered following employment for any claims that occur during the employment period. A claims policy covers the APRN only during the time that the policy is in effect (Wright, 2004). For example, a claim made after employment has ended is not covered by this type of policy. APRNs who change employment should purchase a "tail" policy to cover any claims that occur after the APRN has left that place of employment.

APRNs can protect themselves from potential malpractice claims in several ways. First and foremost, APRNs must practice within their scope of practice and the legal scope as determined by their individual state. Second, APRNs should carry professional liability insurance either through their employer, through personal professional liability insurance, or both. Arguments can be made both ways for whether an APRN should carry both employment and personal liability insurance. For example, if the APRN carries only professional liability insurance through the employer, the policy may not cover private duty, volunteer, or off-duty incidents. Buppert (2006) advises that APRNs read the policy very closely to answer these coverage questions before they arise and recommends that they carry at least $1 million per occurrence in coverage.

An APRN can take several preventive measures to avoid legal or malpractice claims. The importance of thorough and accurate documentation cannot be overemphasized. If ethical or legal issues arise, the APRN should report concerns to the proper persons or authorities. It is also important that APRNs know the roles and responsibilities within their scope of practice. Negligence or malpractice can occur if the APRN does not keep current on standards of practice or treatments. Also, a good patient–client relationship is important. APRNs must also delegate appropriately to avoid claims of negligence. Buppert (2008) offers the following suggestions to avoid malpractice claims:

- Do not offer services or advice to individuals outside of the clinical practice setting.
- Do not offer advice, diagnosis, or treatment outside your scope of practice or expertise.
- Base diagnosis and therapy on evidence-based practice guidelines (if available).
- Refer the patient if the differential diagnoses includes one with high mortality that has not been ruled out.
- Conduct all standard of care screening tests for patient's age, gender, or risk factors and follow through if results are positive.
- Document your actions and process of medical decision making.
- Leave the work setting if unable to practice safely in current environment.
- Purchase your own "occurrence" malpractice insurance policy. (p. 406)

In summary, legal issues related to negligence and malpractice can be a cause of concern and stress for health care providers, including APRNs. APRNs should take preventive measures to limit the risk of having claims filed against them.

PRACTICE ISSUES

There are many practice issues that can be discussed; some have definitive answers, and some do not. Most practice issues have safety, legal, or ethical implications. Some practice issues may resolve as new legislation is passed or new policy is put in place, but other issues may persist and new practice issues will emerge. This section discusses selected practice issues related to innovative technology, billing and reimbursement, blurred practice boundaries, and professional accountability. There are many gray areas in advanced nursing practice; therefore, knowing your legal responsibility, scope of practice, and prescriptive authority is extremely important.

Innovative Health Technology

As health care technology grows exponentially, several issues arise. First, with advancement in treatment modalities, many patients are surviving beyond their prognostic time frames. As these patients survive longer, unanticipated consequences of their treatment may arise. For example, Zakak (2009) raises the possibility of fertility issues in childhood cancer survivors. Therapies used to treat the cancers may have been successful in terms of curing or remitting the cancer but may have eliminated the patient's ability to conceive and later achieve the developmental milestone of parenthood. Anticipating consequences of therapies is essential in providing informed consent and in allowing patients to choose alternative treatments.

Another issue related to innovative technology is the choice of test that is needed to diagnose or follow up on a condition. Perhaps the clinical practice guideline suggests a computed tomography (CT) scan for evaluation of a mass, but a newer technology is developed that may provide better diagnostic information. However, the new technology is much more expensive and puts the patient at a greater radiation risk. Innovative technology might also allow a parent to choose not to treat a child's condition or terminate a pregnancy based on the probability that the child or fetus would not survive (Williams, 2006). Elderly patients may choose not to undergo expensive diagnostic tests or treatment because they have lived a healthy, productive life and are prepared for death. APRNs will face many similar situations that conflict with personal ethical beliefs and must determine whether to support the patient's choice based on the ethical, regulatory, and legal boundaries of their practice.

Off-label use of pharmacologic agents is another example in which the original research submitted to the U.S. Food and Drug Administration (FDA) was for one indication but, through its use, another indication arose. The manufacturer often decides not to go through the process of gaining FDA approval for a second indication. If APRNs were to prescribe the medication for a use other than the approved indication, would prescribing that medication put them at risk for malpractice, even though the use of that medication for the nonapproved indication is common among health care providers?

Billing and Reimbursement Issues

Accurate billing and coding is difficult to learn, but it is extremely important to ensure that the APRN obtains the appropriate reimbursement and does not overbill or underbill the patient. Although APRNs historically underbill for services provided, both underbilling and overbilling are considered fraud. Chapter 11 provides an excellent overview of the reimbursement process, billing, and coding. Ongoing review and continuing education on reimbursement cannot be overemphasized. Some practice issues related to billing and reimbursement arise from shared billing practices or pressure from organizations to bill incident-to for higher reimbursement.

Along the lines of reimbursement is the choice of pharmacologic agents. Pharmacy formularies adopted by insurance companies may insist on a certain pharmacologic agent for a certain diagnostic code. That particular drug may not be the most beneficial for the patient. Prior authorizations can be requested, but they are denied if the generic or formulary equivalent has not been tried for a certain amount of time. If the medication is approved, it is often approved at a higher copay for the patient. The time spent obtaining approval or the time the patient has to spend trying and failing an alternative agent diminishes the quality of care.

Blurred Boundaries

APRNs may be placed in situations in which there is not a clear delineation of role. The APRN needs to feel comfortable when making any decision or engaging in any procedure. For example, an NP whose practice is limited to adults provides care for a 32-year-old mother. The mother asks the NP to assume care for her 10-year-old daughter because she has confidence in the NP and the closest provider for the daughter is 30 miles away. You might argue that when adult-care NPs care for 10-year-olds, they are clearly out of their scope of practice. However, if that 10-year-old were in a life-threatening situation, would the NP be liable for not initiating care?

APRNs may encounter other situations that stretch the limits of educational preparation or that are not clearly defined within the regulatory realm. Hudspeth (2007) discusses balancing the need for adequate educational preparation with the needs of behavior health services. For example, an adult NP or a clinical nurse specialist may have a large percentage of patients with behavior health issues. APRNs will need to determine whether they have adequate preparation to care for these patients or if more education and/or certification is required. Brekken and Sheets (2008) address balancing the need to provide adequate pain management with following regulatory guidelines for controlled substances. A recent random clinical trial demonstrated improved outcomes with providing vocational case management services in primary care to support patients with musculoskeletal problems (Bishop et al., 2014). The cost versus benefit of adding such services is often a difficult decision for providers and managers.

Professional Accountability

APRNs are continually faced with situations that have implications for accountability. Snyder (2005) describes the accountability that occurs when there is failure to accurately assess diminished driving skills in patients with dementia that results in premature or delayed driving cessation. Inaccurate assessment of driving skills can have adverse effects on the patient, family, and on public safety. For example, if a patient is seen by an APRN for evaluation of progressive visual loss and the APRN does not address driving skills, is the APRN accountable or liable for injuries that occur if that patient is involved in a motor vehicle accident following that evaluation?

Another area of accountability relates to identifying incompetence or fraud. If APRNs encounter fraud or an unethical situation, they are faced with "blowing the whistle" or choosing not to take action (Hannigan, 2006). The APRN is responsible for ensuring safe, competent care.

Accountability issues are not limited to advanced nursing practice in the United States. Wiseman (2007) examines accountability of APRNs as they expand their role within the United Kingdom. As new roles develop, it is important to examine them closely within a framework that takes education, legal, and ethical issues into account. This often provides a challenge in health care systems that are beginning to incorporate advanced nursing practice.

The scenarios discussed in this section are laden with ethical, fiscal, and legal implications. The APRN must be adequately prepared to address these issues and have a solid ethical, legal, and professional foundation to make appropriate decisions for the protection and safety of the public.

SUMMARY

This chapter addresses professional issues that influence advanced nursing practice. APRNs may encounter situations that place them at risk for liability claims or regulatory misconduct. It is the responsibility of APRNs to have a full sense of their scope of practice, maintain adequate liability coverage, and practice within the legal authority for their state. Every APRN must understand his or her scope of practice, know the regulations in his or her state, and maintain appropriate certifications to demonstrate competence as an entry-level APRN. As the APRN regulatory model is implemented and titling of APRNs becomes more consistent, there will be less confusion regarding their roles in whatever settings they choose to practice. As more states implement full practice authority for APRNs, they will move from nonlicensed independent practitioners to licensed independent practitioners within health care organizations.

REFERENCES

American Association of Critical-Care Nurses Certification Corporation. (2014). Retrieved from http://www.aacn.org/dm/mainpages/certificationhome.aspx

American Association of Nurse Practitioners. (2011). *AANP comments on the IOM report The future of nursing: Leading change, advancing health.*

American Association of Nurse Practitioners. (2014). 2014 nurse practitioner state practice environment. Retrieved from http://www.aanp.org/legislation-regulation/state-legislation-regulation/state-practice-environment

American Association of Nurse Practitioners Certification Corporation Program. (2014). Retrieved from http://aanpcertification.org

American Nurses Association. (2013). *Title "nurse" protection.* Retrieved from http://www.nursingworld.org/MainMenuCategories/Policy-Advocacy/State/Legislative-Agenda-Reports/State-TitleNurse

American Association of Colleges of Nursing. (2006). *The essentials of doctoral education for advanced practice nurses.* Washington DC: Author.

American Association of Colleges of Nursing. (2009). *Update on the new comprehensive care certification exam.* Retrieved from http://www.aacn.nche.edu/DNP/pdf/CCExamStatement.pdf

American Midwifery Certification Board. (2014). Retrieved from http://www.amcbmidwife.org

American Nurses Credentialing Center. (2014). Retrieved from http://www.nursecredentialing.org

APRN Consensus Workgroup and APRN Joint Dialogue Group. (2008). *Consensus model for APRN regulation: Licensure, accreditation, certification and education.* Retrieved from http://www.aacn.nche.edu/Education/pdl/APRNReport.pdf

Bishop, A., Wynne-Jones, G., Lawton, S. A., van der Windt, D., Main, C., Sowden, G., . . . Forster, N. C. (2014). Rationale, design and methods of the study of work and pain (SWAP): A cluster randomised controlled trial testing the addition of a vocational advice service to best current primary care for patients with musculoskeletal pain. *BMC Musculoskeletal Disorders, 15*(1), 232.

Brekken, S. A., & Sheets, S. V. (2008). Pain management: A regulatory issue. *Nursing Administration Quarterly, 32*(4), 288–295.

Buppert, C. (2006). Questions and answers on malpractice insurance for nurse practitioners. *Medscape.* Retrieved from http://www.medscape.com/viewarticle/520660.

Buppert, C. (2008). Frequently asked questions and answers about malpractice insurance. *Dermatology Nursing, 20*(5), 405–406.

Buppert, C. (2015). *Nurse practitioners business practice and legal guide* (5th ed.). Burlington, MA: Jones & Bartlett Learning.

Cooper E. (1998). Credentialing and privileging nurse-midwives. *Journal of Nursing Care Quality, 12*(4), 30–35.

Duffy, M. (2008). Clinical nurse specialists gain title protection in Pennsylvania. *Clinical Nurse Specialist, 22*(1), 41–43.

Federal Register. (1992). Definition and registration of mid-level practitioners 21 C.F.R. Parts 1301 and 1304. *Federal Register, 57*(146), 33465.

Hannigan, N. S. (2006). Blowing the whistle on health care fraud: Should I? *Journal of the American Academy of Nurse Practitioners, 18*(11), 512–517.

Hudspeth, R. (2007). Balancing need, preparation and scope of practice: Issues impacting behavioral health services by advanced practice registered nurses. *Nursing Administration Quarterly, 31*(3), 264–265.

Institute of Medicine. (2011). *The future of nursing: Leading change, advancing health.* Washington, DC: National Academies Press.

Joint Commission on Accreditation of Health Care Organizations. (2012). *Comprehensive accreditation manual for hospitals: The official handbook (CAMH).* Oakbrook Terrace, IL: Joint Commission Resources.

Jordan, L. M., Ouraishi, J. A., & Liao, J. (2013). The national practitioner data bank and CRNA anesthesia-related malpractice payments. *American Association of Nurse Anesthetists Journal, 81*(3), 178–182.

Klein, C. A. (2003). The scoop on credentialing. *Nurse Practitioner, 28*(12), 54.

Klutz, D. L. (2004). Tort reform: An issue for nurse practitioners. *Journal of the American Academy of Nurse Practitioners, 16*(2), 70–75.

National Association of Clinical Nurse Specialists. (2004). Model rules and regulations for CNS title protection and scope of practice. *Clinical Nurse Specialist, 18*(4), 178–179.

National Association of Clinical Nurse Specialists. (2009). *Core practice doctorate clinical nurse specialist (CNS) Competencies.* Harrisburg, PA: Author.

National Board of Certification and Recertification for Nurse Anesthetists. (2014). Retrieved from http://www.nbcrna.com/Pages/default.aspx

National Certification Corporation. (2014). Retrieved from https://www.nccwebsite.org

National Council of State Boards of Nursing. (2014). *Nurse licensure compact.* Retrieved from https://www.ncsbn.org/nlc.htm.

National Organization of Nurse Practitioner Faculties. (2012a). *Nurse Practitioner Core Competencies.* Washington, DC: Author. Retrieved from http://c.ymcdn.com/sites/www.nonpf.org/resource/resmgr/competencies/npcorecompetenciesfinal2012.pdf

National Organization of Nurse Practitioner Faculties. (2012b). *Criteria for evaluation of nurse practitioner programs.* Washington, DC: Author. Retrieved from http://c.ymcdn.com/sites/www.nonpf.org/resource/resmgr/docs/ntfe-valcriteria2012final.pdf

Nurse Licensure Compact Administrators. (2012). APRN Licensure Compact. Retrieved from http://www.ncsbn.org/APRN_Compact_hx_timeline_April_2012_(2).pdf

Nurse Practitioner Roundtable. (2008). *Nurse practitioner DNP education, certification and titling: A unified statement.* Washington DC: Author.

Oncology Nursing Certification Corporation. (2014). Retrieved from http://www.oncc.org

Orthopaedic Nurses Certification Board. (2014). Retrieved from http://oncb.org/apn-certification

Patient Protection and Affordable Care Act. (2010). PL 111-148. Retrieved from http://housedocs.house.gov/energycommerce/ppacacon.pdf

Pearson, L. J. (2009). The Pearson Report. *The American Journal for Nurse Practitioners, 13*(2), 4–82.

Pearson, L. J. (2014). *2014 Pearson Report.* Burlington, MA: Jones & Bartlett Learning.

Pediatric Nursing Certification Board. (2014). Retrieved from http://www.pncb.org/ptistore/control/index

Phillips, S. J. (2014). 26th annual legislative update: Progress for APRN authority to practice. *The Nurse Practitioner, 39*(1), 29–52.

Smolenski, M. C. (2002). *Playing the credentials game.* Retrieved from http://nursingworld.org/FunctionalMenuCategories/AboutANA/Leadership-Governance/NewCNPE/CNPEMembersOnly/CNPEReferenceDocuments/PlayingtheCredentialsGame.pdf

Snyder, C.H. (2005). Dementia and driving: Autonomy versus safety. *Journal of the American Academy of Nurse Practitioners, 17*(10), 393–402.

Williams, C. (2006). Dilemmas in fetal medicine: Premature application of technology or responding to women's choice. *Sociology of Health and Illness, 28*(1), 1–20.

Wiseman, H. (2007). Advanced nursing practice—the influences and accountabilities. *British Journal of Nursing, 16*(3), 167–173.

Wright, W.L. (2004, September–October). *Liability and malpractice: Everything the NP needs to know.* Presentation given at the National Conference of Gerontological Nurse Practitioners. Phoenix, AZ: Author.

Zakak, N. N. (2009). Fertility issues of childhood cancer survivors: The role of the pediatric nurse practitioner in fertility preservation. *Journal of Pediatric Oncology Nursing, 26*(1), 48–59.

Cheri Friedrich and Linda L. Lindeke

11

REIMBURSEMENT REALITIES FOR THE APRN

Health care is changing, and the advanced practice registered nurses (APRNs) of today are playing meaningful roles in changing systems as they care for individuals and populations. One recent national change is the implementation of the Patient Protection and Affordable Care Act (ACA) that went into effect in 2013 with three primary goals: to improve access, to decrease cost, and to ultimately shift the focus from treatment to prevention, commonly called the Triple Aim. The focus of the Triple Aim is to improve care experiences for individuals, improve health of populations, and lower costs. Health care cost containment is critical yet hard to achieve without decreasing care quality. Factors such as the aging population's need for advanced treatment technologies, chronic diseases, obesity, and genetic advancements affect costs and are all areas where APRNs have practice and leadership opportunities if they understand reimbursement realities.

It is well documented that APRNs provide high-quality, cost-effective care (Newhouse et al., 2011). To ensure that APRN care is recognized, APRN care must to be visible through provider-specific coding and documentation. As reimbursement trends are expected to change from fee-for-service to outcome-based reimbursement, APRNs need to be informed and engaged in reimbursement processes and issues. This engagement should include negotiating contracts, lobbying insurance companies for direct reimbursement, and maintaining strong relationships with clinic administrators and coders. APRNs must understand the changing economics of health care.

ACCESS, QUALITY, AND COST

Health care costs are expected to rise as the population ages, expensive technologies develop, and the prevalence of chronic illness rises (Deloitte, 2014). Employers continue to raise employees' cost sharing for health care by increasing the deductible amounts and copayments for care. Health care spending in 2012 rose more than 3% from 2009 to $2.8 trillion, or $8,233 per person in the United States (Martin, Hartman, Whittle, Catlin, & the National Health Expenditure Accounts Team, 2014). In 2013, those with employer-sponsored health insurance paid an average of $16,351 for family coverage, with additional out-of-pocket expenses for copayments, medications, and other health-related costs (Kaiser Family Foundation, 2013).

Although health care costs continue to increase worldwide, the American health care system remains the most expensive in the world. For example, health care spending exceeded 17% of the United States' gross domestic product (GDP) in 2012, far more than in any other developed country (Martin et al., 2014). This rate is in striking contrast to that of other countries providing a similar quality of health care. For instance, Canada spent 11.2% of its 2013 GDP on health care (Canadian Institute for Health Information, 2013). Factors contributing to higher U.S. costs include a payment system that rewards doing more as opposed to being efficient, an aging U.S. population, and a focus on advancing technologies (Appleby, 2012).

Health care reform efforts are focusing on cost containment, disease prevention, and evidence-based practice as means to address the economic realities. However, there is no "quick fix" for long-standing issues related to health care access, quality, and cost-effectiveness. Health care is costing patients, employers, and payers more each year and has become a very closely watched economic indicator. APRNs must be well informed about the context and specifics of reimbursement to be successful in practice. Federal and state actions influence health care reimbursement in many ways, such as by regulating health care systems, by supporting research, and particularly by financing and delivering health care services. Reimbursement politics are played out in Congress, in state legislatures, and within county governments. Political processes may also take place at APRN work sites as employment agreements and organizational policies are negotiated. APRNs must understand the various health care forces and players, particularly issues related to access, quality, and cost.

Access to care is complex in the United States and is directly related to cost issues. In 2012, about 48 million individuals (15.4%) in the United States lacked insurance coverage and access to health care (U.S. Census Bureau, 2013). To address this national issue of health care access the ACA was signed into law by President Obama on March 23, 2010. The primary goals of the ACA are to expand health coverage, lower health care costs, and shift focus from treatment to prevention (U.S. Department of Health and Human Services [DHHS], 2013). It is expected that with the implementation of the ACA, the numbers of those with insurance will increase.

Approximately 63.9% of individuals with insurance in 2012 were covered by private insurance plans (U.S. Census Bureau, 2013). Americans with insurance continue to have concerns because copayments are increasing and benefits are sometimes limited. Many health plans require referrals and prior authorizations for the more costly health care components.

In addition, some health plans limit patients to seeing only the providers on their salaried staff (staff-model health maintenance organizations, or HMOs) or a contracted list of specialists and agencies (preferred provider organizations, or PPOs). Triage or tiering of clients according to the types and price of coverage offered by employer plans and insurance carriers is a way of limiting health care services. HMOs, self-insured companies, and small businesses may have high deductibles, copayments, and prior authorization procedures that limit choices of providers, procedures, and referrals. Another care model recently introduced along with the implementation of the ACA is that of accountable care organizations (ACOs). ACOs are groups of health care providers and hospitals that come together to give high-quality care to patients (Centers for Medicare & Medicaid Services [CMS], 2013). The goal of this coordinated care is to reduce duplication of services, thereby reducing costs (CMS, 2013).

Many programs attempt to monitor and improve health care quality. One example is the Agency for Healthcare Research and Quality (AHRQ), a federal agency devoted to tracking trends, providing model programs, and researching outcomes. Partnerships of public and private agencies, such as the program Consumer Assessment of Healthcare Providers and Systems (CAHPS), work together to assess care, report system performance, and recommend or fund improvement efforts. A myriad of reports of care outcomes of hospitals, nursing homes, and individual providers is available for comparison. The Commonwealth Fund, the Institute of Medicine [IOM], the Robert Wood Johnson Foundation, the National Committee for Quality Improvement, and National Quality Forum are just a few of the organizations very active in quality improvement efforts. Nurses working toward care improvement are active in all those entities as well as in many professional nursing organizations. APRNs can contribute to these efforts by membership and leadership in these organizations. This active engagement will ensure that APRNs stay abreast of current quality improvement efforts in health care, which can have a direct effect on reimbursement.

U.S. REIMBURSEMENT TRENDS

The U.S. health care delivery system hardly resembles the system in place just a decade ago, and a whole new language has developed that APRNs must understand (Table 11.1). The U.S. health care industry has adopted the bottom line–oriented, profit–loss mentality of the business world, now with the overlay of the law of the land (ACA) as it is being interpreted in each state. As this complexity pervades American health care, APRNs can offer ways of ensuring access and quality of care while keeping costs reasonable for consumers.

Capitated systems (that replace fee-for-service payments) are common in most states. Payers contract with provider groups to pay a per-member amount to cover the cost of member health care services over a certain time period. Services are increasingly delivered in outpatient clinics that

TABLE 11.1 Reimbursement Vocabulary

TERMINOLOGY	DEFINITION
Actual charge	The amount of money a provider charges for a particular service, which may be more than the amount payers approve
Additional benefits	Health care services not covered by Medicare; additional benefits subject to cost sharing by plan enrollees
Adjusted community rating	Premium rates based on regional differences in health care costs; leads to great regional differences in Medicare payment rates to providers
Advanced beneficiary notice (ABN)	A notice that a provider must have Medicare beneficiaries sign when providing a service that Medicare does not consider medically necessary; if the patient does not get an ABN to sign before the service is provided and Medicare does not pay for it, the patient does not have to pay for the service
Affiliated provider	A health care provider or facility that is paid by a health plan to give service to plan members (i.e., a credentialed provider)
Ancillary services	Professional services by a hospital or other inpatient facility (e.g., x-rays, drugs, laboratory services)
Appeal	A formal complaint made to a health plan
Approved amount (or approved charge)	The fee a payer sets as reasonable for a covered service (may be less than the amount charged by the provider)
Balance billing	A situation in which private fee-for-service providers can charge and bill Medicare patients 15% more than the plan's payment
Beneficiary	The name for a person who has health insurance through the Medicare or Medicaid program
Capitation	A per-member amount paid to providers to cover the cost of member health care services for a certain time period
Carrier	A private company that has a contract with Medicare to pay Medicare Part B bills

(continued)

TABLE 11.1 Reimbursement Vocabulary *(continued)*

TERMINOLOGY	DEFINITION
Catastrophic limit	The highest amount of money patients have to pay out of pocket during a certain time period for certain charges
Centers for Medicare & Medicaid Services (CMS)	Federal agency that runs Medicare and works with the states to run Medicaid programs
Consolidated Omnibus Budget Reconciliation Act (COBRA)	A law that makes an employer continue to cover an employee for a period of time after spousal death, job loss, divorce, or hours/benefits reduction; typically requires payment of both employee and employer shares of the premium
Coordination of benefits	Process in which two or more health plans share costs of a claim
Cost sharing	The cost for medical care that patients pay (copayment, coinsurance, deductible)
Covered benefit	A service that is paid for (partially or fully) by a health plan
Diagnosis-related group (DRG)	A payment system begun in 1983 to pay hospitals for health care based on patients' diagnosis, age, gender, and complications; DRGs affect length of hospital stay
Durable medical equipment/goods	Reusable equipment that is ordered for use in the home (e.g., walkers) and paid for under Medicare
Facilities charge	A charge billed to a health plan or provider for the facility in which the service was received; results in two bills (provider bill and facility bill)
Fiscal intermediary	A private company that contracts with Medicare to pay Part A and some Part B bills; located in various regions of the United States
Fraud and abuse	Fraud: to purposely bill for services that were never given or to bill for a service at a higher reimbursement rate than the service produced
	Abuse: payment for items or services that are billed by mistake

(continued)

TABLE 11.1 Reimbursement Vocabulary *(continued)*

TERMINOLOGY	DEFINITION
Health maintenance organization (HMO)/network	A health plan that contracts with group practices of providers to give services in one or more locations
Managed care plan with point-of-service (POS) option	A managed care health plan that lets patients use providers and hospitals outside the plan for an additional cost
Medically necessary services	Services deemed by Medicare to be proper and needed for a medical diagnosis or specific treatment
Medical savings account (MSA)	A Medicare health plan option made up of two parts: (a) Medicare MSA Health Insurance Policy (has a high deductible) and (b) special savings account in which Medicare deposits money to help patients pay their own medical bills
Preferred provider organization (PPO)	A managed care plan in which hospitals and providers belong to a network and contract together with payers/employers to provide services at predetermined rates
Prior authorization	Managed care organization (MCO) approval that is necessary before receiving care from providers who are out of the PPO or not on the staff list (can be verbal or is a written form from the MCO)
Referral	A written document that must be received by a provider before giving care to a health plan beneficiary
Resource-based relative value scale (RBRVS)	A Medicare fee schedule established in 1989 to reimburse providers based on relative work value units (RVUs)

contract with payers for coverage of client groups. Hospital stays (regulated by federally administered diagnostic-related group [DRG] regulations) have been shortened because of the cost, and patients are discharged earlier and sicker than in the past. The amount of health care delivered in outpatient settings continues to grow, likely as a result of health care legislation (Premier, Inc., 2013). Home care services may or may not be available upon discharge, often putting burdens on families and communities to provide care that used to occur in hospitals. Medicare regulations have become more complex, and employer-paid health care benefits, not surprisingly, have become a very contentious issue in labor negotiations.

Prescription drug use has increased, partly due to direct-to-consumer advertising that urges patients to contact their health care providers for the latest "miracle" drug. In an attempt to provide medications while controlling costs, the federal government implemented a voluntary program called Part D of Medicare in 2006 to subsidize prescribed medications for those covered by Medicare who apply for this special program. Part D is a very complex program that is a public–private partnership; it offers the elderly many different plan choices, and the application process is very complex. Opinions are mixed regarding its effectiveness; prescription drug costs continue to be a large part of Medicare expenditures and much lobbying occurs from the pharmaceutical industry. Americans spend about 40% more on pharmaceuticals compared with the next highest spender, Canada (Organization for Economic Co-operation and Development [OECD], 2013).

APRNs can now be directly reimbursed for their services and must be knowledgeable about trends, developments, and proposed payment systems and reimbursement schedules. APRNs will be successful in their practices to the extent that the value of their services is recognized by payers and employers and is equitably rewarded. APRNs must be cost-effective and must track their productivity within complex systems; however, the rapid pace of change in reimbursement legislation, policies, and procedures makes this a daunting task. APRNs can be cost-effective by offering high-quality care, working within health care home models, and managing chronic diseases.

APRNs were not always reimbursed for their services by public and private payers. A series of lobbying efforts at national and state levels occurred over time to make this possible. Federal and state legislation currently regulates APRN reimbursement. For example, the 1997 federal Balanced Budget Act (PL 105-33) provides direct Medicare reimbursement for nurse practitioners (NPs) and clinical nurse specialists (CNSs), effective January 1, 1998. Rules to implement this law were written by the CMS (formerly known as the Health Care Financing Administration [HCFA]) and were finalized in November 1998. These Medicare laws and rules influence the policies of nongovernmental payers, although there is a great deal of variability from state to state. APRNs must carefully monitor CMS activities to ensure that the policies continue to favor APRN reimbursement. The goal is to have provider-inclusive language, meaning that laws and policies do not specifically designate payment to physicians but use the term *providers*, which is inclusive of NPs and CNSs. Terminology in policy and law is an extremely important issue for APRN practice. Since January 2010, nurse-midwives are reimbursed by Medicare at 100% of the physician fee schedule, a major victory for that group of APRNs.

The Health Insurance Portability and Accountability Act (HIPAA), a law passed in 1996 (also sometimes called the Kassebaum–Kennedy law), began the practice of implementing provider-inclusive language in federal law and policy. It expanded health care coverage related to job loss or transfer and provided some patient protection by limiting ways that insurance companies could use preexisting medical conditions to deny health insurance coverage. Although HIPAA generally guarantees the right to renewal of health coverage, it did not supersede states' roles as the primary regulators of health insurance. It standardized health care billing and payment mechanisms across systems, a move that promised to reduce costs once it was fully implemented. As part of that standardization, stringent patient privacy regulations were also instituted. The anticipated cost and quality improvements from HIPAA have not yet been realized, although it has certainly had many positive results. Electronic health records (EHRs) have rapidly been introduced since HIPAA was passed, and there are predictions that in time EHRs will bring about cost savings and quality improvements.

There continues to be significant growth in retail-based health care, which debuted in the early 2000s. Retail-based clinics are called by many names, including convenient care clinics and in-store clinics. Their numbers increase yearly, and one study demonstrated a lower overall cost of health care (Sussman et al., 2014). Medical associations such as the American Academy of Pediatrics have openly stated that the use of retail-based clinics is an inappropriate choice for pediatric care (Laughlin, 2014). These clinics typically employ NPs and have given new visibility to APRN practice. They appear to offer consumers a good-quality alternative to care in ambulatory clinics and emergency departments for commonly occurring complaints.

Another model of care and reimbursement being introduced is termed *medical home*, sometimes referred to as health care home. This payment mechanism aims to reimburse designated practices for care coordination activities. The goal is to deliver community-based, continuous, comprehensive, culturally appropriate health care. Originally developed in pediatrics for children with chronic conditions, this model has been increasingly advocated for all primary care practices. A NP-delivered medical home demonstration project demonstrated feasibility, excellent care outcomes, and patient satisfaction (Palfrey et al., 2004). It has also been shown that this model of care will help meet the expected primary care physician shortage (Auerbach et al., 2013). It is essential that APRNs track medical/health care home models of care and reimbursement policies to ensure that they all contain provider-inclusive language. If not, this model of care will benefit physician practices and either exclude or make invisible the work of APRNs. The cost–benefit of the model is a matter of controversy (Friedberg, Schneider, Rosenthal, Volpp, & Werner, 2014).

Pay-for-performance (also called P4P) is another health care trend that APRNs must carefully track and use to their best advantage. Reimbursement is linked to outcome measures by public and private payers, including the CMS. The goal is to provide incentives for quality care, a worthy aim. However, clinical performance is not easily measured given multifactorial patient outcomes, and P4P has had mixed reviews as a strategy to decrease costs and increase care quality (Chien, Eastman, Li, & Rosenthal, 2012).

REIMBURSEMENT STRUCTURES

Third-Party Payers

APRNs must understand many issues about health care regulation (Figure 11.1), including the relationships among entities that pay for and provide services. For example,

1. For-profit insurance companies known as "indemnity providers" (e.g., Aetna, Prudential)
2. Government payment programs (e.g., Medicare, Medicaid, Tricare/ CHAMPUS, the military health system)
3. Nonprofit corporations (e.g., BlueCross/BlueShield)
4. Self-insuring corporations or coalitions (e.g., union health care plans)

Although payer policies and procedures differ greatly, most are influenced by the CMS Medicare regulations that enact federal legislation. Payers pay fee-for-service bills, the traditional way that health care has been funded. More recently, they pay for health care delivered under service contracts with HMOs and PPOs; provider systems must compete and bid for those contracts, unions participate in the negotiations, and contracts are rebid every few years. Employers typically offer their employees a choice of approved health system plans with which they can contract. Other employers self-insure by directly contracting with provider networks for their employees' care. These competitive contracts are frequently renegotiated in response to rising health care costs. The federal and state interpretations

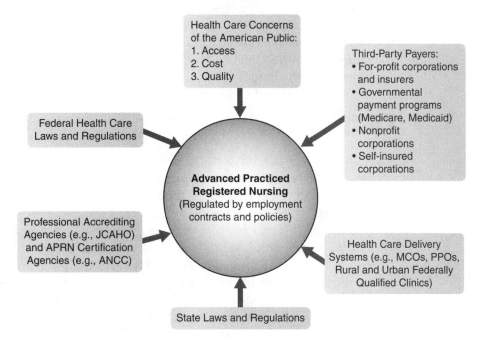

FIGURE 11.1 Reimbursement regulations for APRNs.

of the ACA through state insurance exchanges are dynamic, political, and an area of rapid change. Thus, health care finance is complex and volatile, and provider system costs are under constant review by payers, regulators, and the general public.

APRNs must be individually identified through payer credentialing to obtain reimbursement under their own names. Payer credentialing makes APRNs visible because their contributions can be specifically identified. Although many payers allow APRNs to bill individually, others refuse to reimburse APRN services, even in states with laws that mandate third-party APRN reimbursement. Medicare and Medicaid have moved many clients from fee-for-service payment systems into managed care reimbursement systems, in which case managed care organization (MCO) policies overlay CMS regulations. Therefore, APRNs must be cognizant of the many layers of reimbursement policies and procedures in their state, region, and organization.

Provider Systems

U.S. health care is delivered by many types of providers, each with its own policies, regulations, and practices affecting APRN reimbursement (refer to Table 11.1). These types of providers include:

1. MCOs
2. Managed care networks
3. HMOs
4. PPOs
5. Nurse-managed centers (NMCs)
6. Fee-for-service private practices
7. Home health care agencies
8. Public health agencies
9. Community health centers
10. Federally qualified health centers (FQHCs)
11. Migrant health clinics
12. Indian Health Board (IHB) clinics and hospitals
13. Rural health clinics (RHCs)
14. Retail-based clinics

Some types of FQHCs have policies that mandate APRNs be employed in order for the clinic to receive funding dollars. These regulations were passed based on federal studies that demonstrated APRN safety and cost-effectiveness (Newhouse et al., 2011). FQHCs credential APRNs for reimbursement and hospital privileges, provide them membership on provider panels, and validate their scope of practice. In most other systems, however, APRNs must negotiate for their place and power. APRNs must strive to obtain leadership positions in provider systems so that their contributions to patient outcomes are identified and valued by administrators and payers. Examples of leadership roles include performing administrative functions, participating on policy committees, and conducting research projects.

One way that APRNs have shown leadership and have achieved some level of autonomous practice is through the creation of nurse-managed health clinics (NMHCs). Often serving underinsured and uninsured populations with the associated limitations in funding, NMHCs have new visibility because of their being included in the ACA. Key to their success is the National Nursing Centers Consortium that promotes nurse-led care delivery. Successful NMHCs must have low administrative overhead costs, low fixed costs, and the ability to generate sufficient patient volume. There is increasing evidence that NMHCs offer quality, cost-effective care (Esperat, Hanson-Turton, Richardson, Debisette, & Rupinta, 2012). These outcomes have enabled NMHCs to obtain further grants to expand.

SELECTED ENTITIES AND PROVIDER SYSTEMS

Medicare

Medicare was established in 1965 as part of President Lyndon Johnson's Great Society initiative; its programs are primarily oriented to acute care for the elderly. The goal was to create a safety net for the nation's elderly, who had endured hardships in the world wars and the Depression during the 1930s. Medicare is a two-part, federally funded health care program; approximately 95% of the nation's elderly are enrolled in Medicare Part A. Part A provides hospital insurance that covers inpatient services, up to 100 days in a skilled nursing facility following hospitalization, and some home health care. Although there are no premiums for Part A Medicare, patient cost sharing is required. Cost sharing consists of an annual deductible as well as a payment percentage. Medicare does not cover eye examinations, medications, or long-term nursing care. Medicare Part B pays for physician visits, services and supplies, outpatient services, and home health care, all at rates set by the federal government.

The 1997 Balanced Budget Act (PL 105-33) allows Medicare reimbursement of services provided by NPs and CNSs if the services are reimbursable when provided by a physician and if the services are within the APRN scope of practice. The law removed all restrictions on the practice setting and permitted NPs and CNSs to submit fees for services rendered in hospitals, skilled nursing facilities, nursing homes, comprehensive outpatient rehabilitation facilities, community mental health centers, and rural health centers. Payments for NP and CNS services are discounted, compared with physician reimbursement, to 80% of the lesser of either the actual charge or 85% of the physician fee schedule amount.

NPs and CNSs billing under their own names must complete claim forms (called Form 1500) using their unique national provider identifier (NPI) numbers. These numbers are obtained from the CMS. Established as part of the 1997 legislation, this provider-specific tracking number is used by all systems for administrative and financial transactions.

Some APRNs do not submit claims under their own names, although this practice is typically discouraged by nursing leaders and professional organizations because it implements a system of physician supervision of

APRN practice. In fact, in many states APRNs are actively seeking independent practice. Medicare has a payment system for nursing and physician assistant services rendered under physician supervision called "incident-to" billing. Incident-to billing allows APRNs to bill under physician names for services that are provided as incident-to physician services. Payment then equals 100% of the physician fee schedule.

Although incident-to billing increases the revenue that APRNs can generate under current reimbursement rates, this billing practice raises red flags for fraud and abuse because it is governed by a tangle of federal regulations. APRN-billable activities must be integrated into daily physician practice. Incident-to billing is typically interpreted as implying direct supervision of APRNs by physicians. Supervising physicians must be physically present (although not in the patient examination room) at all times when APRNs are providing billable services, and physicians must perform all the initial patient visits and must establish the plans of care that APRNs then follow. Incident-to billing limits APRN autonomy and may also be very impractical. For example, if the physician leaves the building for lunch or vacation, the APRN could not bill incident-to for patients seen during that time frame. (Note: APRNs could, however, bill for this care under their own names if they were individually credentialed as providers with the payer; the practice would receive 85% of the physician fee if they did so, rather than the 100% incident-to payment.) Incident-to billing makes the contribution of APRNs to the fiscal output of organizations invisible. Billing under their own provider numbers (NPIs) is now strongly encouraged to increase productivity, to avoid the potential for billing fraud, and to permit full utilization of the legal APRN scope of practice.

Another Medicare billing practice incorporates a system that reimburses providers based on relative work value units (RVUs). Established in 1989, the Resource-Based Relative Value Scale (RBRVS) is a system aligned with Current Procedural Terminology (CPT) codes. Each CPT code is assigned a relative dollar value by the CMS based on practice research about work and practice expenses and professional liability insurance costs. Allowable service charges are determined annually by multiplying this RVU by a standard dollar amount conversion factor established by the CMS, based on the CMS's determination of regional cost variations (the geographic adjustment factor, GAF). The CMS publishes its RBRVS annually in the *Federal Register,* and practices then use the RBRVS to determine their fees.

The goal is to have a logical system of national fees set annually in relationship to actual costs and ongoing research. The result is that New York practitioners will have higher Medicare payments than practitioners in Iowa, for example, because it costs more to run a practice in New York than it does in Iowa. With support from the American Nurses Association (ANA), Sullivan-Marx and Maislin (2000) carried out a study comparing NP and family physician RVUs; there was no significant difference between the provider groups. The ANA continues to work with the American Medical Association's (AMA's) Health Professional Advisory Committee on reimbursement issues, including ways to fairly integrate NP billing practices into the RBRVS structure.

The 1997 Balanced Budget Act (BBA) (PL 105-33) provided both access and barriers to Medicare reimbursement for APRNs. During the rule-writing process for this act, the definition of *collaboration* was debated. The primary debate was about the impact of regulatory collaboration language on APRN practice in states where physician collaboration is not required and APRNs practice independently. This contentious issue continues to be closely monitored federally and in each state by APRN professional groups. Because state APRN practice laws by and large determine APRN practice, collaboration is a continuing and important issue for all APRNs. Most contentious was the language in the 1997 BBA that set APRN reimbursement at 85% of the physician rate; this was a compromise, and the bill would not have passed had APRNs not agreed to this requirement. This law still stands today and some believe this keeps health care costs down.

PL 105-33 regulations require that to be credentialed as Medicare providers NPs or CNSs must be master's-prepared registered nurses authorized to practice as NPs or CNSs by the state in which the services are furnished and be certified as NPs or CNSs by recognized national certifying bodies that have established standards. The requirements have been problematic for many CNSs because national certification has not been highly pursued by CNSs in the past, and in some cases no national certification examination exists to reflect their practice specialty. Although CNSs meet the master's degree requirement, certification continues to be an issue of debate within their ranks. CNSs in psychiatry and mental health are an exception because they have pursued reimbursement since the early 1970s and typically are nationally certified.

The rules also contained a time-limited "grandfather" clause to allow certified NPs without master's degrees to obtain provider numbers if they applied before January 1, 1999. In general, PL 105-33 was a victory for NPs and CNSs and met the intent of the law, which was to increase greater consumer access to NPs and CNSs. The legislation lifted some of the barriers to APRN reimbursement.

Medicaid

Medicaid expanded the 1965 federal Medicare system by providing funds for states to pay for health care of low-income groups. Federally supported and state administered, Medicaid covers costs of care for vulnerable groups through programs such as Aid to Families with Dependent Children (AFDC). Low-income elderly persons and some individuals with disabilities are also covered under this program. Medicaid is different from Medicare in that it is a vendor program, meaning that providers offering services to these individuals or families must accept the Medicaid reimbursement as full payment and cannot request copayments from patients. Because Medicaid payments are low (typically less than 50% of submitted bills), many providers (including dentists) restrict the number of Medicaid clients that they serve. Some states enroll Medicaid patients in MCOs by establishing contracts with MCOs in programs called prepaid medical assistance programs (PMAPs).

Section 6405 of the Omnibus Budget Reconciliation Act (OBRA 1989, PL 101-239) authorizes Medicaid payment for services of certified pediatric NPs and certified family NPs. Requirements necessary for reimbursement include possession of a current RN license in the state in which services are provided, and compliance with state APRN Medicaid reimbursement rates, which vary between 70 to 100% of physician fees, depending on the state.

Indemnity Insurers

Indemnity insurers are traditional insurance companies that pay for but do not deliver health care. They typically require an annual deductible that members self-pay; once this deductible is reached, the company will pay 80% of their members' health care costs on a per person, per procedure basis. Reimbursement rates are based on "usual and customary charges," which vary between regions and companies. If provider charges are more than the indemnity insurer allows, patients are responsible to pay the balance. Some indemnity insurance companies will pay for APRN services. APRNs can contact these companies to negotiate for recognition as reimbursable providers.

Managed Care Organizations (MCOs)

Capitated managed care developed rapidly in the 1990s in response to many economic and political forces. One factor was that the U.S. post–World War II baby boom generation began transitioning into middle age, increasing the number of health care consumers. This trend is projected to greatly increase costs, particularly for expensive, emerging technologies. MCOs sell health service packages to employers, individuals, or governmental agencies. Services are provided by the MCO panel of health care providers, who may or may not be MCO employees. APRNs can apply to become primary care providers (PCPs) on MCO provider panels, but this recognition has been slow in coming. MCOs reimburse PCPs using a fee-for-service, a capitated, or a fee-per-member basis, or by using a combination of fee-for-service and capitation.

MCOs are growing rapidly in the United States and are typically large, complex organizations. They stress the importance of health promotion, chronic care management, and patient education, and they typically provide their members with preventive services. They have so far been unable to demonstrate the expected cost savings. Some managed care strategies, such as employing economies of scale in purchasing, centralizing services such as emergency care, and developing systems for referrals and after-hours care have been cost-effective. However, administrative costs are very high.

Managed care is frequently interpreted as "managed costs." Efforts by CMS to uncover fraud in Medicare/Medicaid billing has added to the negative light in which many providers and consumers view MCOs. APRNs are also voicing their discomfort with MCO policies, particularly about the expectations that limit the length of patient visits to

10 to 15 minutes. RVU billing in MCOs is also a system that concerns APRNs who value time and care continuity with their clients. In high-production managed care models, APRNs may not be able to fulfill their responsibilities to prevent illness, coordinate care, and teach patients about their treatment plans.

CNM and CRNA Reimbursement

Certified nurse-midwives (CNMs) successfully obtain third-party reimbursement for their services based on their cost-effectiveness and high level of consumer satisfaction. Excellent research about CNM outcomes is compelling to payers seeking safe care at reasonable cost. In 1973, Washington was the first state to enact laws permitting CNM reimbursement by private and public benefit plans, which opened the door for other states to follow. The American College of Nurse-Midwives (ACNM) provides its members with excellent resources for billing, coding, and reimbursement through its website and publications. State laws and regulations must be in place to support CNM activities, including reimbursement. CNMs and all APRNs must be active in public policy formulation in order to establish favorable legal and regulatory practice climates.

Although few of their clients qualify for Medicare, CMS Medicare regulations restrict midwifery payments to 65% of the physician fee schedule. ACNM is currently lobbying to increase Medicare reimbursement to 97%, in part because Medicare regulations affect all payers in setting this precedent of establishing a widely used payment process. ACNM is also lobbying to have freestanding birth center facility costs covered in state Medicaid regulations. In some systems, CNMs work in incident-to relationships with physicians, which raises the potential for fraudulent claims if all the aspects of incident-to regulations are not strictly followed. Billing under their own names is strongly recommended for all APRNs, including CNMs, so that autonomous practice can provide the best possible care to clients and families.

Despite many difficulties, certified registered nurse anesthetists (CRNAs) have been successful in obtaining third-party reimbursement. OBRA granted CRNAs the right to be directly reimbursed for their services to Medicare recipients. CRNA services are also reimbursed directly by Medicaid and a number of commercial carriers. When both a CRNA and an anesthesiologist participate in the same case, the services of both anesthesia providers can be billed according to the extent of their involvement in the case. Independently billing CRNAs provide savings for government programs and for private payers because they typically charge less than their physician counterparts. Many complex issues regarding CRNA working relationships with physicians (including anesthesiologists) affect their work environments and billing practices. The American Association of Nurse Anesthetists offers CRNAs many reimbursement resources.

DOCUMENTATION AND CODING TO GAIN REIMBURSEMENT

Documentation is the key to reimbursement and must be sufficient to support the level of charge being requested. In addition, APRNs must understand their billing process and be able to use several types of diagnostic and procedure codes. One type of code is called the Health Care Common Procedure Coding System (HCPCS), which assigns a dollar amount to patient care activities. For example, there are HCPCS codes for immunization and wound suturing. Each patient visit is also coded using CPT codes, another part of the uniform coding language. The CPT coding directory covers all possible types of patient–provider interactions. It is owned and updated annually by the AMA and has been adopted by Medicare and other third-party payers (AMA, 2004).

A subgroup of CPT codes includes the Evaluation and Management Codes (E&M Codes), the CPT codes most used by APRNs (typically CPT codes 99201 through 99456). These five-digit codes are based on the levels of history taking and physical examination, complexity of decision making, counseling, and minutes of face-to-face time in each patient encounter. APRNs must distinguish between new patients and established patients in their choice of codes because new patients are reimbursed at a higher rate than established patients. A new patient is a patient who has not received professional services within the past 3 years from a provider in the same specialty in the same practice. Telephone communication, however, is considered a professional service.

In addition to assigning a CPT code on the standard claim forms (Form 1500), APRNs must select appropriate diagnostic codes from the *International Classification of Diseases, 10th Revision, Clinical Modification* (ICD-10). ICD-10 is based on the World Health Organization (WHO) disease classification. The 43rd World Health Assembly endorsed the ICD-10 in May 1990. ICD-10 took effect in the United States in October 2015 and is currently under revision, with an expected release date for ICD-11 in 2018 (WHO, 2015). ICD codes assign symptoms and diseases numeric codes: characters 1 to 3, categories 4 to 6 (etiology, anatomical site, and severity, respectively), and 7 extensions (injuries, fractures, etc.) (CMS, 2014).

Documentation begins with a concise statement of the chief complaint, usually stated in the patient's own words in the medical history (Table 11.2). The classic eight variables should be used to document the chief complaint: location, quality, severity, duration, timing, context, modifying factors, and signs/symptoms. For billing purposes, there are four categories of history taking: problem-focused, expanded problem-focused, detailed, and comprehensive. Each level expands the history according to the level of history taking required to investigate the chief complaint. A problem-focused history consists of the chief complaint and brief history of the present illness (HPI) or problem. An expanded problem-focused history adds a problem-pertinent review of systems (ROS). The ROS has data categories including constitutional, ear/eye/nose/throat, cardiac, respiratory, gastrointestinal, genitourinary, musculoskeletal, skin, breast,

TABLE 11.2 Documentation for Reimbursement

COMPONENT	LEVEL 1	LEVEL 2	LEVEL 3	LEVEL 4	LEVEL 5
History	Minimal	Problem-focused; 1–3 elements in history of present illness (HPI); no review of systems (ROS); no patient/family/social history (PFSH)	Expanded problem-focused; 1–3 HPI elements; ROS for 1 related system; no PFSH	Detailed; 4+ HPI elements; 3+ chronic conditions; ROS for 2–9 systems; 1+ items of PFSH	Comprehensive; 4+ HPI elements; 3+ chronic conditions; ROS for 10+ systems; 1+ items from 2+ of 3 PFSH areas
Examination	Minimal	Problem-focused; 1–5 elements of body or organ system examination	Expanded problem-focused; 6–12 examination elements of body or systems	Detailed; 12–18 examination elements of body or systems	Comprehensive; 18+ examination elements in at least 9 systems of body areas
Decision-making examples	Minimal	Straightforward	Low complexity (e.g., routine medications; occupational/physical therapy; intravenous [IV] lines)	Prescribed medications; magnetic resonance imaging (MRI); closed reduction of fracture	Medications; monitor medications; resuscitate; refer for major surgery
Risk	Minimal	Minimal	Low	Moderate	High
Time	5 minutes	10 minutes	15 minutes	25 minutes	40 minutes

neurologic, psychiatric, endocrine, hematology/lymphatic, and allergic/ immune. The detailed level extends the HPI and ROS and adds a pertinent past/family/social history (PFSH). The PFSH consists of three components: past history with illnesses, operations, injuries, and treatments; family history of relevant diseases; and an age-appropriate review of past and current social activities. If a PFSH is on the chart from an earlier encounter, it does not need to be restated, but it must be documented that the PFSH was reviewed with the patient and updated. The comprehensive history involves an extended HPI, complete ROS, and complete PFSH.

The physical examination follows a similar pattern with the same names for the four levels. The problem-focused examination is limited to the affected body area or organ system. The expanded problem-focused examination adds examination of other symptomatic or related systems. The detailed examination is similar but more detailed, and the comprehensive examination is a complete single-system or multisystem examination.

The levels of decision making refer to the complexity of establishing the diagnosis or treatment plan and are influenced by the number of possible diagnoses or management options, the size and complexity of the medical record, tests or other information that must be reviewed and analyzed during the visit, the risk of significant complications, morbidity or mortality, and the diagnostic procedures and management options.

There are four categories of decision making: straightforward, low complexity, moderate complexity, and high complexity. Straightforward decision making, the first level, involves a minimal number of diagnoses or options, minimally complex data, and a minimal risk of complications. Low complexity increases those components to a limited level from the minimal level. The moderately complex level involves multiple diagnoses or options, moderate complexity of data, and a moderate risk of complications. The high complexity level is an encounter that deals with an extensive number of diagnoses or options, extensive complexity of data, and a high risk of complications.

Four additional components can be used to alter the coding, which include counseling, coordination of care, complexity of the presenting problem, and amount of time spent with the patient. To use those elements, careful documentation is necessary. The time category can include face-to-face time, plus review of the patient chart, writing of notes, and communicating with other professionals and patient family members. Time is the key billing factor to use if counseling and coordination of care exceeds 50% of the total visit time.

APRNs can bill for services rendered in nursing homes and skilled nursing facilities. They can also bill for hospital services as long as they are not employees of the hospital. There are three levels of encounters in those settings: detailed, detailed-comprehensive, and comprehensive, each with corresponding required components. Another way to bill is using three categories of subsequent nursing facility care (one-problem history, expanded focus, and detailed). Physicians are allowed to bill Medicare for 12 nursing home client visits per year; NP/physician teams are allowed 18 visits per year. APRNs also can bill for their services in emergency departments using special codes that are appropriate to that setting.

Some specific pointers regarding documentation are important. When a diagnosis is uncertain, coding the presenting symptom is advisable, such as "pain" or "fever." Listing "rule out" differential diagnoses on the encounter form is not acceptable, nor are the terms *possible* or *suspected*. *Abnormal* is not an acceptable term without further description; however, *normal* and *negative* are allowed. A checklist with positive items further explained is also acceptable. All laboratory test and radiographic requests must be justified to Medicare in terms of the medical necessity of their charges.

An example of a satisfactory way to document with billing based on time would be: "Total time, 25 minutes; counseling, 15 minutes; discussed results of tests, provided three options for treatment; follow-up in 3 months." To document care coordination, chart notes might say: "Spent 25 minutes reviewing medications with family and explaining laboratory tests; appointments coordinated for return visit in 3 months; public health nurse contacted regarding need for medication supervision." An APRN can list multiple codes for a single visit and can bill for both an evaluation and management (E&M) visit and a procedure (e.g., examination with suture removal). In complex patients, APRNs can bill for two services in one visit (a general well examination and an acute asthma visit, for example) if a special modifier is used in addition to the two sets of coding and documentation; patients might have to pay two copayments in that circumstance.

Organizations must submit bills quickly because there is typically a 3-month turnaround time from the payers, which affects revenue flow. It is important to remember that the amounts billed out may be very different from the amounts collected from payers. For example, in many states Medicaid pays less than 50% of typical billed amounts.

Health care organizations employ coding specialists and hire consultants to conduct audits and teach staff about these important issues. Consultants often find that organizations are undercoding for their services. Coding too high (called upcoding) can trigger Medicare fraud investigations. Medicare carriers expect to see a bell-shaped curve with most visits at the CPT code 99213 level (problem-focused history, expanded problem-focused examination, low-complexity decision making). However, this is problematic for practices that provide a great deal of care to patients with complex or chronic illnesses.

Most organizations design a superbill for processing claims that incorporates all of the coding information in one place, including procedures, facility charges, vaccines, E&M codes, ICD-10 codes, and any other relevant information. The document trail must be available for internal and external audit purposes. APRNs must communicate regularly with billing, coding, and audit staff and must participate in regular revision of the superbill. The increasing use of computer-based charting is leading to more standardization of these processes and forms.

Inadequate documentation and coding result in loss of revenue to organizations (and therefore to providers), inability to track outcomes of care, and possible penalties if audits turn up discrepancies. Inadequate documentation also leaves APRNs vulnerable in legal investigations. Thorough, accurate documentation provides an auditable evidence trail for reimbursement.

Documentation also is used to audit care quality. Some MCOs and PPOs reward practices and providers for complying with established practice protocols and standards as part of their quest to implement best-practice, evidence-based care. APRNs must be cognizant of coding requirements and provide documentation that reflects the excellence of their care.

CONCLUSION

U.S. health care has undergone tremendous change during recent decades. For example, DRGs were put in place to control costs as part of a prospective payment system. DRGs decreased hospital stays, causing an explosion in the need for skilled nursing facilities (SNFs), home health care programs, and increased patient visits to outpatient clinics. With health care costs burgeoning, APRNs are cost-effective providers of quality patient care. To prove the affordability and quality of their care, however, APRNs must be visible to payers and consumers. Visibility is enhanced when APRNs obtain their own provider numbers, lobby for direct reimbursement from insurance companies, document appropriately, and accurately speak the language of coding and billing. Furthermore, APRNs become visible as they develop strong relationships with administrators and billing staff and track their billing and collections outcomes. APRNs must share their reimbursement expertise with each other in order to raise the performance of all APRNs. APRNs who are not well informed about their practice revenue generation are at a great disadvantage in determining their fiscal impact on systems.

APRNs typically individually negotiate their own employment contracts, a process greatly strengthened by having productivity and financial data. In addition, tracking APRN cost-effectiveness, productivity, and fiscal outcomes is essential to the entire nursing profession as it makes nurses' work visible in the bottom line of organizations. The ANA and other nursing professional organizations have long lobbied for direct reimbursement for health care and continue to pursue the goal of making nursing's contribution visible in overall cost analyses. Measuring care outcomes is one of nursing's highest priorities.

APRNs were traditionally educated to provide care closely aligned to specific settings. Now they face the additional challenge of understanding multiple systems that change rapidly and reimbursement policies that constantly evolve. APRNs must not only practice competently but also must understand health care economics. Therefore, basic and continuing education of APRNs is essential, and nurse educators and administrators must understand and teach about APRN reimbursement. Educational content on leadership, financial management, politics, and health policy is essential to keep APRNs' place at the table where decisions are made, policies are developed, and systems are designed.

Lobbying at various legislative levels is also crucial for APRN reimbursement. There is a pressing need for consistent payment policies across states that are reflected in federal laws and regulations. Legislative and regulatory goals include:

- Legislation requiring APRN payments that are on par with physicians (the "equal pay for equal work" principle).
- Laws that ensure public access to APRN care (e.g., changes to the Employee Retirement Income Security Act of 1974 [ERISA] that exempts self-insured organizations from state regulation and allows them to be more restrictive than regulated organizations).
- Laws requiring payers to credential and list APRNs as licensed independent providers (LIPs), thus placing APRNs on MCO provider panels as specialty and primary care providers (PCPs). (Research must continue to examine the characteristics, quality, and cost/benefit ratio of APRN care. APRN care that is evidence-based should be carefully studied to document its specific components and outcomes, including fiscal outcomes.)
- Study of regulatory compliance as well as the effectiveness of various methods of educating APRNs about these vital issues.

In conclusion, APRNs must understand the realities of health care reimbursement to be effective providers and leaders in health care.

REFERENCES

American Medical Association (AMA). (2004). *The official industry CPT® code book.* Chicago, IL: Author.

Appleby, J. (2012). Seven factors driving up your health care costs. *Kaiser Health News.* Retrieved from http://www.kaiserhealthnews.org/stories/2012/october/25/health-care-costs.aspx

Auerbach, D. I., Chen, P. G., Friedberg, M. W., Reid, R., Lau, C., Buerhaus, P. I., & Mehrotra, A. (2013). Nurse-managed health centers and patient-centered medical homes could mitigate expected primary care physician shortage. *Health Affairs (Millwood), 32*(11), 1933–1941. doi:10.1377/hlthaff.2013.0596

Canadian Institute for Health Information (CIHI). (2013). *National health expenditure trends 1975–2013.* Ottawa, Canada: Author.

Centers for Medicare & Medicaid Services. (2013). Accountable care organizations. Retrieved from http://www.cms.gov/Medicare/Medicare-Fee-for-Service-Payment/ACO

Centers for Medicare & Medicaid Services. (2014). Road to 10: The small physician practice's route to ICD-10. Retrieved from http://www.roadto10.org/icd-10-basics

Chien, A., Eastman, D., Li, Z., & Rosenthal, M. (2012). Impact of a pay for performance program to improve diabetes care in the safety net. *Preventive Medicine, 55,* S80–S85.

Deloitte. (2014). 2014 global health care outlook: Shared challenges, shared opportunities. Retrieved from https://www2.deloitte.com/content/dam/Deloitte/global/Documents/Life-Sciences-Health-Care/dttl-lshc-2014-global-health-care-sector-report.pdf

Esperat, M., Hanson-Turton, T., Richardson, M., Debisette, A., & Rupinta, C. (2012). Nurse-managed health centers: Safety-net care through advanced nursing practice. *Journal of the American Association of Nurse Practitioners, 24*(1), 24–31.

Friedberg, M., Schneider, E., Rosenthal, M., Volpp, K., & Werner, R. (2014). Associate between participation in a multipayer medical home intervention and changes in quality, utilization and cost of care. *Journal of the American Medical Association, 311*(8), 815–825. doi:10.1001/jama.2014.353

Kaiser Family Foundation. (2013). Employee health benefits: 2013 annual survey. Retrieved from http://kaiserfamilyfoundation.files.wordpress.com/2013/08/8466-employer-health-benefits-2013_summary-of-findings1.pdf

Laughlin, J. (2014). AAP principles concerning retail-based clinics. *Pediatrics.* Retrieved from http://pediatricsde.aap.org/pediatrics/march_2014?pg=117#

Martin, A., Hartman, M., Whittle, L., Catlin, A., & the National Health Expenditure Accounts Team. (2014). National health spending in 2012: Rate of health spending growth remained low for the fourth consecutive year. *Health Affairs, 33*(1), 67–77.

National Center for Health Statistics. (2012). *Classification of diseases, functioning and disability: International classification of diseases, tenth revision, clinical modification* (ICD-10-CM). Retrieved from http://www.cdc.gov/nchs/icd/icd10cm.htm

Newhouse, R., Bass, E., Steinwachs, D., Stanik-Hutt, J., Zangaro, G., Heindel L., . . . Fountain, L. (2011). Advanced practice nurse outcomes 1990–2008: A systematic review. *Nursing Economics, 29*(5), 1–22.

Organization for Economic Co-operation and Development (OECD). (2013). Health at a glance 2013: OECD indicators, OECD publishing. Retrieved from http://dx.doi.org/10.1787/health_glance-2013-en

Palfrey, J., Sofis, L., Davidson, E., Liu, J., Freeman, L., & Ganz, M. (2004) The pediatric alliance for coordinated care: Evaluation of a medical home model. *Pediatrics,* 113(Suppl.), 1507–1516.

Premier, Inc. (2013). *Providers projecting significant inpatient to outpatient admission shift in 2013.* Retrieved from http://issuu.com/premiercs/docs/eo_spring2013

Sullivan-Marx, E., & Maislin, G. (2000). Comparison of nurse practitioner and family physician relative work values. *Journal of Nursing Scholarship, 32,* 71–76.

Sussman, A., Dunham, L., Snower, K., Hu, M., Matlin, O., Shrank, W., . . . Brennan, T. (2014). Retail clinic utilization associated with lower total cost of care. *The American Journal of Managed Care, 19*(4), 148–158.

U.S. Census Bureau. (2013). *Income, poverty, and health insurance coverage in the United States: 2012.* Retrieved from http://www.census.gov/prod/2013pubs/p60-245.pdf

U.S. Department of Health and Human Services. (2013). *Key features of the Affordable Care Act.* Retrieved from http://www.hhs.gov/healthcare/facts/timeline/index.html

World Health Organization (WHO). (2015). *International classification of diseases.* Retrieved from http://www.who.int/classifications/icd/en

Karen S. Feldt

12

ETHICAL ISSUES IN ADVANCED PRACTICE NURSING

Advanced practice registered nurses (APRNs) are active in a variety of clinical, educational, and executive roles, with varying degrees of involvement in and influence over clinical practice. As part of their professional role, APRNs must be able to recognize ethical conflicts and serve as mediators or resources for patients, families, or other nurses who are struggling with ethical dilemmas. The new doctorate of nursing practice (DNP) requirement will expand the knowledge required and the role of APRNs in a variety of settings. Ulrich and colleagues (2006) found that 25% of the nurse practitioner (NP) and physician assistant (PA) respondents they studied felt isolated in making ethical decisions, and 68% of them expressed the need for more ethics training. Understanding the application of ethical constructs and theories is essential for APRNs as they address complex health issues and manage ethical conflicts in research and business arenas (Peirce & Smith, 2008).

APRNs are confronted with a variety of everyday ethical conflicts, including:

1. Patient or family conflicts when the prognosis or goals of care are unclear (Dubler, 2011; Laabs, 2005; Ulrich et al., 2010; Wiegand, 2003)
2. Family conflicts when surrogates are not honoring the patient's advance directives or when there is uncertainty over the aggressiveness of care in pediatric or terminally ill patients who lack decisional capacity (Dubler, 2011; Laabs, 2005; Peirce & Smith, 2008; Ulrich et al., 2010; Volker, Kahn, & Penticuff, 2004)
3. Clients whose care is compromised because of inadequate funding by insurers or inadequate personal or public resources (Baum, Gollust, Goold, & Jacobson, 2007; Browne & Tarlier, 2008; Laabs, 2005; Ulrich et al., 2006)

4. Concerns about privacy and confidentiality of information in the era of human genomics and protected health information in the electronic medical record (Badzek, Henaghan, Turner, & Monsen, 2013; Demiris, Oliver, & Courtney, 2006; Peirce & Smith, 2008; Ulrich et al., 2010)
5. Conflicts between insurer/payer system guidelines and the perceived most appropriate care (Laabs, 2005; Ulrich et al., 2006; Ulrich & Soeken, 2005)
6. Unethical practices of health care colleagues or demands by employers for coding or billing practices that may be questionable or fraudulent (Peirce & Smith, 2008; Laabs, 2005; Hannigan, 2006: Ulrich et al., 2010)
7. Undue influence or conflict of interest in prescribing because of pharmaceutical promotions or use of pharmaceutical samples (Crigger, 2005; Erlen, 2008)
8. Struggles with pain management and opiate prescribing practices for patients in chronic pain (Fontana, 2008)

Research exploring nursing ethics for APRNs has also addressed areas such as respect for human dignity (Kalb & O'Connor-Von, 2007; Ulrich et al., 2010) and the ethical problems encountered by APRNs related to client care and organizational–industrial issues (Hannigan, 2006; Laabs, 2005, 2007; Ulrich & Hamric, 2008; Ulrich & Soeken, 2005). This chapter reviews basic ethics definitions, discusses keys to application of ethical guidelines for APRN challenges, and briefly defines and critiques the current ethical decisional frameworks.

ETHICAL CONCEPTS AND DEFINITIONS

The term *ethics* is used broadly to understand and examine the moral life, and the norms, social customs, and rules that define society's conceptions of right and wrong. Ethical theories organize concepts or principles into a framework that can be used to approach ethical conflicts. Consequentialist theories identify an action as right or wrong based on the outcome or consequences of that action (Beauchamp & Childress, 2009). The *ends* (or consequences, if they are good consequences) justify the *means* (or the action taken). The action considered morally right is the action that produces the best overall result. Utilitarianism, perhaps the most well known of the consequentialist theories, identifies the principle of utility as the fundamental and only principle of ethics (Beauchamp & Childress, 2009). Nurses who follow this theory would take the action that produces the greatest good for the greatest number. For example, APRNs who embrace this theory might work to shape public funding to address preventive measures or access to basic health care issues for larger populations rather than high-cost interventions for individuals (Baum, Gollust, Goold, & Jacobson, 2007; Browne & Tarlier, 2008).

Deontologic theories differ widely from consequentialist theories. These theories, based on the works of Immanuel Kant, identify actions as morally right or wrong in relation to underlying moral principles

(Frankena, 1988). Kant requires that all actions meet the Categorical Imperative: One ought never to act except in such a way that one can also will that action to become a universal law (Beauchamp & Childress, 2009; Frankena, 1988). In other words, actions must be reasoned through to determine whether we would want all others to take that same action in all cases of that kind. Kantian ethics require the test of universalizability in all ethical decisions. For example, an APRN may believe that lying to a patient would be wrong in every case (universalizable veracity). The APRN would be morally conflicted when a family requests that he or she hide the truth from the patient because of the family concern for that patient's emotional status.

The application of bioethical theories to clinical situations originated when acute care medical technology advances made it possible to preserve life without consideration to the quality of the life preserved (Dierckx de Casterle, Roelens, & Gastmans, 1998; Dubler, 2011). Bioethicists implemented ethical theories with a principlist approach as a way to examine ethical conflicts. This rule-based deontologic approach to ethical problem solving uses the specific bioethical principles of autonomy, beneficence, nonmaleficence, justice, and rules of veracity, confidentiality, and fidelity (Beauchamp & Childress, 2009). Bioethicists encourage specific decisional strategies to apply this principlist theory to clinical situations (Fiester, 2007). APRNs soon discover that ethical principles can conflict and compete and become the basis for ethical dilemmas in clinical situations. For example, a client may refuse to follow up by getting a necessary diagnostic test (autonomy) even though obtaining an accurate diagnosis and appropriate treatment for a recurring problem may benefit the client's health (beneficence) (Dubler, 2011; Fiester, 2007).

There are other ethical theories that may be relevant and helpful guides to health care practitioners. Virtue ethics offers a framework that provides a warmer interpersonal view of ethical decisions compared with the calculated reasoning that Kantian principles require. Virtue ethics examines the character traits that affect a person's judgment and actions and dispose that person to act in accordance with professional guidelines (Beauchamp & Childress, 2009; Gillon, 2003). The American Nurses Association (ANA) *Code of Ethics* (ANA, 2015) is a good example of incorporating virtue ethics into the ethical and legal obligations of the nursing profession (Exhibit 12.1). Respectfulness and integrity are identified in this code and have been examined as an important part of ethics education for APRNs (Kalb & O'Connor-Von, 2007; Peirce & Smith, 2008).

Beauchamp and Childress (2009) refer to virtues of compassion, discernment, trustworthiness, faithfulness, and integrity as character traits that would produce correct actions in health professionals. Laabs (2007) describes a theory of maintaining moral integrity in the face of moral conflict as the key process that NPs use to manage the ethical issues encountered in primary care practices.

EXHIBIT 12.1 ANA Code of Ethics

---

1. The nurse practices with compassion and respect for the inherent dignity, worth, and unique of attributes of every person.
2. The nurse's primary commitment is to the patient, whether an individual, family, group, or community.
3. The nurse promotes, advocates for, and protects rights, the health, and safety of the patient.
4. The nurse has the authority, accountability, and responsibility for nursing practice; makes decisions; and takes action consistent with the obligation to promote health and to provide optimal care.
5. The nurse owes the same duties to self as to others, including the responsibility to promote health and safety, preserve wholeness of character and integrity, maintain competence, and continue personal and professional growth.
6. The nurse, through individual and collective effort, establishes, maintains, and improves the ethical environment of work setting and conditions of employment that are conducive to safe, quality health care.
7. The nurse, in roles and settings advances the profession through research and scholarly inquiry, professional standards development, and the generation of both nursing and health policy.
8. The nurse collaborates with other health professionals and the public to protect human rights, promote health diplomacy, and reduce health disparities.
9. The profession of nursing, collectively through its professional organizations, must articulate nursing values, maintain integrity of the profession, and integrate principles of social justice into nursing and health policy.

Source: American Nurses Association (ANA; 2015).

ETHICAL ISSUES VERSUS LEGAL ISSUES

Before discussing a decisional framework for ethical issues, it is important to identify the difference between ethical and legal issues. Ethics can guide the development and enforcement of laws. However, ethics and legal issues can conflict. Some actions that are perfectly legal may be perceived as immoral or unethical (e.g., capital punishment). Other actions that are illegal in many states could be viewed as moral by some people (e.g., physician-assisted suicide or voluntary euthanasia for terminally ill patients). Ethical concepts or principles are not black and white and should not be approached as "taking sides." Ethics reflect social customs and rules and are influenced by them. Ethical principles may be applied differently as scientific advances, and social mores alter the way society views these norms.

APRNs should be aware of the legal rules that govern professional practice so that they can act in an ethical manner (Peirce & Smith, 2008).

For example, laws concerning patient referrals (the Stark Act) and whistle-blowing (False Claims Act of 1986) provide a legal basis or framework for professional behavior while clearly defining behavior that is fraudulent and illegal. APRNs should follow the laws on scope of professional practice within their state; know legal guidelines regarding professional courtesy, kickbacks, and noncompetition agreements; and understand the Health Insurance Portability and Accountability Act (HIPAA) (Peirce & Smith, 2008). Although laws guide professional ethical behavior, APRNs must recognize that there are situations in which an action is legally correct but still creates a moral conflict. If ethical issues are confused with legal issues, APRNs may only seek to understand the law and legal liability of a situation without fully identifying the ethical implications (see Cases 1 and 2). As these cases indicate, the APRN needs to resolve ethical conflicts. In case 1, the conflict is between confidentiality of patient information and the APRN's obligation for beneficence and protection of other vulnerable adults. In Case 2, the practice had addressed the legal aspects of billing; however, the APRN will need to resolve the ethical conflict between the obligation for beneficence for elderly clients and the financial accounting that is required to maintain the business aspects of the practice.

Nurses who are strongly influenced and focused on the legal aspects of an ethical conflict may come to a premature solution or conclusion about which actions to take. This approach may leave the underlying ethical conflict unresolved and create lingering internal misgivings.

KEYS TO APPLYING ETHICAL GUIDELINES

APRNs must have the foundation to understand, identify, and work through issues that affect all the aspects of practice. APRNs should embrace the reasoned, decision-making approaches, virtues, and relational guidelines that help them sort through the multitude of complex ethical issues that confront them in practice (Dubler, 2011; Ulrich & Hamric, 2008). Nurse ethicists have developed decisional tools to assist nurses in applying bioethical principles. One example of a decisional tool to assist nurses in applying bioethical principles was developed by Calabro and Tukoski (2003) to assist NPs in resolving ethical conflicts. They identify several steps to participative ethical decision making. These include (a) identifying the ethical dilemma, (b) delineating the variables in the dilemma (persons involved, time frame for decision), (c) assessing the NP's perspective, (d) assessing the patient's perspective, (e) sharing the assessment and exchanging goals in a participative way, (f) identifying a mutually acceptable ethical framework, and (g) identifying a potential solution.

Unfortunately, this decisional model has an underlying assumption that compromises its applicability to ethical dilemmas. The model assumes that there can be a shared style of analysis and problem solving to the ethical issue between health care professionals and patients (Botes, 2000). The real world of clinical care can be marked by cultural or educational differences and language barriers that can create huge gaps in comprehension, precluding any reasoned discussion. The idea that a "consensus" may be reached ignores the APRN's ethical obligation to remain a neutral mediator while exploring a patient's decision (Dubler, 2011). Calabro and Tukoski's model (2003) requires the professional and the patient to identify a mutually acceptable ethical framework, a challenging and onerous approach. There may be marked differences in socioeconomic, educational, and cultural backgrounds of patients and health care professionals facing these ethical situations. These underlying differences affect the patient's understanding of potential outcomes of treatment decisions.

A second problem with this decisional model is that it is based on an approach that values individual autonomy (a deeply embedded Western cultural principle). Gillon (2003) argues that autonomy is a necessary component of all of the basic biomedical principles and must be the guiding principle for all ethical decisions. However, this principle takes on far less importance in some cultures, where the good to the family or community may be more valued than individual autonomy (Gillon, 2003). Patients, who are limited in their ability to grasp the full implications of their "autonomous" decision, may insist on continuing treatment long after it is considered futile (Dubler, 2011). Principle-oriented frameworks ignore the role of individual character in ethical deliberations and leave out the texture of the lived experience of each of the individuals. The principle-oriented framework in its assumption of a rational, reasoned approach neglects the importance of the style of communication, personal attributes of the nurse, the nonverbal connections, and the interpretation of the meaning of the problem by the patient or family (Dierckx de Casterle, Roelens, & Gastmans, 1998; Gadow, 1989). Other critics of this principlist approach argue that the paradigm is limited in the range of moral considerations that can be accommodated. These critics argue that the use of principles cannot adequately address the complexity of ethical situations that arise in clinical care (Dubler, 2011; Fiester, 2007).

Third, these decisional models assume that there is some certainty regarding the treatment possibilities or outcomes in health care. NPs and clinical nurse specialists will continuously be faced with the uncertainties of treatments and outcomes. For example, will this cancer treatment put the patient into remission, or will it weaken the patient's immune system so that he or she cannot recover? Occasionally an APRN provides information to a patient as that person is sorting through tough treatment decisions, only to find that the patient responds physiologically completely differently than was expected. Fiester (2007) acknowledges the moral challenge of unexpected outcomes and offers a commonsense moral obligation to apologize when our professional guidance has led to unnecessary treatment or suffering.

Fourth, principled decision-making frameworks assume that ethical decision making is a reasoned process made within a structured group by participants who are well informed about ethical principles. It is just as likely that ethical dilemmas are resolved in a moment of uncertainty with less than adequate information, leaving APRNs and patients to sort through the process at a later date or not at all. Acute changes in patient status happen quickly; sometimes they are completely unanticipated. Clinical nurse specialists (CNSs) and NPs often deal with families who must struggle with making a decision for a sick family member who lacks decisional capacity for the first time in that family member's life. These families need a supportive presence and reminders of the personhood of the patient. Families often are afraid of making a "wrong" decision for a loved one and decide to do many things that the person may not have done (Dubler, 2011; Laabs, 2005). These overwhelming crises make reasoning through an ethical process unlikely or difficult at best.

Finally, the decisional frameworks assume that health care organizations or working conditions allow time and supportive resources for a logical, participatory, reasoned model of decision making (Botes, 2000; Dubler, 2011; Peirce & Smith, 2008). In some settings, APRNs may be left out of the decision-making loop at a critical time. Not all APRNs are able to quickly identify the process required for ethical decisions. In nonhospital care settings, ethics committees and ethics experts are less common. Practitioners with ethical concerns are more likely to get referred to a risk manager in a clinic setting (who will identify legal concerns, not ethical processes) for assistance with ethical conflicts.

REST'S FOUR-COMPONENT MODEL

Rest and Narvaez (1994) identified four integrated abilities that determine moral behavior by health professionals. These conditions or components offer guidelines that allow for more than application of bioethical principles and include the virtue ethics and interpersonal qualities that can assist in resolving ethical conflicts.

The first condition is *ethical sensitivity*, or the ability to see things from the perspective of others. Rather than focusing on one's own views, a person with greater ethical sensitivity can interpret a situation from other points of view and show sensitivity to the feelings and reactions of others. Dubler (2011) defines a bioethics mediator as one who recognizes that there are always multiple options for the plan of care, rather than advocating for only their own perception of the best plan. On a clinical level, an advanced practice nurse who is ethically sensitive seeks information and listens carefully. Cameron (2004) identifies ethical listening as paying full attention in order to hear an ethical problem in what someone says. This active ethical listening involves being compassionate, establishing rapport, using open-ended statements, and encouraging the person to examine the conflict on a deeper level. Ethical listening requires the professional to avoid lecturing, giving advice, or correcting comments so that the person feels free to talk openly and move closer to a resolution. Advanced practice nurses who use ethical listening skills become skilled at uncovering underlying ethical conflicts that require resolution. Peirce and Smith (2008) state that DNP APRNs must demonstrate ethical sensitivity and knowledge of research ethics, clinical ethics, business ethics, and laws that influence practice.

The second component of the four-component model is *moral judgment.* Moral judgment requires knowledge of concepts, codes of conduct, and ethical principles, and helps to identify the guidelines that support a decision. APRNs should be familiar not only with the ANA's *Code of Ethics* (ANA, 2001) and ethical theories and principles, but also the research that helps guide clinical decisions. Dubler (2011) identifies that if health professionals are to assist patients in decision making, they must develop mediator skills, learn to remain neutral, listen to the patient, and identify conflicts and decisional barriers. APRNs should practice teaching skills that allow them to present the potential risks and benefits of treatments using evidence-based findings in a neutral manner.

The third component of Rest's model is *moral motivation,* that is, the difference between knowing the right thing to do and making it a priority. Moral motivation has to do with the importance given to competing choices. Deficiencies in moral motivation occur when personal values compete with concerns for doing what is right. An NP who decides to spend less time with each patient so that she can get a bonus for having the highest number of patients billed per month may be overlooking important clinical needs at the patients' expense (Ulrich et al., 2006). This behavior demonstrates a deficiency in moral motivation. A nursing administrator who decides to staff short so that her department will exceed budget goals (giving her an administrative bonus) has a problem with moral motivation.

The fourth component of Rest's model is *moral character.* This component requires APRNs to persist and have courage in implementing their skills. Bebeau (2002) writes, "A practitioner may be ethically sensitive, may make good ethical judgments, and place a high priority on professional values; but if the practitioner wilts under pressure, is easily distracted or discouraged, or is weak willed, then moral failure occurs" (p. 287). Nurses in advanced practice roles should identify how they would carry out a specific moral action in the clinical setting. Clinical situations will expose them to a variety of problems that may require ethical action. For example, when a nurse manager identifies clinically incompetent or negligent performance of a staff nurse but decides not to report it because the staff nurse is not under her direct report, that manager is missing an important ingredient in ethically sound advanced practice.

SUMMARY: ETHICAL DECISION MAKING

Two ethical decision-making frameworks have been discussed as guides for APRNs. Although nurses may be most familiar with the bioethical principles, the principle-oriented frameworks are not as well equipped to address the many everyday ethical issues in health care that are not about life-and-death decisions. These day-to-day decisions may be best served by Rest's four-component model that identified the need to ensure heightened ethical sensitivity and ethical implementation.

APRNs are entering an ever more complex world of practice. As they become aware of the role of ethical behavior and choices in their clinical world, they need to consider ethical approaches to the research and business aspects of their practices (Peirce & Smith, 2008). APRNs can work to improve their awareness of ethical clinical issues by active ethical listening. Education about ethical theories and principles should include skilled practice for becoming neutral mediators with clients, to fully understand the patient's view and understanding. In examining their own professional conduct, APRNs can better understand the choices that compete with the ethical decisions they make.

As information technology explodes in this decade, patient privacy and confidentiality become increasingly important. The consideration of ethics in information sharing is essential. APRNs must become astute to the financial accounting and billing practices of clinical practices. APRNs who work in research settings should conduct themselves ethically in the management of research data, privacy, and confidentiality and be aware of the potential for conflict of interest in industry-supported research.

CASE STUDIES

Case 1

Frank Jones and his wife lived in retirement housing. His wife was recently transferred from the "memory care" section of the retirement community to a local nursing home that provides skilled care. Staff members noted that Mr. Jones has continued to visit "memory care" after his wife's discharge and was making suggestive sexual comments to other residents in memory care. He was found nude in a female resident's room making advances that were clearly distressing and unwanted by the female resident. Police were called, the incident was reported to adult protection, and Mr. Jones was discharged from the community. The victim's family decided not to press charges against Mr. Jones if he was discharged from the community. A week after discharge, the director of the retirement community received a call from another retirement community with questions about Mr. Jones's background, including his reason for moving. Mr. Jones and his daughter had not signed a release of records form. The assisted living facility's lawyer said that, from a legal standpoint, because no charges were pressed against the man, it was "as if the incident didn't occur" and the community had no legal obligation to disclose. The APRN who provided primary care to the residents on the dementia unit was uncomfortable with this lack of disclosure to the new community. Discuss the ethical obligation to respect resident confidentiality as it conflicts with the ethical obligation to warn a new community about potential risks to other vulnerable adults.

Case 2

J. R. is an adult NP in a rural clinical practice attached to a small hospital that serves a lot of elderly clients. While completing her basic examination for her clinic visits she frequently finds that her clients are in need of a simple procedure (e.g. skin biopsy). However, the business manager for the clinic requires that patients be rescheduled for any additional procedures. That way they can be billed separately for each primary concern (hypertension management) and each procedural issue (skin biopsy). The clinic is able to capture greater income for two separate visits. The administrator says, "We can't keep you on staff if you don't generate enough visits." Although J. R. understands that it is perfectly legal to bill the visits in this manner, she is conflicted about the undue pressure to create more bills. She feels it is unfair to her elderly clients who must arrange transportation to return to the clinic. Identify the nature of the ethical conflict and actions you would take.

REFERENCES

American Nurses Association (ANA). (2015). *Code of ethics for nurses with interpretive statements* (p. v). Silver Spring, MD: Author.

Badzek, L., Henaghan, M., Turner, M., & Monsen, R. (2013). Ethical, legal, and social issues in the translation of genomics into health care. *Journal of Nursing Scholarship, 45*(1), 15–24. doi:10.1111/jnu.12000

Baum, N. M., Gollust, S. E., Goold, S. D., & Jacobson, P. D. (2007). Looking ahead: Addressing ethical challenges in public health practice. *Global Health Law, Ethics and Policy, 35*(4), 657–667.

Beauchamp, T. L., & Childress, J. F. (2009). *Principles of biomedical ethics* (6th ed.). New York, NY: Oxford University Press.

Bebeau, M. J. (2002). The defining issues test and the four component model: Contributions to professional education. *Journal of Moral Education, 31*(3), 271–295.

Botes, A. (2000). An integrated approach to ethical decision-making in the health team. *Journal of Advanced Nursing, 32*(5), 1076–1082.

Browne, A. J., & Tarlier, D. S. (2008). Examining the potential of nurse practitioners from a critical social justice perspective. *Nursing Inquiry, 15*(2), 83–93.

Calabro, M. D., & Tukoski, B. (2003). Participative ethical decision making. *Advance for Nurse Practitioners, 11*(6), 83–89.

Cameron, M. E. (2004). Ethical listening as therapy. *Journal of Professional Nursing, 20*(3), 141–142.

Crigger, N. J. (2005). Pharmaceutical promotions and conflict of interest in nurse practitioner's decision making: The undiscovered country. *Journal of the American Academy of Nurse Practitioners, 17*(6), 207–211.

Demiris, G., Oliver, D. P., & Courtney, K. L. (2006). Ethical considerations for the utilization of telehealth technologies in home and hospice care by the nursing profession. *Nursing Administration Quarterly, 30*(1) 56–66.

Dierckx de Casterle, B., Roelens, A., & Gastmans, C. (1998). An adjusted version of Kohlberg's moral theory: Discussion of its validity for research in nursing ethics. *Journal of Advanced Nursing, 27,* 829–835.

Dubler, N. N. (2011). A "principled resolution": The fulcrum for bioethics mediation. *Law and Contemporary Problems, 74*(3), 177–200. Retrieved from http://scholarship.law.duke.edu/lcp/vol74/iss3/8

Erlen, J. A. (2008). Conflict of interest. *Orthopaedic Nursing, 27*(2), 135–138.

Fiester, A. (2007). Viewpoint: Why the clinical ethics we teach fails patients. *Academic Medicine, 82*(7), 684–689.

Fontana, J. S. (2008). The social and political forces affecting prescribing practices for chronic pain. *Journal of Professional Nursing, 24*(1), 30–35.

Frankena, W. K. (1988). *Ethics* (2nd ed.). Englewood Cliffs, NJ: Prentice-Hall.

Gadow, S. (1989). An ethical case for patient self-determination. *Seminars in Oncology Nursing, 5*, 99–101.

Gillon, R. (2003). Ethics needs principles: Four can encompass the rest, and respect for autonomy should be "first among equals." *Journal of Medical Ethics, 29*, 307–312.

Hannigan, N. (2006). Blowing the whistle on healthcare fraud: Should I? *Journal of the American Academy of Nurse Practitioners, 18*, 512–516.

Kalb, K. A., & O'Connor-Von, S. (2007). Ethics education in advanced practice nursing: Respect for human dignity. *Nursing Education Perspectives, 28*(4), 196–202.

Laabs, C. A. (2005). Moral problems and distress among nurse practitioners in primary care. *Journal of the American Academy of Nurse Practitioners, 17*(2), 76–83.

Laabs, C. A. (2007). Primary care nurse practitioners' integrity when faced with moral conflict. *Nursing Ethics, 14*(6), 795–809.

Peirce, A. G., & Smith, J. A. (2008). The ethics of curriculum for doctor of nursing practice programs. *Journal of Professional Nursing, 24*(5), 270–274.

Rest, J., & Narvaez, D. F. (Eds.). (1994). *Moral development in the professions: Psychology and applied ethics.* Hillsdale, NJ: Lawrence Erlbaum Associates.

Ulrich, C. M., & Soeken, K. L. (2005). A path analytical model of ethical conflict in practice and autonomy in a sample of nurse practitioners. *Nursing Ethics, 12*(3), 305–315.

Ulrich, C. M., Danis, M., Ratcliffe, S. J., Garrett-Mayer, E., Koziol, D., Soeken, K. L., & Grady, C. (2006). Ethical conflicts in nurse practitioners and physician assistants in managed care. *Nursing Research, 55*, 391–401.

Ulrich C. M., & Hamric. (2008). What is so distressing about moral distress in advanced nursing practice? *Clinical Scholars Review, 1*(1), 5–6. doi:10.1891/1939-2095.1.1.5

Ulrich, C. M., Taylor, C., Soeken, K., O'Donnell, P., Farrar, A., Danis, M., & Grady, C. (2010). Everyday ethics: Ethical issues and stress in nursing practice. *Journal of Advanced Nursing, 66*(11), 2510–2519. doi:10.1111/j.1365-2648.2010.05425.x

Volker, D. L., Kahn, D., & Penticuff, J. H. (2004). Patient control and end of life care, part I: The advanced practice nurse perspective. *Oncology Nursing Forum, 31*(5), 945–953.

Wiegand, J. (2003). Treatment dilemmas in neonatology. *Advance for Nurse Practitioners, 11*(5), 59–61.

Kathryn A. Blair

13

EVIDENCE-BASED PRACTICE: STAYING INFORMED AND TRANSLATING RESEARCH INTO PRACTICE AND POLICY

More than a decade ago the Institute of Medicine (IOM) recommended evidence-based practice (EBP) as a core competency (IOM, 2001). EBP is the process of using current research to guide patient care while incorporating patient values and clinical decision making. With the advent of the Patient Protection and Affordable Care Act (ACA) and the formation of Patient-Centered Outcomes Research Institute, advanced practice registered nurses (APRNs) are critical in the transformation of health care delivery systems. As a member of the health care team, APRNs play important roles in patient care, community engagement, and policy development. If an APRN is going to be a competent clinician and participate in redesigning the health care system, then he or she must become a consumer of and/or participant in research. The APRN not only has to be familiar with current research but also must be able to translate the research into practice.

When examining published research, clinicians need to be aware that there is, on average, a 15-month lag time from completed research outcomes to publication and a 6- to 13-year delay for inclusion in databases and systematic reviews (e.g., Cochrane; Green, 2014). Some studies have reported that the typical time from bench research to implementation into practice is 15 to 20 years (Carpenter et al., 2012; Squires et al., 2011), culminating in only 14% of research that actually reaches clinical practice (Green, 2014).

With an average of 1,800 research papers and 55 randomized control trials (RCTs) published daily or more than 500,000 publications annually (Blair, 2009; Meats, Brassey, Heneghan, & Glasziou, 2007), staying up to date can be challenging for the busy clinician. One source argued that the average family practice clinician would have to spend a minimum of

TABLE 13.1 Examples of E-Mail Updates

Healthcare Update News Service	admin@healthcareupdatenewsservice.com
MDLinx Family Med	newsletter@newsthree.mdlinx.com
Medscape Special Report	Medscape_Special_Report@mail.medscape.com
Consultant360	newsletters@consultant360.com
MedPage Today	daily.headlines@medpagetoday.com
Merck Medicus	MerckMedicus@1merck.com
DocGuide	webmaster3@docguide.com
Total E-Clips	totaleclips@fbresearch.org
Physician's First Watch	FirstWatch@jwatch.org
ADVANCE for Nurses	advancefornurses@emedia.advanceweb.com
Food and Drug Administration	http://www.fda.gov/AboutFDA/ContactFDA/StayInformed/GetEmailUpdates/default.htm
Agency for Healthcare Research and Quality	http://www.ahrq.gov
Centers for Disease Control and Prevention	http://www.cdc.gov/Other/emailupdates/
Practice-Based Research Networks	PBRNLIST@list.ahrq.gov

20 hours a day to stay current (Majid et al., 2011). Although not a perfect solution, e-mail updates can assist the APRN in addressing this complex problem. Table 13.1 provides examples of e-mail updates that provide weekly or daily clinical updates.

In addition to e-mail updates, there are online subscriptions such as Up-To-Date that are updated frequently and provide clinicians with latest evidence-based treatment recommendations. APRNs can also enlist the support of a medical librarian to assist in finding topics of interest. The majority of providers do not know how to search for information that supports clinical decision making (Majid et al., 2011). Developing collaborative relationships with medical librarians can enhance this skill so that retrieval of evidence is easy and the accumulation of useless information and wasted time is avoided. Other strategies to manage the overwhelming amount of new evidence include access to evidence-based journals, which typically scan multiple journals for relevant research or organizing interprofessional journal clubs where recent research can be discussed.

TRANSLATING RESEARCH INTO PRACTICE

The translation of research into practice requires the integration of three processes: disseminating research evidence to the clinician, critically analyzing such evidence, and applying such evidence to practice. The latter two steps are embedded in EBP and are discussed later in this chapter.

Historically, there have been several models (diffusion, systematic reviews, industrial commodity, system engineering, and social innovation) that were developed to explain how research evidence reaches the clinician and to identify how this evidence translates into practice (Scott, 2007). The early *diffusion model* depicts information from journals and conferences as being transferred by "osmosis." The stronger the evidence, the more likely it was that research would filter down to the practitioner and find its way into practice. Unfortunately, this method did not assist the clinician in applying the evidence to the clinical arena.

Systematic reviews, meta-analyses, and clinical guidelines were developed to simplify the process. Experts would analyze and summarize the research and make recommendations, thus facilitating the application of the evidence into practice. Some practitioners resisted the application of guidelines because there was not always consensus among experts and some clinicians believed the guidelines were prescriptive and did not allow for patient variability.

The *industrial commodity approach*, like clinical practice guidelines, was an effort to distribute information and improve its use in clinical practice. Health care industry stakeholders (e.g., regulatory and insurance agencies) used case reviews, audits, and educational outreach programs to change clinical practice. Change was sometimes avoided because providers thought they were no longer in control of health care decisions.

Systems engineering, the utilization of early electronic information systems to improve access to information, did not interface well with clinical practices; their reliability came into question, and individual adoption of this methodology was limited. Recently this model has received a great deal of attention (Squires et al., 2011).

Social innovation, examines the motivators of behavior change within social systems, utilizing the characteristics of change and social learning to distribute new information and facilitate its application to practice. In essence, this model assesses the provider's readiness for change and tailors an educational program and materials with this variable in mind. Additionally, opinion leaders, peer networks, and key players in social networks (e.g., patients, insurers, administrators) are used to influence provider behavior. Interestingly, there is strong evidence that patient-mediated interventions or patient/consumer education is a powerful motivator for change.

In general, the failure of these models to change practice may be related to the "disconnect" between research and implementation into practice. Some research is not clinically relevant, and other research is preliminary or done with unsound methodology (Dogherty, Harrison, Graham, Vandyk, & Keeping-Burke, 2013). When the research is clinically relevant and methodologically sound, there can still be separation between research and practice. Several variables such as sample characteristics, the lack of comparisons, and the feasibility of the interventions contribute to the failure of adopting and applying research evidence to practice. From a clinician's viewpoint, "the right patients," or representative patients (e.g., ethnic and racial minorities, the underserved), are often excluded from clinical trials (Koh et al., 2010), and most intervention trials are all or none (e.g., treatment versus placebo) rather than comparisons of less expensive alternatives.

One missing component in the aforementioned models is *knowledge translation,* which is described as a "dynamic and iterative process that includes synthesis, dissemination, exchange, and ethically-sound application of knowledge to improve the health" (Menear, Grindrod, Clouston, Norton, & Légaré, 2012, p. 623). Knowledge translation enables the clinician to view the research from a socioeconomic and cultural perspective rather than from a disease state. Furthermore, it facilitates the application of research to practice.

Another factor that may be absent is the flow of information. Typically, research flows from the researcher to the clinician when it should be bidirectional (Carpenter et al., 2012). Practitioners should be active in identifying salient issues found in clinical practice that researchers should address. Researchers should seek input from clinicians to design research studies to examine relevant questions and models for implementation.

Another component is the disconnect between the community-based physician and academic research centers. However, in 2000, Congress charged the Agency for Healthcare Research and Quality (AHRQ) with assisting in the development of primary care practice-based research networks (PBRNs) to close the "reality gap" between the clinical evidence and what clinicians and patients want to know (AHRQ, 2012; Carpenter et al., 2012). PBRNs are collaborative relationships between academic centers and community-based practitioners. Although PBRNs are primarily comprised of physician networks, APRN networks also exist (American Academy of Nurse Practitioner Network for Research, Advanced Practice Nurse-Ambulatory Research Consortium, and Advanced Practice Nurse Research Network, www.ahrq.gov). PBRNs are a source for ongoing health services research, clinical research, and prevention research that is specific to a community or state. These forums for research improve its relevance to patients and clinicians and ease the transfer of clinical data into clinical practice.

Finally, with a refinement and resurgence in the use of information, technology systems may facilitate the transfer of research and guide implementation into practice. Recently, expansion of the utilization of electronic medical records and Web 2.0 applications can be the new tools for the transfer of research to practice to providers and consumers (Bernhardt, Mays, & Kreuter, 2011). Web 2.0 technologies have the capability to share information through electronic messaging, video conferencing, and blogs. Social networking (Twitter, wikis, Facebook, LinkedIn, etc.) is another Web 2.0 application that can connect clinical researchers, clinicians, consumers, and policy makers (Bernhardt et al., 2011).

EVIDENCE-BASED PRACTICE

EBP is the integration of research and clinical judgment that is used to evaluate and manage patient issues (Sackett, Rosenberg, Gray, Haynes, & Richardson, 1996). The key elements of EBP are clinically relevant research that is patient-centered and clinical judgment that includes clinical expertise and incorporates the patient-specific characteristics and preferences.

EBP is not a "cookbook" approach to care, nor was it designed as a health care cost-cutting tool (Sackett et al., 1996). EBP does not replace clinical judgment; however, EBP can direct health care policy.

EBP has been reviewed and discussed in health care delivery systems for several decades, yet it is still shrouded in controversy. Some argue that the best evidence is not always relevant to a given patient or practice and that it cannot replace clinical decision making (Avorn & Fischer, 2010; Ubbink, Guyatt, & Vermeulen, 2013). This argument is flawed: EBP is the template for making clinical decisions, not a prescription for patient care. Clinical experience is not usurped by research; rather, the research evidence serves as a complement or adjunct to the clinician's judgment.

Assimilating EBP into health care, the practitioner incorporates five steps: (1) ask the question, (2) collect data, (3) critically assess the research, (4) integrate the findings into practice, and (5) evaluate the outcomes of the decision that was made (Cleary-Holdforth & Leufer, 2008). The health care provider does not have to follow each step. For example, the clinician identifies the question, but systematic reviews or practice guidelines have completed the synthesis of the literature. An essential role for today's APRN is the implementation of the research findings into practice.

Characteristics of the Question or Clinical Problem

Identifying the problem or defining the question is the beginning of the exploratory process. Although several models exist to formulate the question with clarity, the simplest approach is PICO (population/problem, intervention, comparison interventions, and outcomes; Cleary-Holdforth & Leufer, 2008). *Population/problem* refers to the patient or condition of interest. As clinicians begin to formulate the question, they must identify the most important characteristics of the patient (e.g., age, race, gender) or the attributes of the condition that will be examined in the research.

Intervention searches for the answers to what the clinician desires to do, such as identifying prognostic indicators, drug therapy, or diagnostic tests to be performed. *Comparison* addresses alternative therapies (e.g., differences between two drugs) or approaches (e.g., diagnostic test options), although in some cases there is no need for comparisons or alternative options. *Outcome* answers what is to be accomplished and what the effect (positive or negative) of the intervention will be.

Sources of Answers

When the practitioner has clearly articulated the question, the next step is to look for answers. Several electronic databases, such as the Cumulative Index of Nursing and Allied Health Literature (CINAHL), MEDLINE, Database of Abstracts of Review of Effects (DARE), the Cochrane Library, and others, can be useful tools in searching for information.

The value of the Internet cannot be overstated. There are several reliable sources of clinical guidelines and systematic reviews. Refer to Table 13.2 for a listing of these resources and Web addresses.

Evaluation of Research

After locating the answers or the evidence that addresses the question as defined by the clinician, the final step is a critical assessment of the research. This step is probably the most difficult element of the process.

TABLE 13.2 Systematic Reviews and Clinical Guidelines

AHRQ	www.ahrq.gov/clinic/epcix.htm
Bandolier	www.medicine.ox.ac.uk/bandolier/
Clinical Evidence	www.clinicalevidence.bmj.com/ceweb/ index.jsp
Cochrane Database of Systematic Reviews	www.cochrane.org/reviews/
Database of Abstracts of Review of Effects (DARE)	www.crd.york.ac.uk/crdweb/
Turning Research into Practice (TRIP)	www.tripdatabase.com/index.html
U.S. National Guideline Clearinghouse	www.guideline.gov
U.S. Preventive Services Task Force (USPSTF)	www.ahrq.gov/clinic/uspstfix.htm
Health Evidence/McMaster University	www.health-evidence.ca/
Bibliomap and DoPHER (Database of Promoting Health Effectiveness Reviews), Evidence for Policy and Practice Information Centre	www.eppi.ioe.ac.uk/cms/Default. aspx?tabid=185

To understand the relevance and validity of research, the practitioner must be familiar with the levels of research studies. The hierarchy of research for interventions moves from RCTs, often viewed as providing the best evidence, to expert opinion, the least favored, or lowest on the continuum. Exhibit 13.1 illustrates the hierarchy of intervention studies.

The RCT-N of one (each subject is studied in both the intervention and control groups and therefore serves as his or her own control) is the gold standard for clinical research (Miser, 2006b). The next level includes integrative studies, which summarize and draw conclusions from a series of primary studies. These integrative studies can be nonsystematic (written by an expert in the area of interest; the least favorable approach), or the more precise systematic reviews that include meta-analyses and clinical practice guidelines. The third and fourth levels include RCTs conducted at multiple centers and at a single center, respectively. Cohort, case control, cross-sectional, case report, case series, and finally expert opinion are the remaining levels of research (Miser, 2006b).

This hierarchy may not be appropriate for questions that are focused on diagnosis or screening, prognosis, or causation. For example, if the practitioner is interested in the prognosis, the most appropriate study design would be a longitudinal cohort study. If causation is the issue, then a cohort or case control study would be the preferred design (Miser, 2006a).

Although RCTs are viewed by many as the gold standard in clinical decision making, the contributions of qualitative studies should not be devalued. Qualitative data are needed to answer questions of why, how, and when and are seldom included in RCTs in enough detail to apply an intervention consistently (Wilson & Fridinger, 2008).

The internal validity of the research depends on a critical analysis of the intent of the research and the methodology used to examine the results; external validity, in contrast, is assessed by answering the question of generalizability to a larger population (Miser, 2006a). From this analysis, the clinician can then discern the relevance of the evidence as it relates to a specific patient, population, or problem.

Exhibit 13.1 HIERARCHY OF INTERVENTION STUDIES

RCT*-N of 1	Highest
Integrative studies meta-analysis	
Systematic reviews, multicenter RCTs	
One-site RCT, observational studies	
Cohort studies (longitudinal)[†]	
Case control studies (retrospective)	
Cross-sectional studies (prevalence)	
Case reports/series	
Expert opinion	Lowest

---

*Randomized control trials.
[†]Cohort studies can also be prospective or retrospective.

BARRIERS TO TRANSLATING RESEARCH
INTO PRACTICE AND POLICY

The obstacles that prevent the translation of research into practice are many and complex. These barriers can be summarized into two categories: individual characteristics and systems or organizational factors.

Individual barriers that have been reported include insufficient knowledge about the research process, lack of competence in reading and evaluating research or scientific articles and reports, lack of time, lack of knowledge of statistical analyses, and sometimes lack of authority to change practice (Ubbink et al., 2013; Weng et al., 2013). Organizational or system barriers that have been described are lack of access to research, inadequate resources to implement change, and lack of support from staff and colleagues (Ubbink et al., 2013; Weng et al., 2013).

Individual Characteristics

APRNs prepared at the master's level and doctorate of nursing practice (DNP) level are taught to critique research, initiate EBP initiatives, and translate findings into practice; however, educational preparation alone does not seem to be sufficient to result in the application of research into practice. Some studies suggest that attitudes toward EBP may be as important as educational preparation in the implementation of research into practice (Stokkel, Olsen, Espehaug & Nortvedt, 2014; Ubbink et al., 2013).

Clinical information must filter down to individual clinicians and cross disciplines (Newhouse, 2008). The lack of interprofessional collaboration compromises research efforts between disciplines (e.g., biological sciences and physical sciences) and prevents the transmission of research data from one discipline to another. Although the different interests among various health care disciplines are justified, the artificial boundaries and turf issues created by different professions impede the flow of information and obscure the one commonality or unifying factor that should be improving patient care.

System/Organizational Barriers

Many health care institutions, whether they are hospitals or primary care clinics, frequently spend resources on acquiring and using new and innovative medical equipment and developing new procedures to improve patient care. Failure to invest in human technology such as the development of behavioral interventions, prevention strategies, or quality improvement programs or the failure to develop processes that support nurses and others in the evaluation of interventions and policy development are examples of implementation failure (Rangachari, Rissing, & Rethemeyer, 2013). Without infrastructure support, nurses, particularly APRNs, may perceive that they do not have the authority or organizational support to develop or evaluate new models of care.

Although many institutions have adopted electronic technology in their medical records with the intent of consolidating patient information and reducing errors, little technology is incorporated into the systems that directly access the clinical research or clinical practice guidelines that may improve patient care. Computer information systems that are integrated into electronic medical records are often underused, in part because practicing clinicians are often not engaged in the development of these systems.

SOLUTIONS: A ROLE FOR APRNs

The solutions for translating research into practice and policy are as diverse and multifaceted as the barriers. Proposed solutions can be examined at three levels: the micro level (individual clinician and patient), the meso level (systems or organizations), and the macro (economic and political) solutions (Scott, 2007).

Micro-Level Solutions

Possible solutions for addressing the barriers to translating research into practice on the micro level require an examination of patient and clinician perspectives. Although much of the previous discussion has focused on the practitioner, a brief discussion of the patient's interface with the clinician's decision making is in order.

Patient Perspective

From the patient's perspective, the clinician is a repository of information, and the underlying assumption is that the clinician's expertise is based on current and accurate information. The role of the clinician is to present the relevant information, risks, and benefits of interventions so that the patient can make an informed decision. Often, this information is complex and is presented in a way that does not empower the patient to participate in the decision-making process (Col, 2005). Ultimately, the result of this type of interaction leads to miscommunication and withdrawal of the patient from active participation.

APRNs are skilled in the art of communication and have a fundamental understanding of adult learning principles. With this skill set, APRNs can reduce the flow of misinformation by serving as interpreters of information from lay media sources or other health care professionals. Informed patients can make appropriate health care decisions and can become participants in their own health care.

Practitioner Perspective

From a practitioner's perspective, the failure to use research to guide practice is governed by attitudes about research and its relevance to clinical practice. To increase the relevance of research, the patient population's needs should be the driving force for the research agenda. As articulated earlier, the flow of information should be bidirectional between the researcher and clinician. APRNs should be the link between the researcher and the patient population. They should assist the researcher design studies that answer clinical questions that are relevant to patients and clinicians. APRNs play a vital role in implementing new interventions or guidelines; therefore, they should be active participants in constructing and testing implementation models and delivery systems (Kottke et al., 2008). Furthermore, the APRN needs to recognize that when there are gaps in the evidence, the patient's exposure to unnecessary risks and expenditures increases.

Clinical faculty or preceptors, who are often practicing APRNs, can have a profound influence on APRN students' opinions about research and its relationship to practice (Jeffers, Robinson, Luxner, & Redding, 2008). When EBP is incorporated into clinical experiences, attitudes are changed, and the APRN students' skills in research translation and utilization are increased (Singleton, 2008; Singleton & Levin, 2008).

Translating research into practice requires changes not only in attitudes but also in behavior. Most models for clinical practice change, such as Promoting Action on Research in Health Services, Rosswurm and Larrabee's Model for Change to Evidence-Based Practice, or the Iowa Model of Evidence-Based Practice (Eastwood, O'Connell, & Gardner, 2008), advocate the development of collaborative interprofessional teams to promote changes in practice. The members of these teams are variable and dependent on the practice site, the expertise of the individual members, and the current problem or patient issue being examined.

For many years, APRNs have been the bridge between nursing, medicine, and other health care professionals and patients. APRNs should assume a major role in interprofessional collaborative teams. They can serve as mentors for nursing staff and allied health care professionals in the implementation of EBP and can function as the translators or interpreters of research in these teams.

Meso-Level Solutions

Application of evidence into nursing or clinical practice is unlikely unless it is integrated into workflow (Bakken et al., 2008). Institutional support for the integration of research into practice can come through the development of computer information systems (CIS). Information systems that provide immediate access to databases with synopses of best evidence that is relevant and has undergone critical review are necessary for practitioners to make informed or evidence-based choices. CIS with embedded guidelines can prompt the clinicians to integrate EBP into clinical decision making.

The development of CIS should be a collaborative effort between the clinicians and the institution rather than the institution purchasing a system that may or may not meet the needs of the practitioner. APRNs who have been prepared at the DNP level or who have expertise in informatics have the skills necessary to be members of the CIS design team. If they are not directly involved in CIS design, APRNs should work with institutions when decisions are being made to purchase or design informatics systems for enhancing clinical services.

Institutional investment in human capital is important if research is to be translated into clinical services. This investment includes such activities as training staff, cultivating and supporting research implementation, mentoring, and providing resources (time and fiscal support) for developing a research agenda.

Armed with the knowledge of health care systems, APRNs can function as change agents within organizations. They have the leadership skills to garner institutional support, engage the stakeholders, and institute changes that support EBP at all levels of care delivery.

As computer information systems develop, best practices are becoming integrated into some of these systems. As clinical doctoral programs develop, APRNs will be more knowledgeable about information systems and can participate in their development.

Macro-Level Solutions

Health care providers do not function in a vacuum. Practitioners must function within an economic and political system. Health care is governed by the "cost of doing business." When they are considering the adoption of new practices, clinicians are forced to consider the cost to the patient. Obviously, if the cost exceeds the patient's resources, often the intervention will not be followed or will be unsuccessful. Even if the evidence supports a new technology or drug, the feasibility is determined by the economic impact.

The issue of cost transcends the individual patient and permeates all health care delivery systems. On a systems level, administrators have to evaluate the fiscal impact of new interventions. Administrators must weigh the new method against the old and determine the added value of the new treatment plan. If APRNs believe that a new intervention is in the best interest of patient care, these clinicians must be prepared to evaluate the cost–benefit ratio of new practice.

APRNs should also become astute fiscal managers. They must appreciate that EBP does not suggest that all new evidence can or should be the standard of care. Most APRNs have been trained to focus on the delivery of care to the individual patient; however, in the current health system, with its limited resources, the emphasis must shift to a population perspective and cost containment.

Politicians are not health care experts and rely on multiple sources for information regarding EBP. In general, the goals of the politician are to allocate limited resources to accomplish the greatest good and to regulate health care systems and providers to protect the public from harm.

As members of the nursing profession and as part of the largest health care provider network, APRNs have considerable political clout and should use this power to influence politicians. When advocating for the adoption of new evidence, the APRN must be mindful of the goals of the policy makers.

SUMMARY

Becoming competent practitioners requires not only the acquisition of clinical skills but the ability to use research to guide practice. With the proliferation of new evidence, APRNs must be able to critically analyze and evaluate the evidence and appraise its utility. Applying the skills acquired during their educational experience, APRNs can and should become the translators of research into practice and policy.

APRNs have the skill set to understand the research process, and they are effective change agents. Therefore, they are in the position to identify the determinants of the clinician's and patient's behaviors and to design models that will not only facilitate the transfer of knowledge into clinical practice but assist in the implementation process. APRNs, particularly those prepared at the clinical doctorate level, can become interpretive researchers or context adaptors (Chelsa, 2008). This role consists of applying new interventions designed in academic research centers to primary care clinics.

Even when research is adapted to the primary care setting, there is no guarantee that this will facilitate implementation. As discussed earlier, the models that currently exist to promote adoption and implementation of research into practice are inadequate. The evidence is clear that provider education, computerized clinical support, and financial incentives have minimal or modest effect on increasing the use of EBP. The answer may be in using the best of all models and formulating a new paradigm to bridge the gap between research and practice.

The DNP expands the APRN's skill set to include becoming a change agent, understanding and developing informatics systems, and appreciating the operations of health care systems. Therefore, APRNs prepared at the doctoral level are in the position to expand and put into operation the previously discussed systems engineering and social innovation models for the dissemination and application of research. In this way, they can further elaborate the translation of research into practice.

As APRNs assume leadership roles in health care, they should become proactive in removing the barriers to translating research into practice. Now and in the future, APRNs can and should be the innovators in health care delivery systems through research.

REFERENCES

Agency for Healthcare Research and Quality. (December 2012). *Primary care practice-based research networks: An AHRQ initiative.* Retrieved from http://www.ahrq.gov/research/findings/factsheets/primary/pbrn/index.html

Avorn, J., & Fischer, M. (2010). "Bench to behavior": Translating comparative effectiveness research into improved clinical practice. *Health Affairs, 29*(10), 1891–1900. doi:10.1377/hlthaff.2010.0696 http://content.healthaffairs.org/content/29/10/1891.full.html

Bakken, S., Currie, L. M., Lee, N., Roberts, W. D., Collins, S. A., & Cimino, J. J. (2008). Integrating evidence into clinical information systems for nursing decision support. *International Journal of Medical Informatics, 77*(6), 413–420.

Bernhardt, J. M., Mays, D., & Kreuter, M. W. (2011). Dissemination 2.0: Closing the gap between knowledge and practice with new media and marketing. *Journal of Health Communication, 16,* 32–44. doi:10.1080/10810730.2011.593608

Blair, K. A. (2009). Staying up to date: Quick resources and email alerts. *Topics in Advanced Practice Nursing eJournal, 9*(3) Retrieved from http://www.medscape.com/viewarticle/707581

Carpenter, W. R., Meyer, A., Wu, Y., Qaqish, B., Sanoff, H. A., Goldberg, R. M., & Weiner, B. J. (2012). Translating research into practice: The role of provider-based research networks in the diffusion of an evidence-based colon cancer treatment innovation. *Medical Care, 50*(8), 737–748. Retrieved from http://www.lww-medicalcare.com

Chelsa, C. A. (2008). Translational research: Essential contributions from interpretive nursing science. *Research in Nursing and Health, 31,* 381–390.

Cleary-Holdforth, J., & Leufer, T. (2008). Essential elements in developing evidence-based practice. *Nursing Standard, 23*(2), 42–43.

Col, N. F. (2005). Challenges in translating research into practice. *Journal of Women's Health, 14*(1), 87–95.

Dogherty, E. J., Harrison, M. B., Graham, I. D., Vandyk, A. D., & Keeping-Burke, A. (2013). Turning knowledge into action at the point-of-care: The collective experience of nurses facilitating the implementation of evidence-based practice. *Worldviews on Evidence-Based Nursing, 10*(3), 129–139.

Eastwood, G. M., O'Connell, B., & Gardner, A. (2008). Selecting the right integration of research into practice strategy. *Journal of Nursing Quality Care, 23*(3), 258–265.

Green, L. (2014). Closing the chasm between research and practice: Evidence of and for change *Health Promotion Journal of Australia, 25,* 25–29. Retrieved from http://dx.doi.org/10.1071/HE13101

Institute of Medicine (IOM). (2001). *Crossing the quality chasm: A new health system for the 21st century.* Washington, DC: National Academies Press.

Jeffers, B., Robinson, S., Luxner, K., & Redding, D. (2008). Nursing faculty mentors as facilitators for evidence-based nursing practice. *Journal of Staff Development 24*(5), E8–E12.

Koh, H. K., Oppenheimer, S. C., Massin-Short, S. B., Emmons, K. M., Geller, A. C., & Viswanath, K. (2010). Translating research evidence into practice to reduce health disparities: A social determinants approach. *American Journal of Public Health, 100*(S1), S72–S80. doi:10.2105/AJPH.2009.167353

Kottke, T. E., Solberg, L. I., Nelson, A. F., Belcher, D. W., Caplan, W., Green, L. W.,…Woolf, S. H. (2008). Optimizing practice through research: A new perspective to solve an old problem. *Annals of Family Medicine, 6*(5), 459–462.

Majid, S., Foo, S., Luyt, B., Zhang, X., Theng, Y. L., Chang, Y. K., & Mokhtar, I. A. (2011). Adopting evidence-based practice in clinical decision making: Nurses' perceptions, knowledge, and barriers. *Journal of the Medical Library Association, 99*(3), 229–236. doi:10.3163/1536-5050.99.3.010

Meats, E., Brassey, J., Heneghan, C., & Glasziou, P. (2007). Using the Turning Research into Practice (TRIP) database: How do clinicians really search? *Journal of the Medical Library Association, 95*(2), 156–163.

Menear, M., Grindrod, K., Clouston, K., Norton, P., & Légaré, F. (2012). Advancing knowledge translation in primary care [commentary]. *Canadian Family Physician, 58,* 623–627.

Miser, W. F. (2006a). An introduction to evidence-based medicine. *Primary Clinical Office Practice, 33,* 811–829.

Miser, W. F. (2006b). Finding the truth from medical literature: How to critically evaluate an article. *Primary Care Clinical Office Practice, 33,* 839–862.

Newhouse, R. (2008). Evidence based behavioral practice: An exemplar of interprofessional collaboration. *Journal of Nursing Administration, 38*(10), 414–416.

Rangachari, P., Rissing, P., & Rethemeyer, K. (2013). Awareness of evidence-based practices alone does not translate to implementation: Insights from implementation research. *Quality Management in Health Care, 22*(2), 117–125. doi:10.1097/QMH.0b013e31828bc21d

Sackett, D. L., Rosenberg, M., Gray, J. A., Haynes, R. B., & Richardson, W. S. (1996). Evidence-based medicine: What it is and what it isn't. *British Medical Journal, 312,* 71–72.

Scott, I. A. (2007). The evolving science of translating research evidence into clinical practice. *ACP Journal Club, 146*(3), 9–11.

Singleton, J. (2008). Strategies for learning evidence-based practice: Critically appraising clinical practice guidelines. *Journal of Nursing Education, 47*(8), 380–383.

Singleton, J., & Levin, R. (2008). Strategies for learning evidence-based practice: Critically appraising clinical practice guidelines. *Journal of Nursing Education, 47*(8), 380–383.

Squires, J. E, Hutchinson, A. M., Boström, A. M., O'Rourke, H. M., Cobban, S. J., & Estabrooks, C. A. (2011). To what extent do nurses use research in clinical practice? A systematic review. *Implementation Science, 6,* 21–32. Retrieved from http://www.implementationscience.com/content/6/1/21

Stokkel, K., Olsen, N. R., Espehaug, B., & Nortvedt, M. W. (2014). Evidence based practice beliefs and implementation among nurses: A cross-sectional study. *BioMed Central Nursing, 13*(8). Retrieved from http://www.biomedcentral .com/1472-6955/13/8; doi:10.1186/1472-6955-13-8

Ubbink, D. T., Guyatt, G. H., & Vermeulen, H. (2013). Framework of policy recommendations for implementation of evidence-based practice: A systematic scoping review. *British Medical Journal Open, 3.* doi:10.1136/bmjopen-2012-001881

Weng, Y. H., Kuo, K. N., Yang, C. Y., Lo, H. L., Chen, C., & Chiu, Y. W. (2013). Implementation of evidence-based practice across medical, nursing, pharmacological and allied healthcare professionals: A questionnaire survey in nationwide hospital settings. *Implementation Science, 8*(112). Retrieved from http://www.implementationscience.com/content/8/1/112

Wilson, K. M., & Fridinger, F. (2008). Focusing on public health: A different look at translating research into practice. *Journal of Women's Health 17*(2), 173–179.

Vicki J. Brownrigg

14

HEALTH INFORMATION TECHNOLOGY FOR THE APRN

Advanced practice registered nurses (APRNs) must be knowledgeable users of health information technology (HIT) to ensure high-quality, efficient care and be familiar with the terms *health information technology, certified electronic health records, meaningful use,* and *telehealth* (Curtis, 2010). However, many APRNs and other providers remain uncertain about what HIT means for them, their practices, and their patients.

Although HIT can be traced to the 1960s, when computers were initially introduced into health care (Saba & Westra, 2011), it did not receive widespread attention until the release of the Institute of Medicine (IOM) Quality Series in 2000 (IOM, 2000). Subsequent IOM reports concluded that increased use of technology is essential to ensure high-quality, safe patient care (IOM, 2001, 2011).

Propelled by the publication of the early IOM reports, HIT entered the national health care dialogue in 2004 when President George W. Bush signed an executive order mandating electronic health records (EHRs) for most Americans by 2014. Congress strengthened this directive with passage of the Health Information Technology for Economic and Clinical Health (HITECH) Act in 2009 as part of the American Recovery and Reinvestment Act (ARRA). HITECH provided $27 billion in incentives during a 10-year period of time for providers and hospitals to adopt EHRs and use them meaningfully (Blumenthal & Tavenner, 2010). However, meaningful use requirements for securing HITECH incentives continue to perplex many providers. Important questions remain on what is required and whether most providers and hospitals can realistically meet the criteria for meaningful use within the mandated time frames (Conn, 2014; Marcotte et al., 2012).

Although a number of definitions of HIT exist (see Exhibit 14.1), the element common to each definition is an explicit or implicit reference to information. The term *informatics* refers to the discipline of study concerned with electronic information (Healthcare Information and Management

Systems Society Government Relations [HiMSS], 2010), and HIT is the operationalization of this discipline. It is the documentation, storage, utilization, sharing, and analysis of health information for the benefit of those entrusted to the care of health care providers. Information technology provides the mechanism that allows health care providers to effectively and efficiently store and access needed information when caring for a single patient, groups of patients, or entire populations.

HIT is not simply the entry of patient information into an EHR. The importance of HIT lies in how the information is used after it has been entered into the patient record. If the information is used only to record a single patient's health status and treatment, a paper document serves the purpose. However, as the IOM quality reports conclude, simply documenting the information is no longer sufficient (Blumenthal & Tavenner, 2010; IOM, 2001, 2011). For example, the APRN can access real-time information to systematically track patient progress over time, compare the effectiveness of different treatment modalities across a group of patients, or analyze the outcomes of treatments provided by health care providers across multiple disciplines. The ability to obtain this level of information from paper charts or EHRs without interoperability capabilities is at best cumbersome and, at worst, impossible.

This chapter discusses HIT competencies for nurses and APRNs as well as common information management resources that APRNs are using or are likely to encounter in the near future. The chapter also includes a discussion of select HIT controversies and failures. HIT related terms are introduced throughout the chapter with initial reference to these terms presented in italics. Definitions of terms are in Exhibit 14.1.

HIT COMPETENCIES FOR NURSE PRACTITIONERS (NPs)

Leaders in nursing informatics have developed and revised competencies for nurses since 1995, when the American Nurses Association (ANA) published its initial definition of *nursing informatics* and identified eight standards of practice (ANA, 2008). ANA then developed 16 standards based on a Delphi study by Staggers, Gassert, and Curran (2002) that identified 305 informatics competencies (ANA, 2008). Curran (2003) modified the initial list of 305 nursing informatics competencies into 32 informatics competencies. These competencies are directly applicable to APRNs and are listed in Exhibit 14.2.

Nursing informatics competencies were further modified in 2009 by the Technology Informatics Guiding Education Reform (TIGER) initiative. The TIGER initiative grew from a 2006 summit where nursing leaders representing practice, education, and administration met to discuss HIT in nursing. Given the charge to "define the minimum set of informatics competencies that all nurses need to succeed in practice or education in today's digital era" (TIGER, 2009, p. 5), the TIGER Competencies Collaborative (TICC) synthesized the existing competencies into a single, comprehensive set of informatics competencies reflecting 21st century technology. The

Exhibit 14.1 HIT DEFINITIONS

Term	Abbreviation	Description
Analytics	—	"The systematic use of data combined with quantitative as well a qualitative analysis to make decisions" (Simpao, Ahumada, Gálvez, & Rehman, 2014, p. 44).
Clinical decision support	CDS	"(1) An application that uses preestablished rules and guidelines that can be created and edited by the health care organization and integrates clinical data from several sources to generate alerts and treatment suggestions. (2) Computer system designed to help health professionals make clinical decisions" (HiMSS, 2010, p. 21).
Electronic health record	EHR	"A longitudinal electronic record of patient health information produced by encounters in one or more care settings. Included in this information are patient demographics, progress notes, problems, medications, vital signs, past medical history, immunizations, laboratory data, and radiology reports. The EHR automates and streamlines the clinician's workflow. The EHR has the ability to generate a complete record of a clinical patient encounter, as well as supporting other care-related activities such as decision support, quality management, and outcomes reporting" (HiMSS, 2010, p. 119).
Health information exchange	HIE	"The sharing action between any two or more organizations with an executed business/legal arrangement that have deployed commonly agreed-upon technology with applied standards, for the purpose of electronically exchanging health-related data between the organizations" (HiMSS, 2010, p. 57).

(continued)

Exhibit 14.1 HIT DEFINITIONS *(continued)*

Term	Abbreviation	Description
Health information technology	HIT, Health IT	*"Health information technology* is an all-encompassing term referring to any technology that captures, processes, and stores health information" (Marcotte et al., 2012, p. 11). "HIT makes it possible for health care providers to better manage patient care through secure use and sharing of health information. HIT includes the use of electronic health records (EHRs) instead of paper medical records to maintain people's health information" (ONC, 2012).
Informatics	—	"The discipline concerned with the study of information and manipulation of information via computer-based tools" (HiMMS, p. 62).
Interoperability	—	"The ability of different operating and software systems, applications, and services to communicate and exchange data in an accurate, effective, and consistent manner" (HiMSS, 2010, p. 201).
Mobile health	mHealth	"Application of mobile technology either by consumers or providers, for monitoring health status or improving health outcomes, including wireless diagnostic and clinical decision support" (Kumar et al., 2013, p. 228)
Nursing informatics	NI	"The specialty that integrates nursing science, computer science, and information science in identifying, collecting, processing, and managing data and information to support nursing practice, administration, education, and research and to expand the knowledge of nursing" (ANA, 2008, p. 1).

(continued)

Exhibit 14.1 HIT DEFINITIONS *(continued)*

Term	Abbreviation	Description
Patient portal	—	"Provider-tethered applications that allow patients to electronically access health information that is documented and managed by a health care institution" (Ammenwerth, Schnell-Inderst, & Hoerbst, 2012, p. 1).
Personal health records	—	"Electronic application(s) through which individuals can maintain and manage their health information (and that of others for whom they are authorized) in a private, secure, and confidential environment" (HiMSS, 2010, p. 104).
Security	—	"Measures and controls that ensure confidentiality, integrity, availability, and accountability of the information processed and stored by a computer" (HIMSS, 2010, p. 119).
Store and forward	—	"Transmission of static images or audio–video clips to a remote data storage device from which they can be retrieved by a medical practitioner for review and consultation at any time" (HIMSS, 2010, p. 126).
Telehealth	—	"Using communications networks to provide health services including, but not limited to, direct care, health prevention, consulting, and home visits to patients in a geographical location different than the provider of these services" (HiMSS, 2010, p. 130).

TIGER competencies are placed within three major categories: (a) basic computer competencies, (b) information literacy, and (c) information management (see Exhibit 14.2).

Exhibit 14.2 COMPARISON BETWEEN TIGER AND NP NURSING INFORMATICS COMPETENCY STANDARDS

TIGER Competencies (2009)	NP Informatics Competencies (Curran, 2003)
BASIC COMPUTER COMPETENCIES	
Concepts of information and communication technology	Accesses shared data sets
Using the computer and managing files	Extracts data from clinical data sets
Word processing	Uses applications to format and present data and information
Spreadsheets	Uses interactive communication devices with patients and other health care providers
Using databases	Performs basic troubleshooting in applications
Presentations	
Web browsing and communication	
INFORMATION LITERACY	
Determine the nature and extent of the information needed	Extracts selected literature resources and integrates them to a personally usable file
Access needed information effectively and efficiently	Is knowledgeable regarding optimal search strategies to locate clinically sound and useful studies from information resources
Evaluate information and its sources critically and incorporate selected information into his or her knowledge base and value system	Identifies, evaluates, and applies the most relevant information
Individually or as a member of a group, use information	Synthesizes best evidence

(continued)

Exhibit 14.2 COMPARISON BETWEEN TIGER AND NP NURSING INFORMATICS
COMPETENCY STANDARDS *(continued)*

TIGER Competencies (2009)	**NP Informatics Competencies (Curran, 2003)**
Evaluate outcomes of the use of information	Evaluates health information on the Internet using a structured critique format
	Assists patients in using databases to make informed decisions

INFORMATION MANAGEMENT

Concepts

Verbalize the importance of health information systems to clinical practice	Converts information needs into answerable questions
Have knowledge of various types of health information systems and their clinical and administrative uses	Describes general applications, systems to support clinical care
	Describes general applications available for research
	Incorporates structured languages into practice
	Understands the principles of data display to facilitate analysis

Due Care

Ensure confidentiality of protected patient health information when using health information systems under his or her control	Promotes the integrity of nursing information and access necessary for patient care within an integrated computer-based patient record
Ensure access control in the use of health information systems under his or her control	Describes ways to protect data
Ensure the security of health information systems under his or her control	Acts as an advocate of system users including patients and colleagues
	Applies the principles of data integrity, professional ethics, and legal requirements for patient confidentiality and data security

(continued)

Exhibit 14.2 COMPARISON BETWEEN TIGER AND NP NURSING INFORMATICS
COMPETENCY STANDARDS *(continued)*

TIGER Competencies (2009)	NP Informatics Competencies (Curran, 2003)
User Skills	
Have the user skills as outlined in direct care component of the HL7 EHRS model, which includes all the ECDL–health user skills of navigation, decision support, output reports, and more	Critically analyzes data, information, and knowledge for use in site-specific, evidence-based practice
	Uses applications to aggregate and analyze data for forecasting accreditation, clinician value, nurse-sensitive outcomes, evidence-based practice, and quality improvement
	Uses decision support systems, expert systems, and aids for differential diagnosis
	Provides for efficient data collection
	Uses data and statistical analyses to describe and evaluate practice
	Designs and uses database reports
	Demonstrates knowledge and clinical decision-making processes within site-specific practice
	Converts data into information and then knowledge
	Discusses the impact of computerized information management on the role of the nurse
	Evaluates the appropriateness of the monitoring system for the type of data needed
	Evaluates computer-assisted instruction (CAI) as a teaching tool

Information Literacy

With the increase in published research reports, practice guidelines, and professional web-based resources, the volume of information available to guide APRN practice is growing at an unprecedented rate. Fortunately, the technology and the tools are available for locating, organizing, and managing information allowing APRNs to provide safe and effective, evidence-based patient care. APRNs can access this wealth of information from a variety of sources such as advanced database search engines, national practice guideline databases, and proprietary consumer health websites.

Literature Databases

Because of the unparalleled rate of newly published articles available both in print and electronically, APRNs must be able to access recent literature through a variety of professional sources. For this reason, bibliographic databases have become increasingly important to APRNs in both practice and academic settings. PubMed and the Cumulative Index to Nursing and Allied Health Literature (CINAHL) are two important bibliographic databases for health care providers. Although there is a degree of overlap in the search results obtained from the two databases, each has a unique purpose and contributes equally to APRN practice. It is therefore a common strategy to search both databases when seeking health care information.

PubMed (available at www.ncbi.nlm.nih.gov/pubmed/) is the database of biomedical journal citations and abstracts created by the U.S. National Library of Medicine (NLM). The largest component of PubMed is MEDLINE (Medical Literature Analysis and Retrieval System Online), which indexes the biomedical literature from 1949 to the present. PubMed includes citations for articles that have been published but not yet included in MEDLINE indexes. PubMed also includes additional citations for some life sciences journals that are beyond the scope of MEDLINE. PubMed indexing uses medical subject headings (MeSH) terms, and the PubMed website includes a MeSH browser that enables users to locate search terms related to their topic of interest. PubMed provides links to full-text articles when they are available. To assist those not familiar with database searches, the PubMed website includes short tutorials and resources helpful for novice users.

CINAHL is owned and operated by EBSCO Publishing and is available through most medical and nursing libraries as well as many public libraries. This bibliographic database indexes the nursing and allied health literature from 1982 to the present using CINAHL subject headings that were developed to reflect nursing and allied health terminologies. In addition to journal articles, CINAHL includes dissertations, book chapters, nurse practice acts, and audiovisual materials. Many full-text articles are available through CINAHL.

Other bibliographic databases may also be very useful in specific circumstances. For example, PsycINFO, a database produced and copyrighted by the American Psychological Association, provides relevant results if the information needed is in the domain of psychology. The Cochrane

Library can be searched if a rigorous review of the existing literature about a specific topic is required. The Cochrane Library is a subscription service available through most medical and nursing libraries. Access to Cochrane systematic review abstracts and summaries is available free of charge at www.cochrane.org/reviews.

Clinical Information Resources and Clearinghouses

Many public and commercial resources are available to help APRNs find answers to clinical questions. The National Guideline Clearinghouse (NGC) is an online repository of evidence-based guidelines for clinical practice. Maintained by the Agency for Healthcare Research and Quality (AHRQ), the NGC provides access to guidelines from a variety of authoritative sources that are critically reviewed and updated regularly. Special features of the website include side-by-side display of guidelines for comparison, annotated bibliographies associated with each guideline, and the ability to download guidelines to handheld devices (e.g., smartphones and tablets). The NGC is available without charge at www.guideline.gov. Like the bibliographic databases described earlier, the NGC website includes instructions and tips for searching the database.

Additional practice guidelines developed and published by professional and governmental organizations are available on specific organization or government websites. Frequently accessed clinical practice guideline websites for chronic conditions include:

- The American Diabetes Association Clinical Practice Recommendations: care.diabetesjournals.org/content/36/Supplement_1
- Guidelines for Diagnosis and Management of Asthma: www.nhlbi.nih .gov/health-pro/guidelines/current/asthma-guidelines/index.htm
- 2014 Evidence-Based Practice Guideline for the Management of High Blood Pressure in Adults: Report From the Panel Members Appointed to the Eighth Joint National Committee (JNC 8): http://jama.jamanetwork. com/article.aspx?articleid=1791497
- Global Strategies for Diagnosis, Management, and Prevention of COPD: www.goldcopd.org/guidelines-resources.html
- Guide to Clinical Preventive Services: Recommendations of the U.S. Preventive Services Task Force: www.ahrq.gov/professionals/clinicians-providers/guidelines-recommendations/guide/index.html

Commercially Available Information Resources

Numerous commercial resources that provide quick and simple access to peer-reviewed articles and evidence-based material are available to health care providers. These provide APRNs with concise overviews, management, and follow-up guidelines. These resources are available online or as a download to mobile devices and smartphones. Examples of commercial resources include UpToDate, MD Consult, and Nursing Consult.

Information Management

The TIGER competencies define information management as "a process consisting of (a) collecting data, (b) processing the data, and (c) presenting and communicating the processed data as information or knowledge" (TIGER, n.d., p. 11). EHRs are the primary source of stored information that is discussed in this chapter; however, it is important to note that other sources of data also contribute to information management in health care. Among other sources of stored data not discussed in this chapter include the Centers for Medicare & Medicaid Services (CMS), the Centers for Disease Control and Prevention (CDC), and National Public Health databases.

Electronic Health Record (EHR)

The EHR is a specific application within the broader category of HIT. It is a data repository that allows health care providers to access a complete collection of patient information using a single resource (see Exhibit 14.1). The EHR often provides the structure for other HIT functions designed to improve patient safety and outcomes such as computerized practitioner order entry (CPOE), clinical decision support (CDS), *interoperability, health information exchanges* (HIE), and quality improvement (QI).

The 2004 mandate for widespread adoption of EHRs was based on the premise that using the technology would "improve health outcomes by improving quality and efficiency of care, enhancing patients' engagement in their care, and building an infrastructure to digitally exchange health information" (Marcotte et al., 2012, p. 731). Although some evidence exists to support this premise of improved health outcomes (Buntin et al., 2011; King, Patel, Jamoom, & Furukawa, 2014), other studies suggest the adoption of EHRs and HIT alone is not sufficient to improve patient outcomes (Bowman, 2013; Romano & Stafford, 2011; Zhou et al., 2009).

To enhance patient safety and health care efficiency, the HITECH Act not only requires the adoption of EHRs but also mandates that providers show evidence of meaningful use (MU) of the technology by meeting specific objectives during three stages (Marcotte et al., 2012). Each stage of MU includes and expands upon the preceding stage and requires progressively higher levels of technology. Stage 1 objectives emphasize functionality and building an EHR structure capable of capturing required data. Stage 2 builds upon the first stage by underscoring development and application of clinical processes such as integration of laboratory results into the EHR, *clinical decision support* (CDS), and providing increased patient accessibility to the EHR. Stage 3 objectives are expected to require measurement and documentation of improvement in patient and population health outcomes as well as evidence of increasing interoperability (Marcotte et al., 2012). Stage 1 criteria were finalized in 2010 with hospitals and providers beginning to receive incentive payments in 2011. Stage 2 criteria were finalized in 2012 with full implementation extended from 2014 to 2016 due to difficulties encountered by eligible providers and hospitals in achieving the mandated elements (HiMSS, 2014). Stage 3 requirements are anticipated to be released during the first half of 2015 with implementation beginning in 2017 for those who have participated in stage 2 for a minimum of 2 years (HiMSS, 2014). Detailed overviews of stages 1 and 2 criteria are available on the CMS website at www.cms.gov/Regulations-and-Guidance/Legislation/EHRIncentivePrograms/Meaningful_Use.html.

Personal Health Record (PHR)

PHRs are EHRs owned and maintained by consumers. Although the exact definition of PHRs continues to evolve (Jordan-Marsh, 2011), they are generally described as repositories for health data contributed by the consumer and providers. PHRs include tools that allow consumers to become more engaged in their own health care decisions (Koeniger-Donohue, Kumar, Hawkins, & Stowell, 2014). The American Medical Informatics Association (AMIA) and the American Health Information Management Association (AHiMA) differentiate the PHR from the EHR based upon who controls the record, with the consumer maintaining control of the PHR (Jordan-Marsh, 2011).

PHRs can be divided into comprehensive and focused health records. The comprehensive PHR includes information similar to that found in the EHR maintained by health care providers and ideally includes interoperable features capable of importing data from the EHR. Focused PHRs are customized to maintain information related to specific health problems. Microsoft HealthVault and Google Health are examples of comprehensive, proprietary PHRs that are currently available.

Clinical Decision Support Systems (CDSSs)

CDSSs integrate information about a particular patient with a knowledge base from a variety of sources to generate patient-specific alerts and recommendations designed to aid the provider or patient in making health-related decisions (HiMSS, 2010; Hunt, Haynes, Hanna, & Smith, 1998). Bright et al. (2012) classified CDSSs into three categories: classic, information retrieval tools, and knowledge sources.

Classic CDSSs are those systems that automatically provide patient-specific alerts and treatment recommendations based upon preprogrammed criteria (Bright et al., 2012). The classic CDSSs are often an element of EHRs and are commonly related to drug dosages, treatment interactions, and alerts related to patient diagnoses, age, allergies, and potential drug duplications. The second type of CDSSs described by Bright et al. (2012) are "information retrieval tools," the prototype of which is the *infobutton*. Infobuttons are often embedded within EHRs or clinical information systems to assist providers in retrieving online information based upon the context of specific patient and/or provider attributes (Del Fiol et al., 2012). "Knowledge resources," the third type of CDSSs, are point-of-care products that allow the health care provider to obtain pertinent information related to the care of the patient at hand. Knowledge resources differ from the other CDSS categories in that the health care provider, not the CDSS, must apply the information accessed from the CDSS to the specific attributes of the patient. Examples of knowledge resources include proprietary products such as UpToDate, Epocrates, and Lexicomp, as well as numerous low-cost and free apps developed by government agencies and professional health care organizations. These resources are designed to be accessed quickly and used at the point of care. They are often available online or by using wireless mobile devices (mHealth CDSS).

The IOM report *Crossing the Quality Chasm* (IOM, 2001) identified CDSSs as a key approach to enhancing the quality of patient safety and improving patient outcomes by providing access to evidence-based recommendations at the point of care. There is some evidence that the projection made in the IOM reports was correct and CDSSs can be effective in improving the quality of either provider processes and/or patient outcomes (Bright et al., 2012; Jaspers, Smuelers, Vermeulen, & Peute, 2011; Robbins et al., 2012; Roshanov et al., 2011). However, recent systematic reviews of CDSSs indicate the results of randomized controlled trials investigating CDSSs are mixed, demonstrating some improvement in provider processes but limited evidence of improved patient outcomes (Bright et al., 2012; Jaspers et al., 2011; Roshanov et al., 2011).

Telehealth

The terms *telemedicine* and *telehealth* are often differentiated into whether health care providers use the technology as a means of interaction with patients (telemedicine) or consumers use the technology to access health information (telehealth) (Kvedar, Coye, & Everett, 2014; Sprague, 2014). However, because this differentiation between telemedicine and telehealth is not universally defined, for the purposes of this chapter, the more encompassing term of *teleheath* will be used in reference to the use of telecommunications in health care (see Exhibit 14.1).

Telehealth can be divided into three categories: interactive videoconferencing, store and forward (asynchronous) technology, and remote patient monitoring. Interactive videoconferencing uses live video between providers and patients, most often for specialty consultations. The technology brings the expert to the patient and primary care provider, eliminating distance as a barrier to accessing specialty medical care. Psychiatry, dermatology, and cardiology are examples of specialty consultations routinely conducted via teleheath. Project ECHO (Extension for Community Healthcare Outcomes) is a highly acclaimed telehealth project that was adopted in New Mexico to provide specialty care to patients with chronic hepatitis C in remote areas of the state. It has now spread to other regions of the United States and encompasses other chronic illnesses. This program uses videoconferencing to provide a venue for specialists and primary care providers to meet virtually to discuss specific patient cases. The interaction provides two advantages by simultaneously providing remote specialty consultations and primary care provider education on specialty care of patients with chronic illness. Other examples of telehealth videoconferencing include its use in emergency departments (EDs) and intensive care units (ICUs) for direct access to specialist care. The Veterans Administration (VA) and Department of Defense have extensive telehealth videoconferencing programs throughout the United States and abroad.

Store and forward telehealth is used for consultations in which simultaneous participation of two or more health care providers is not required. Radiology is currently the most common store and forward telemedicine specialty practice. Radiographs are digitized, transmitted, and read at a distance. The practice is often used when a radiologist is not on site in health care facilities that use outside specialty radiologists (Thrall, 2007). Other store and forward telemedicine specialties include ophthalmology and dermatology.

The third common type of telehealth is *remote monitoring*, which allows remote observation of patient status using technology. Telemonitoring equipment available for use in the home includes scales, blood pressure monitors, pulse oximeters, glucose monitoring equipment, electrocardiograph monitoring equipment, and peak flow meters, all used to monitor patients from a distance.

The VA and home health agencies have been using remote monitoring successfully for many years and have demonstrated the value of telemonitoring in the home. Patients are instructed in the use of a variety of devices that connect to a central system to monitor their health conditions. For example, measurements taken using the remote monitoring equipment automatically transmit through a phone line to a central server, which is then accessed by a nurse monitoring a patient caseload. The advantage of the system is that the nurse monitors the patient daily, allowing recognition of subtle changes in the patient's condition from the uploaded data. The nurse can then contact the patient and other health care providers as needed. Studies have found the monitoring process to be very effective in decreasing hospital days and clinic visits (Dang, Dimmick, & Kelkar, 2009).

Mobile Health (mHealth)

mHealth, a subset of telehealth, is the use of mobile or wireless devices by health care providers and/or health care consumers (see Exhibit 14.1). Mobile technology provides a system to continuously monitor patient health status, provides communication between two or more health care providers, provides communication between patients and HPCs, promotes healthy lifestyles, and enhances management of chronic disease (Klonoff, 2013; Kumar et al., 2013). Examples of mHealth devices include smartphones, tablets, personal digital assistants (PDAs), patient monitoring devices, wearable health devices, and laptop computers. Stand-alone patient monitoring devices, such as wearable appliances that continuously track specific health parameters (e.g., pulse, blood pressure and blood glucose) and transmit this information to health care providers, are becoming widely available (Klonoff, 2013). Similar commercial technology for download to smartphones, tablets, and PDAs is being developed and marketed at exponential rates with the reported number of health and medical apps increasing from 1,000 to 20,000 between 2011 and 2013 (HiMSS, 2013).

Health Professional mHealth CDSSs

Health care providers are increasingly using mobile devices to access CDSSs. Popular proprietary CDSS programs such as UpToDate, Epocrates, and Lexicomp were discussed previously. These programs provide a thorough review of the most recent information on disease processes, diagnostics, and treatment choices. Other mobile CDSS apps provide easy access to patient-specific recommendations simply by entering a few quick keystrokes, eliminating the need to search through pages of algorithms and clinical practice guidelines. One such program is the AHRQ electronic preventive services selector (ePSS) software that is available for download to Android, iOS, BlackBerry, and Windows devices at no cost. The software provides instant access to U.S. Preventive Services Task Force (USPSTF) recommendations for specific patients based upon provider input into drop-down boxes of patient age, sex, pregnancy status, tobacco use, and sexual activity status. Similar free apps are available from the CDC for selection of contraceptive methods based upon patient health conditions. Other apps are available for a small price from reputable health care associations such as one from the Society for Lower Genital Tract Disorders that provides immediate access to the Updated Consensus Guidelines for Managing Abnormal Cervical Cancer Screening Tests and Cancer Precursors. A full discussion of available mHealth CDSS apps is beyond the scope of this chapter. The reader is encouraged to search government and professional health care websites if interested in mHealth apps that provide quick access to treatment guidelines.

Consumer mHealth CDSSs

Continuous patient monitoring devices with embedded decision support that automatically analyzes patient data and provides immediate treatment advice to the patient are rapidly being implemented in the care of patients with diabetes and other chronic illnesses. Using mHealth technology, the health care provider can preprogram these devices with decision support advice individualized to the patient.

Like all HIT applications, rigorous research is needed to determine the safety and efficacy of mHealth CDSSs (Klonoff, 2013; Kumar et al., 2013; Silberman & Clark, 2012; van Heerden, Tomlinson, & Swartz, 2012). This is especially important in the use of consumer mHealth CDSSs, where it is essential that the reliability of the monitoring devices is established before widespread use to ensure patient safety. Rigorous investigation of mHealth has been met with unique challenges, however, because the devices and apps quickly become obsolete as newer technology is developed and marketed (Kumar et al., 2013).

Consumer Engagement

Consumer engagement is increasingly becoming a national priority for changing the health care landscape. It is asserted that improved patient engagement will result in improved patient outcomes and enhancement of the health of the nation (Ammenwerth et al., 2012; Goldzweig et al.,

2013). Two examples of patient engagement, PHRs and mHealth, have previously been discussed. A third mechanism for patient engagement is the increasing use of patient portals. Often provided through EHRs and maintained by health care organizations, these web-based applications enable the consumer to carry out simple tasks, including ordering prescription refills, requesting an appointment, and sending questions to a health care provider. Patient portals allow consumers to view parts of their records under certain circumstances. For example, some laboratory values may be shown to the consumer immediately, primarily those that require little interpretation and are familiar to consumers, such as cholesterol level. Other laboratory results might be revealed to the patient after review and interpretation by the provider. Still others might never be available through the web-based application due to privacy concerns, such as the results of an HIV test or genetic screening result. Overall, consumer response to patient portals has been positive although there is little evidence at this time to support the assertion that patient portals affect patient outcomes (Ammenwerth et al., 2013).

Analysis of Health Information

Recent data indicate that 78% of all office-based physicians in the United States are using EHRs (Hsiao & Hing, 2014) and 93% of all nonfederal hospitals in the United States have certified EHR technology (Charles, Gabriel, & Furukawa, 2014). This widespread adoption of EHRs has resulted in a massive accumulation of complex patient data that are collectively referred to as "big data" (Simpao, Ahumada, Gálvez, & Rehman, 2014). Because of the enormous amount of available data, traditional analytic programs are insufficient, resulting in a need for new, advanced data analysis methods. To meet this new demand, analytics programs (see Exhibit 14.1) are being deployed to systematically integrate data from various different, seemingly incongruent sources to guide decision making across health care (Simpao et al., 2014).

Predictive analytics is the technology that promises to accomplish the goals of improved patient outcomes at lower costs. *Predictive analytics* is defined as "the use of electronic algorithms that forecast future events in real time" (Cohen, Amarasingham, Shah, Xie, & Lo, 2014, p. 1139). Although widely used in other industries such as business, finance, and retail, predictive analytics is relatively new to health care. Early applications in large inpatient settings include analytics for predicting patients at high risk for adverse and/or high-cost events such as cardiopulmonary arrest or readmissions. These predictions assist in allocating or reallocating resources to patients at greatest risk for adverse events (Cohen et al., 2014). Suggested future applications of predictive analytics in the hospital setting include patient triage and prediction of patients at risk for rapid deterioration in their condition (Bates et al., 2014).

As the field of predictive analytics evolves, the APRN can expect to see its use in primary care settings in addition to the acute care hospitals. This will lead to greater accuracy in making diagnostic and treatment decisions based on data from millions of patients throughout the world. Decisions on when it is safe to follow the patient in the primary care setting and when patients should be referred to specialists can be guided by the information obtained through predictive analytics. It is likely that as the use of predictive analytics matures, new and unforeseen uses will also emerge.

Current HIT Controversies and Failures

Despite the rapid growth in HIT, controversies remain in the adoption rates and outcomes associated with the technology. On the short list of these controversies are problems with interoperability and privacy and security concerns. These issues must be addressed and solutions found before the APRN can fully experience the long-term benefits of HIT.

Sharing of information across health care systems is paramount to the transformation of U.S. health care into a system with improved outcomes and decreased costs (Le, 2013). Interoperability provides a mechanism for sharing of patient information among providers, health care systems, third-party payers, and consumers. The Office of the National Coordinator for Health Information Technology (ONC, 2014) has contended that interoperability is the foundation necessary for realization of the HIT benefits that have long been espoused. However, interoperability and sharing of patient information has been slow. Recent surveys found only 14% of physicians shared data electronically with providers outside of their office (Furukawa et al., 2014) and only 10% of health care providers were participating in health information exchanges (Adler-Milstein, Bates, & Jha, 2013). Another survey found that a majority of physician respondents indicated that health information exchange will positively affect patient care, care coordination, and cost of care (Bipartisan Policy Center, 2012). Cost and financial sustainability were the primary concerns cited by providers regarding their participation and ability to share health information. These concerns must be addressed to ensure full-scale interoperability and realization of the projected benefits of HIT.

Patient privacy and security of health care information is an area of concern increasingly being voiced among HIT experts. Recent data from the U.S. Department of Health and Human Services (DHHS) show security breaches in health care have increased 138% from 2012 (McCann, 2014). A study reported by Degaspari in 2013 showed widespread breaches in electronic medical records with 94% of respondent health care organizations reporting at least one data breach and 45% reporting a minimum of five breaches in the 2 years before the study. Moreover, respondents indicated minimal ability to discover all data breaches. It is important to note, however, that most data breaches have not been the result of electronic hacking. The vast majority of breaches were the result of the loss or theft of encrypted mobile devices and computers. Unauthorized access was the second leading occurrence, and hacking accounted for only 6% of data breaches (McCann, 2014).

To protect electronic information from security breaches, the DHHS requires an authorized testing and certification body (ATCB) to certify all EHRs. Before granting certification, the ATCB attests that the EHR meets security requirements in seven areas: access control, emergency access, automatic log-off, audit log, integrity, authentication, and general encryption (Office of Inspector General [OIG], 2014). However, in a 2014 audit, the OIG found that EHR certification does not necessarily ensure security and protection of patient information. Specifically, the audit found procedures were not in place for follow-up evaluations to ensure that previously certified EHRs continued to meet the security standards. The audit found an ACTB training program was not in place to ensure competency of personnel (OIG, 2014). Based on the OIG report, new safeguards are being implemented to update ATCB procedures to address these issues.

CONCLUSION

HIT resources and tools are available to help health care providers and consumers locate and manage information, support decision making, and improve safety. Recognizing the need for information and knowing about resources that can help to provide relevant information are vital skills for APRNs. By keeping abreast of technology, APRNs will be able to benefit from HIT tools, resources, and innovations.

HIT is being developed at an unprecedented rapid pace; the resources described in this chapter should be viewed only as a representative sample of the informatics tools available to APRNs, not as an exhaustive list. New resources are constantly being developed, and the reader is encouraged to use this chapter as a starting point for considering HIT resources for practice. Many mechanisms for staying abreast of current technology, such as professional development and APRN journals, provide opportunities to learn about and evaluate new innovations as they become available.

Acknowledgment

The author acknowledges the contributions of Jane Peace and Pamela Scheibel to this chapter in the previous edition.

REFERENCES

Adler-Milstein, J., Bates, D. W., & Jha, A. K. (2013). Operational health information exchanges show substantial growth, but long-term funding remains a concern. *Health Affairs, 32*(8), 1486–1492.

Adler-Milstein, J., DesRoches, C., Furukawa, M., Worzala, C., Charles, D., Kravolec, P., … Jha, A. (2014). More than half of U.S. hospitals have at least a basic EHR, but stage 2 criteria remain challenging for most. *Health Affairs.* doi:10.1377/hlthaff.2014.0453

American Nurses Association (ANA). (2008). *Nursing informatics: Scope and standards of practice.* Silver Spring, MD: Author.

Ammenwerth, E., Schnell-Inderst, P., & Hoerbst, A. (2012). The impact of electronic patient portals on patient care: A systematic review of controlled trials. *Journal of Medical Internet Research, 14*(6), e162. doi:10.2196/jmir.2238

Bates, D., Saria, S., Ohno-Machado, L., Shah, A., & Escobar, G. (2014). Big data in health care: Using analytics to identify and manage high-risk and high-cost patients. *Health Affairs (Project Hope)*, *33*(7), 1123–1131. doi:10.1377/hlthaff.2014.0041

Bipartisan Policy Center. (2012). *Clinician perspectives on electronic health information sharing for transitions of care*. Washington, DC: Author.

Blumenthal, D., & Tavenner, M. (2010). The "meaningful use" regulation for electronic health records. *New England Journal of Medicine*, *363*(6), 501–504.

Bowman, S. (2013). Impact of electronic health record systems on information integrity: Quality and safety implications. *Perspectives in Health Information Management*, *101c*, 1–19.

Bright, T., Wong, A., Dhurjati, R., Bristow, E., Bastian, L., Coeytaux, R.,…Lobach, D. (2012). Effect of clinical decision-support systems: A systematic review. *Annals of Internal Medicine*, *157*(1), 29–43. doi:10.7326/0003-4819-157-1-201207030-00450

Bryan, C., & Boren, S. A. (2008). The use and effectiveness of electronic clinical decision support tools in the ambulatory/primary care setting: A systematic review of the literature. *Informatics in Primary Care*, *16*(2), 79–91.

Buntin, M., Burke, M., Hoaglin, M., & Blumenthal, D. (2011). The benefits of health information technology: A review of the recent literature shows predominantly positive results. *Health Affairs (Project Hope)*, *30*(3), 464–471. doi:10.1377/hlthaff.2011.0178

Charles, D., Gabriel, M., & Furukawa, M. F. (2014, May). *Adoption of electronic health record systems among U.S. non-federal acute care hospitals: 2008-2013*, ONC Data Brief, no. 16. Washington, DC: Office of the National Coordinator for Health Information Technology.

Cohen, I., Amarasingham, R., Shah, A., Xie, B., & Lo, B. (2014). The legal and ethical concerns that arise from using complex predictive analytics in health care. *Health Affairs (Project Hope)*, *33*(7), 1139–1147. doi:10.1377/hlthaff.2014.0048

Conn, J. (2014, January 20). EHR adoption rate slows, with physicians facing big hurdles for meeting stage 2, survey finds. *Modern Healthcare*. Retrieved from http://www.modernhealthcare.com/article/20140120/NEWS/301209957

Curran, C. R. (2003). Informatics competencies for nurse practitioners. *AACN Clinical Issues*, *14*(3), 320–330.

Curtis, J. (2010). Implementation of health information technology. *Journal for Nurse Practitioners*, *6*(3), 228–229.

Dang, S., Dimmick, S., & Kelkar, G. (2009). Evaluating the evidence base for the use of home telehealth remote monitoring in elderly with heart failure. *Telemedicine Journal and E-Health: the Official Journal of the American Telemedicine Association*, *15*(8), 783–796. doi:10.1089/tmj.2009.0028

Degaspari, J. (2013). Providers face uphill battle on data breaches. Healthcare organizations need a new approach in dealing with this pervasive and costly problem. *Healthcare Informatics: The Business Magazine for Information and Communication Systems*, *30*(1), 52.

Del Fiol, G., Huser, V., Strasberg, H., Maviglia, S., Curtis, C., & Cimino, J. (2012). Implementations of the HL7 context-aware knowledge retrieval ("Infobutton") standard: Challenges, strengths, limitations, and uptake. *Journal of Biomedical Informatics*, *45*(4), 726–735. doi:10.1016/j.jbi.2011.12.006

Furukawa, M., King, J., Patel, V., Hsiao, C., Adler-Milstein, J., & Jha, A. (2014). Despite substantial progress in EHR adoption, health information exchange and patient engagement remain low in office settings. *Health Affairs*. doi:10.1377/hlthaff.2014.0445

Goldzweig, C., Orshansky, G., Paige, N., Towfigh, A., Haggstrom, D., Miake-Lye, I.,...Shekelle, P. (2013). Electronic patient portals: Evidence on health outcomes, satisfaction, efficiency, and attitudes: A systematic review. *Annals of Internal Medicine, 159*(10), 677–687. doi:10.7326/0003-4819-159-10-201311190-00006

Healthcare Information and Management Systems Society (HiMSS). (2010). *HiMSS dictionary of healthcare information technology terms, acronyms and organizations* (2nd ed.). Chicago, IL: Author.

Healthcare Information and Management Systems Society (HiMSS). (2013). *Personal health information—paradigm for providers and patients to transform healthcare through patient engagement.* Retrieved from http://www.himss.org/ResourceLibrary/GenResourceReg.aspx?ItemNumber=22235

Healthcare Information and Management Systems Society Government Relations (HiMSS). (2014, September 4). *CMS finalizes regulation with relief for meaningful use providers in 2014.* Retrieved from http://www.himss.org/News/NewsDetail.aspx?ItemNumber=32878

Hsiao, C., & Hing, E. (2014). Use and characteristics of electronic health record systems among office-based physician practices: United States, 2001–2013. *NCHS Data Brief,* (143), 1–8.

Hunt, D. L., Haynes, R. B., Hanna, S. E., & Smith, K. (1998). Effects of computer-based clinical decision support systems on physician performance and patient outcomes: A systematic review. *Journal of American Medical Association, 280*(15), 1339–1346.

Institute of Medicine Committee on Quality of Health Care in America. (2000). *To err is human: Building a safer health system.* Washington, DC: National Academies Press.

Institute of Medicine Committee on Quality of Health Care in America. (2001). *Crossing the Quality Chasm: A New Health System for the 21st Century.* Washington, DC: National Academies Press.

Institute of Medicine Committee on Quality of Health Care in America. (2011). *Health IT and patient safety: Building safer systems for better care.* Washington, DC: National Academies Press.

Jaspers, M., Smuelers, M., Vermeulen, H., & Peute, L. (2011). Effects of clinical decision-support systems on practitioner performance and patient outcomes: A synthesis of high-quality systematic review findings. *Journal of the American Medical Informatics Association: JAMIA, 18*(3), 327–334. doi:10.1136/amiajnl-2011-000094

Jordan-Marsh, M. (2011). *Health technology literacy: A transdisciplinary framework for consumer-oriented practice.* Sudbury, MA: Jones & Bartlett Learning.

King, J., Patel, F., Jamoom, E., & Furukawa, M. (2014). Clinical benefits of electronic health record use: National findings. *Health Services Research, 49* (1, pt. 2), 392–404. doi:10.1111/1475-6773.12135

Klonoff, D. (2013). The current status of mHealth for diabetes: Will it be the next big thing? *Journal of Diabetes Science and Technology, 7*(3), 749–758.

Koeniger-Donohue, R., Kumar Agarwal, N., Hawkins, J. W., & Stowell, S. (2014). Role of nurse practitioners in encouraging use of personal health records. *Nurse Practitioner, 39*(7), 1–8. doi:10.1097/01.NPR.0000450743.39981.93

Kumar, S., Nilsen, W., Abernethy, A., Atienza, A., Patrick, K., Pavel, M.,...Swendeman, D. (2013). Mobile health technology evaluation: The mHealth evidence workshop. *American Journal of Preventive Medicine, 45*(2), 228–236. doi:10.1016/j.amepre.2013.03.017

Kvedar, J., Coye, M., & Everett, W. (2014). Connected health: A review of technologies and strategies to improve patient care with telemedicine and telehealth. *Health Affairs, 33*(2), 194–199. doi:10.1377/hlthaff.2013.0992

Le, P. (2013). Strategic interoperability unleashing the full potential of EHRs. *Health Management Technology, 34*(10), 16.

Marcotte, L., Seidman, J., Trudel, K., Berwick, D., Blumenthal, D., Mostashari, F., & Jain, S. (2012). Achieving meaningful use of health information technology: A guide for physicians to the EHR incentive programs. *Archives of Internal Medicine, 172*(9), 731–736. doi:10.1001/archinternmed.2012.872

McCann, E. (2014, February 6). HIPAA data breaches climb 138 percent. *Healthcare News*. Retrieved from http://www.healthcareitnews.com/news/hippa-data-breaches-climb-138-percent

Office of Inspector General (OIG), Department of Health and Human Services. (2014). *The Office of the National Coordinator for Health Information Technology's Oversight of the Testing and Certification of Electronic Health Records*. Retrieved from https://oig.hhs.gov/oas/reports/region6/61100063.pdf

Office of the National Coordinator for Health Information Technology (ONC). (n.d.). Home page. Retrieved from http://healthit.hhs.gov/portal/server.pt/community/healthit_hhs_gov__home/1204

Office of the National Coordinator of Health Information Technology (ONC). (n.d.). *Benefits of electronic health records (EHRs)*. Retrieved from http://www.healthit.gov/providers-professionals/benefits-electronic-health-records-ehrs

Robbins, G., Lester, W., Johnson, K., Chang, Y., Estey, G., Surrao, D., . . . Freedberg, K. (2012). Efficacy of a clinical decision-support system in an HIV practice: A randomized trial. *Annals of Internal Medicine, 157*(11), 757–766. doi:10.7326/0003-4819-157-11-201212040-00003

Romano, M., & Stafford, R. (2011). Electronic health records and clinical decision support systems: Impact on national ambulatory care quality. *Archives of Internal Medicine, 171*(10), 897–903. doi:10.1001/archinternmed.2010.527

Roshanov, P., Misra, S., Gerstein, H., Garg, A., Sebaldt, R., Mackay, J., . . . Haynes, R. (2011). Computerized clinical decision support systems for chronic disease management: A decision-maker-researcher partnership systematic review. *Implementation Science: IS*, 692. doi:10.1186/1748-5908-6-92

Saba, K., & Westra, B. (2011). Historical perspectives of nursing informatics. In V. K. Saba & K. A. McCormick (Eds.), *Essentials of nursing informatics* (5th ed., pp. 11–29). New York, NY: McGraw-Hill.

Silberman, M. J., & Clark, L. (2012). M-health: The union of technology and health care regulation. *Journal of Medical Practice Management, 28*(2), 118–120.

Simpao, A., Ahumada, L., Gálvez, J., & Rehman, M. (2014). A review of analytics and clinical informatics in health care. *Journal of Medical Systems, 38*(4), 45. doi:10.1007/s10916-014-0045-x

Sprague, N. (2014, April 11). Telehealth: Into the mainstream? *National Policy Forum*. Retrieved from http://www.nhpf.org/library/details.cfm/2960

Staggers, N., Gassert, C., & Curran, C. (2002). A Delphi study to determine informatics competencies for nurses at four levels of practice. *Nursing Research, 51*(6), 383–390.

The TIGER Initiative (TIGER). (2009). *Informatics competencies for every practicing nurse: Recommendations from the TIGER Collaborative.* TIGER Summit website. Retrieved from http://www.thetigerinitiative.org/docs/TigerReport_InformaticsCompetencies_001.pdf

Thrall, J. (2007). Teleradiology. Part I. History and clinical applications. *Radiology, 243*(3), 613–617.

von Heerden, A., Tomlinson, M., & Swartz, L. (2012). Point of care in your pocket: A research agenda for the field on m-health. *Bulletin of the World Health Organization, 90*(5), 393–394.

Zhou, L., Soran, C., Jenter, C., Volk, L., Orav, E., Bates, D., & Simon, S. (2009). The relationship between electronic health record use and quality of care over time. *Journal of the American Medical Informatics Association: JAMIA, 16*(4), 457–464. doi:10.1197/jamia.M3128

PART III: TRANSITIONS TO THE ADVANCED PRACTICE ROLE

Kathryn A. Blair and Patricia A. White

15

SCHOLARSHIP OF PRACTICE AND PROFESSIONALISM

HISTORICAL PERSPECTIVE

Riley, Beal, Levi, and McCausland (2002) outlined the importance of the concept of scholarly practice for the nursing profession. Many nurse leaders have called for links between practice and scholarship (Diers, 1995; Meleis, 1987), and rather than espouse a model that emphasizes a purely academic approach to scholarship, they developed a model that emphasizes a practice approach to scholarship. Research on this domain explored clinical scholarship from the perspectives of practicing nurses (Riley, Beal, & Lancaster, 2008; Riley & Beal, 2013).

Although advanced practice nursing has explored the concept of novice nurse practitioner adjustment to the new role, there has been little in-depth exploration of the concept of clinical scholarship. Earlier work by Brykczynski (1989) addressed clinical judgment and nurse practitioner practice. Her research highlighted the essential elements involved in the day-to-day practice of nurse practitioners and provided additional understanding of the complexities of providing care in a variety of settings. The knowledge development embedded in the practice of advanced practice nursing and the role development processes identified in her study also added to the understanding of clinical scholarship for advanced practice. Advanced practice role transition and the importance of mentoring have continued to be studied in the advanced practice literature. However, these concepts have not been linked explicitly to the concept of clinical scholarship. The research on clinical scholarship with nurses that is identified in this chapter has important relevance for advanced practice registered nurses (APRNs).

Model for Clinical Scholarship

In response to the need for greater understanding and perspectives on the meaning of scholarship in nursing, leading nurse educators developed the *universal model of nursing* scholarship and identified four domains: *knowing, teaching, practice,* and *service* (Riley et al., 2002). This model is unique to nursing as a practice discipline; it is comprehensive in its design and identifies a range of scholarly activities relevant to nurses in a variety of settings. The Universal Model of Nursing scholarship identifies components of scholarship including service, education, knowledge development, and practice. This model on scholarly practice has been expanded to include practicing nurses' descriptions of scholarly practice (Riley & Beal, 2013, Riley, Beal, & Lancaster, 2008, Riley, Beal, Levi, & McCausland, 2002.). Although the research by Riley and colleagues has been conducted on practicing nurses, it has great potential for application to advanced practice nursing.

Definition of Scholarly Practice

Riley, Beal, and Lancaster (2008) offer a definition of scholarly practice based on their research that states, "Scholarly nursing practice is defined as a multidimensional way of thinking about practice that includes role attributes of *active learner, out-of-the box thinker, passionate about nursing, available,* and *confident,* and the role processes of *lead, give care, share knowledge, evolve,* and *reflect*" (p. 17). These role attributes and processes are outlined in Figure 15.1. This diagram highlights the many dimensions of the role of clinical scholar and the complexities involved in role enactment.

Four themes emerge in the model and include role identification in providing care, role evolution, reflective practice, and leadership. *Role identification* incorporates immersion in care, vigilance, and prioritizing the relationships involved in patient care. *Role evolution* includes the openness to learning from patients and families, advancing knowledge acquisition, and staying abreast of current evidence. The third theme of *reflection in practice* is reported as a multidimensional concept that allows nurses opportunities to consider anticipatory thinking about potential issues that could arise in practice. The fourth component of the model is identified as the nurse as a *leader* that was further developed in the areas of nurses looking to develop other nurses. This dimension of practice is often omitted in the discussions of role development, and identifying this component of scholarly practice requires additional exploration.

Early career perspectives concerning clinical scholarship suggest that nurses identify a very complex process of role development (Riley & Beal, 2013). As nurses become comfortable with clinical competence and decision-making skills, they develop an awareness of what expert scholarly practice embodies and an awareness of a goal that they are working toward (Riley & Beal, 2013).

Experienced acute care nurses identified components of scholarly practice with themes that were different from those for less experienced nurse. These nurses identified expert practice as involving less cognitive effort in the technical aspects of care, allowing for more focus on reflection and relationships with patients, families, and team members. Expert nurses view their professional identity as active

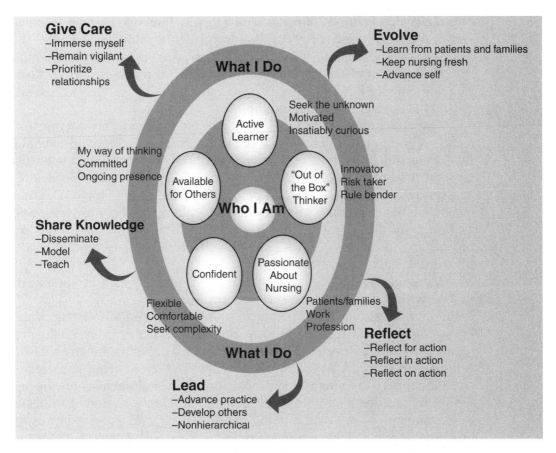

FIGURE 15.1 The scholar in nursing practice. *Source:* Riley, Beal, & Lancaster (2008).

learner, out-of-the-box thinker, passionate about nursing, available, and confident. In addition, expert nurses characterized their roles as leading, caring, sharing knowledge with others, evolving, and reflecting on practice (Beal et al., 2008).

Experienced nurses highlight the ongoing challenges faced in their role. Their descriptions of providing care reflected a process of developing relationships with patients and families as an essential component of providing expert care as well as vigilance in identifying patient needs. Reflection was characterized by reflection on action, reflection in practice, and reflection for action. *Reflection on action* offered opportunities to critique clinical situations that had occurred to learn how to use their experiences to improve patient care. *Reflection in action* provided the opportunities to synthesize information about the patient while providing care. *Reflection for action* helped prepare for possibilities that might require action and provided an additional dimension to the concept of reflection (Beal et al., 2008).

The personal and professional characteristics that the nurses identified in their descriptions of novice and expert practice highlighted a dimension of practice that continues to enrich and inspire them to share with others, and to continually seek opportunities to further develop in their role. This research also provides additional depth to the understanding of the ongoing development of the roles of both the novice and expert nurse scholar. The refinement of these concepts of role attributes as well as processes is critical in our ongoing understanding.

The aforementioned model identifies the evolution of moving from technological practice to scholarly practice. The question remains: What is the scholarship of practice or scholarly practice? And what defines a nurse scholar? A scholar can be defined as person who has done advanced study in a special field and is a learned person (Merriam-Webster, 2011). "Other characteristics of scholars are that they typically know how to speak with authority, and are articulate in both written and oral communication" (Conrad & Pape, 2014, p. 88). An APRN who clearly articulates with authority fits the definition of a scholar.

Many of the day-to-day activities of the APRN, such as staying up to date with current guidelines or practice recommendations and participating in professional organizations, can be considered scholarship if this knowledge is transferred to others to improve practice or to enrich the profession (Conrad & Pape, 2014.) The role of scholar does not mean an APRN is limited to writing or presenting as a means of transferring knowledge. Additional roles demonstrating scholarly activity include teacher (preceptor, formal academic appointment, or staff educator), leadership roles in local state and/or national nursing organizations, and expert witness for litigation or policy development (Conrad & Pape, 2014; Lusk, 2014).

Before proceeding it is important to clarify that staying current or engaging in clinical practice is not sufficient to warrant being called a scholar. A scholar of nursing practice is one who contributes to the implementation of evidence-based clinical practices, comparative effectiveness research, quality improvement exercises, and translational research (Honig, Smolowitz, & Larson, 2013). Membership in a professional organization without engagement is not being a scholar. The scholar is a member but also uses membership and participation to foster policy or clinical changes.

SCHOLARSHIP OF PRACTICE: APRN FACULTY

When scholarship of practice is discussed, most of the dialogue addresses faculty practice and its role in the tripartite mission of colleges and universities. Is faculty practice scholarship? The question has been the angst of many APRN faculty. To maintain APRN certification, the APRN faculty member must practice. The function of faculty practice is to maintain clinical competence, provide a source of professional development, and facilitate the linkage between theory and practice. Faculty practice is the bridge between the academic and clinical arenas (Premji et al., 2011).

Scholarship of practice also applies to the practicing APRN with or without an academic appointment. Scholarship of practice should be incorporated into the APRN professional role (Thomas, 2012). For APRNs to be taken seriously by the greater health care system, they must participate in the scholarship of practice. The question continues to arise: What is the scholarship of practice?

Scholarship of practice fits with Boyer's models (1990), the scholarship of integration and/or application. The scholarship of integration refers to the interpretation of research across disciplines. In other words, it answers the question, "What does this mean?" The scholarship of application "applies" the current evidence to real-world situations. This form of scholarship answers the question, "How does this knowledge help individuals or institutions?" (Boyer, 1990, p. 21).

The scholarship of practice requires building nursing knowledge, interpretation and/or application of the evidence, knowledge transfer, connecting academic research to practice, and practice-based research (Wilkes, Mannix, & Jackson, 2013). Dissemination or knowledge transfer can take many forms, such as presentation at local, state, national, or international forums; scholarly writing or publication; web-based teaching modules; and staff education (Bosold & Darnel, 2012).

The scholarship of practice suggests that knowledge should come from collaboration between the researcher and clinician (Peterson, McMahon, Farkas, & Howland, 2005). Universities often fail to address those issues that are salient to the clinician and community (Crist, 2010). The relationship between the APRN and researcher is synergistic, and partnerships should be developed as well as encouraged. The role of the APRN is critical to guiding the researchers' questions, making the evidence relevant to the patient or community, and/or translating the evidence into practice.

With clarity of definitions and roles of the scholar and scholarship of practice, why do many APRNs not see themselves as scholars or not engage in scholarly activities? Most APRNs perhaps see themselves as "doers," not scholars (Lusk, 2014). Perhaps they lack the skill to conduct or translate research, feel their work is "not good enough," their writing skills are lacking, or the process takes too long. This mentality indirectly lessens APRNs' credibility in the health care system. Another concern for APRNs is that scholarship of practice often goes unrewarded in the clinical setting (Robert & Pape, 2011). Therefore, the motivation to become an active scholar is lacking.

So how does the APRN become a scholar? The APRN may have questions that arise from clinical practice, such as clinical situations, clinical guidelines, or policy issues. These questions can be examined with the current evidence. APRN graduates have the skills to interpret and evaluate current evidence and practice guidelines. The doctorate of nursing programs (DNPs) are designed to expand this knowledge to provide leadership for practice improvement, quality, and safety (Brown & Crabtree, 2013). An APRN who is unsure of his or her ability to evaluate research or outcomes or implement change can work with researchers. If an APRN is a preceptor, a student–practitioner research partnership under the guidance of a faculty researcher can be formed (Crist, 2010).

When an APRN institutes changes in practice, measures outcomes, serves as an expert in a particular area, or has learned the "tricks of the trade," these accomplishments should be shared with colleagues in both an informal and formal way. One way to share information is through publication. Publications can take the form of blogs, web-based activity, journals, and editorials in local papers, and so on. Perhaps the easiest way to begin the publication process is when one is in graduate school and uses the scholarly paper or DNP capstone project to develop a manuscript along with a faculty mentor.

GUIDELINES FOR PUBLICATION AND PRESENTATION

This section provides the APRN with some tips for presentation and writing. Writing or presenting is a means to let your "voice" be heard. In an advanced practice role, the APRN must include professional writing and presenting as an integral part of his or her identity. By not valuing, practicing, and developing these skills while in graduate school, it is easy to slide down the slippery slope into a technical conceptualization of the role rather than professional ideation.

All APRNs will move from novice to expert; however, there are periods of transitions as one moves through the process of becoming an expert. For example, Bridges (1991) described a reorientation phase as a final step in transition. In reorientation, nurses in advanced practice roles redefine themselves as leaders. With this new identity, publishing and presenting are critical leadership actions. It is through dissemination that others' thinking and acting are influenced—and that is leadership.

Health care professionals read the professional literature and attend conferences for a reason, and one needs to identify such a reason. Begin with an issue or question from the reader's/audience's perspective. Ask, why would they want to know this? This may be a methodology, a population-specific intervention, a program, or clinical insight. The unique idea may relate to direct patient care, to a resource issue, or to collaboration within the unit or larger system of health care.

The writer/presenter persuades the reader/audience by writing or presenting in a simple and concise format. The goal is to have readers/audience become as interested as you are in the topic you are presenting. *Know your audience.* The content or topic will be presented differently for different audiences. For example, presenting to APRNs in a clinical arena may be different from presenting to a nurse educator/researcher or to a nonnurse audience.

Identify a journal or other forum for your topic. One should explore the journals and sources of information that are or were used in graduate school. Review the section "information to authors" or "manuscript guidelines." These guidelines are found in the print journals or online. If presenting at a conference, there is typically a conference theme. Reviewing topics and abstract guidelines is a must because the manuscript types or presentations that are accepted by the journal/conference are delineated (e.g., practice focus, research, literature reviews, policy, opinion pieces). Skimming articles in a recent issue or reviewing topics covered in a previous conference to examine style, tone, research base, and intended audience will help you decide whether the manuscript/presentation seems to fit. Finally, the journal's/conference's information for authors/presenters will identify the specific writing/presentation format (e.g., PowerPoint, poster, workshop, roundtable discussion).

Selecting a journal or conference that is peer reviewed is a basic criterion, especially for those in academic positions. In the peer-review process, two or three content and/or method experts provide a double-blind review to assist the journal editor or conference planners in making recommendations to the authors/presenters. The peer-review process ensures that a minimum standard of quality exists in the published literature or conference. For beginning writers/presenters, however, it may be advantageous to select local, state, or regional newsletters or other nonpeer-reviewed publications/conferences. Generally, there is a faster turnaround time to dissemination, and the submission process is less complex.

Once a conference or journal is selected, you need to organize your thoughts, and this can be done by drafting an outline of the major ideas you are interested in conveying to the reader/audience. The structure must be organized so that the reader/audience can move quickly and easily through the article or presentation. If the reader/audience is struggling to stay with you in format, language, or organization, the message may be lost no matter how notable the content; cognitive leaps and disorganization prevent the reader/audience from "getting it."

To help the reader/audience "get it," the use of transition is helpful. The first sentence of each paragraph should be designed as a bridge sentence or link content together by articulating the connections. Do not assume the reader or audience has the same level of expertise that the author or presenter has on the topic.

There are many handbooks for writers beginning the scholarly publication process. Dexter (2000) describes writing tips, including strategies to enhance clarity, precision, accuracy, logic, and depth. For beginning writers, the following may be helpful: (a) use an outline to plan and organize the paper; (b) after setting aside a manuscript, read it out loud (grammar problems, incomplete sentences, long sentences or paragraphs will be more easily heard than seen); and (c) paraphrase and use references precisely. In addition, Silvia (2007) has a bright and practical little book that stresses the need for a weekly writing schedule, how to address common writing barriers, and specific motivational tools. If a structured week-by-week approach appeals to you, Belcher's (2009) book helps academic authors overcome anxieties, learn a particular feature of a strong manuscript every week, and send their own work to a journal at the end of 12 weeks.

Collaborating with others or choosing a mentor is a strategy for beginners to bolster their confidence. By obtaining feedback from a coauthor/mentor, writing/presentation skills will expand. In addition, scheduled timelines with others provide structure, and brainstorming and dialogue enrich the process. However, multiple authors/presenters require consensus building, and blending different writing or presenting styles may be more time consuming. Another word of caution: Clearly determine author/presenter order (primary, secondary, etc.) at the outset, based on agreed-upon contributions and responsibilities.

Precise adherence to the manuscript guidelines or the organization's call for abstracts, particularly page limits or word counts, format, and content focus, is essential. A response from the journal editor after manuscript submission can vary from 6 weeks to nearly a year. Following the ethics of publishing, a manuscript can be submitted to only one journal at a time. The editor's response also may vary; he or she compiles the peer reviewers' appraisals and then typically decides to (a) publish as is, (b) reconsider after suggested revisions, or (c) not publish. Conference abstract submissions have deadlines, and they are either accepted or rejected. One strategy that increases your chances is to submit the abstract for podium or poster. This way a reviewer may say the abstract is not accepted for podium presentation but would be more appropriate for poster presentation.

With both manuscript and abstract submission, rejection is a possibility. Recognizing that everyone has a "pink slip" in their file, mentors are invaluable in helping one stand back up, dust oneself off, revise, reshape, and resubmit.

Delineating a professional development plan is part of the APRN's evolution as an emerging scholar. Career goals around employment, position, setting, and client population are highlighted in each individual plan. As one develops a scholarship of practice, it is helpful to develop an area of expertise early in one's advanced practice career. This area of expertise is then sustained throughout one's career and is the basis for a scholarship of practice.

Acknowledgment

The authors acknowledge the contributions of Cecelia R. Zorn who contributed to this chapter in the previous edition.

REFERENCES

American Psychological Association. (2009). *Publication manual of the American Psychological Association* (6th ed.). Washington, DC: Author.

Beal, J., Riley, J., & Lancaster, D. L. (2008). Essential elements of an optimal clinical practice environment. *The Journal of Nursing Administration, 38*(11), 488–493.

Belcher, W. L. (2009). *Writing your journal article in twelve weeks: A guide to academic publishing success.* Thousand Oaks, CA: Sage Publications.

Bosold, C., & Darnell, M. (2012). Faculty practice: Is it scholarly activity? *Journal of Professional Nursing, 28*(2), 90–95. doi:10.1016/j.profnurs.2011.11.003

Boyer, E. (1990). *Scholarship reconsidered: Priorities of the professoriate.* Princeton, NJ: The Carnegie Foundation for the Advancement of Teaching.

Bridges, W. (1991). *Managing transitions: Making the most of change.* Reading, MA: Addison-Wesley.

Brykczynski, K. A. (1989). An interpretive study describing the clinical judgment of nurse practitioners. *Research and Theory for Nursing Practice, 3*(2), 75–104.

Brown, M. A., & Crabtree, K. (2013). The development of practice scholarship in DNP programs: A paradigm shift. *Journal of Professional Nursing, 29,* 330–337. doi:10.1016/j.profnurs.2013.08.003

Conrad, P. L., & Pape, T. (2014). Roles and responsibilities of the nursing scholar. *Pediatric Nursing, 40*(2), 87–90.

Crist, P. A. (2010). Adapting research instruction to support the scholarship of practice: Practice-scholar. *Partnerships Occupational Therapy in Health Care, 24*(1), 39–55. doi:10.3109/07380570903477000

Dexter, P. (2000). Tips for scholarly writing in nursing. *Journal of Professional Nursing, 16*(1), 6–12.

Diers, D. (1995). Clinical scholarship. *Journal of Professional Nursing, 11*(1), 24–30.

Honig, J., Smolowitz, J., & Larson, E. (2013). Building framework for nursing scholarship: Guidelines for appointment and promotion. *Journal of Professional Nursing, 29,* 359–369. doi:10.1016/j.profnurs.2012.10.001

Lusk, P. (2014). Clinical scholarship: Let's share what we are doing in practice to improve outcomes. [Editorial]. *Journal of Child and Adolescent Psychiatric Nursing, 27,* 1–2.

Meleis, A. (1987). Re-visions in knowledge development: A passion for substance. *Scholarly Inquiry for Nursing Practice: An International Journal, 1*(1), 5–19.

Merriam-Webster Online Dictionary. (2011). Scholar [def.]. Retrieved from http://www.merriam-webster.com/scholar

Peterson, E. W., McMahon, E., Farkas, M., & Howland, J. (2005). Completing the cycle of scholarship of practice: A model for dissemination and utilization of evidence-based interventions. *Occupational Therapy in Health Care, 19*(1/2), 31–46. doi:10.1300/J003v19n01_04

Premji, S. S., Lalani, N., Ajani, K., Akhani, A., Moez, S., & Dias, J. M. (2011). Faculty practice in a private teaching institution in a developing country: Embracing the possibilities. *Journal of Advanced Nursing, 67*(4), 876–883. doi:10.1111/j.1365-2648.2010.05523.x

Riley, J. M., & Beal, J. A. (2013). Scholarly nursing practice from the perspectives of early-career nurses. *Nursing Outlook, 61*(2), E16–E24.

Riley, J., Beal, J. A., & Lancaster, D. (2008). Scholarly nursing practice from the perspectives of experienced nurses. *Journal of Advanced Nursing, 61*(4), 425–435.

Riley, J. M., Beal, J., Levi, P., & McCausland, M. P. (2002). Revisioning nursing scholarship. *Journal of Nursing Scholarship, 34,* 383–389.

Robert, R. R., & Pape, T.M. (2011). Scholarship in nursing: Not an isolated concept. *Medical Surgical Nursing, 20*(1), 41–44.

Silvia, P. J. (2007). *How to write a lot: A practical guide to productive academic writing.* Washington, DC: American Psychological Association.

Thomas, T. (2012). Overcoming barriers to scholarly activity in a clinical practice setting. *American Journal of Health-System Pharmacy, 69,* 465–467. doi:10.2146/ajhp110290

Wilkes, L., Mannix, J., & Jackson, D. (2013). Practicing nurses perspectives of clinical scholarship: A qualitative study. *BioMed Central Nursing, 12,* 21. doi:10.1186/1472-6955-12-21

Shirley E. Van Zandt

16

EMPLOYMENT STRATEGIES FOR THE APRN

The transition to a new advanced practice registered nurse (APRN) role includes looking for a new job. Some APRNs have a position waiting for them for which they have prepared by completing their educational program, but most APRNs are reentering the job market with a new identity. The job market is different for APRNs. Rather than working for large organizations, many APRNs are looking for positions in smaller and independently owned organizations. Some strategies that have worked in previous jobs searches may prove helpful, and others may not. The key element is to recognize that you will be changing your professional role from a registered nurse to an APRN. The evolution of your role can be exciting, challenging, and ultimately rewarding, but it can be also be time consuming, mentally demanding, and occasionally frustrating. This chapter addresses strategies that APRNs can use to find employment and to position themselves for successful career development.

IMPACT OF THE HEALTH CARE SYSTEM ON APRN EMPLOYMENT

Recent developments in the health care environment have resulted in APRNs becoming major players in the redesign of health care delivery systems. The Patient Protection and Affordable Care Act (ACA; U.S. Department of Health & Human Services [DHHS], 2010) has put renewed focus on the role of APRNs in meeting the health care needs of Americans. Initiatives focused on population-based health promotion will provide new employment opportunities for APRNs. In addition, programs to increase funding for education and loan repayment programs will encourage APRNs to practice in underserved areas. Exhibit 16.1 lists some of the programs that offer loan repayment.

The Institute of Medicine's (IOM, 2010) *The Future of Nursing: Leading Change, Advancing Health* highlighted the need for expansion of the role of

Exhibit 16.1 LOAN REPAYMENT PROGRAMS

- Indian Health Service
- U.S. Public Health Service Commissioned Corps
- National Health Service Corps
- Nurse Corps Loan Repayment Program

nurses in the health care system. Specifically related to APRNs, the report's first and third key messages addressed improving the health care system and the health of Americans by enabling APRNs to function to their full capacity.

> *Key Message #1:* Nurses should practice to the full extent of their education and training.
> *Key Message #3:* Nurses should be full partners, with physicians and other health professionals, in redesigning health care in the United States. (IOM, 2010)

These two recommendations place APRNs in an unprecedented position to become active participants in the redesign of health care and to seek and negotiate employment in settings that will utilize their skills effectively.

Having a basic understanding of the health care delivery system enables APRNs to anticipate career opportunities and match their career goals with the available jobs. Identifying the realities of the practice setting and the health care system is crucial in making the APRN marketable and attractive to employers. APRNs must be able to articulate these developments to prospective employers. APRNs may need to be able to articulate the effects of the ACA in their practice setting, and be aware of changes in billing and coding that could affect the practices they would like to work in.

Public acceptance of expanded roles of nurses continues to grow in part as a result of the recent changes in the proposed health care delivery systems. Predictions are positive that more APRN positions will be available (Auerbach, 2012; Hethcock, 2014). Exhibit 16.2 provides a list of the trends in the current health care environment.

UNDERSTANDING THE MARKETPLACE AND MARKETING THE APRN ROLE

APRN roles can be very different depending on the specialty (certified nurse-midwife, nurse practitioner, clinical nurse specialist, certified registered nurse anesthetist) and the type of organization and its mission. The APRN's marketing plan should be based on the market for the APRN specialty in the community where a position is being sought. The APRN specialty may be in high demand and the role well understood, or in low demand because the role is unknown or misunderstood, or in no demand in

Exhibit 16.2 CURRENT TRENDS IN THE HEALTH CARE ENVIRONMENT

- Efforts to control health care costs
- Consumer and payer demands for care that is safe, of high quality, accessible, equitable, effective, and individualized
- Increased competition among providers for market share
- Use of evidence-based systems to guide clinical interventions and analyze outcomes
- Reduction or increased accountability for use of acute care services
- Increasing focus on primary care
- Increased use of alternative, complementary, and nontraditional therapies
- Greater demand for chronic care services, especially for an aging population
- Development of service models to address increasing ethnic diversity
- Increased efforts to develop interdisciplinary team care models, rather than independent practice models
- Rapid growth of medical and pharmaceutical technology
- Expansion of electronic information systems for service delivery, outcomes analysis, and cost control
- Contraction of the overall job market, with increasing competition for desirable positions

an area that has never used an APRN with these skills. Sometimes APRNs are in high demand, but that demand is based on inaccurate expectations.

Success in a competitive marketplace is dependent on the ability of APRNs and employers to identify and match their needs with each other's skills. As in marketing to sell products or services, the process for an APRN involves identifying what a future employer wants or needs, offering a service to meet that need, and then communicating with the prospective employer how the APRN can meet the need. Marketing is about establishing a relationship between the APRN and the employer that demonstrates the competence, necessity, and value of APRN services in meeting the needs of the client (Dayhoff & Moore, 2004).

APRNs will have diverse prospective employers and will need to market themselves and the APRN role with diverse types of information. An APRN's current employer may want to grow or diversify services. Health care consumers or patients, the community, and other health care providers may be the customers for entrepreneurial or independent practice ventures. Whatever the target market, the characteristics of potential clients should be examined. Geographic, demographic, economic, and psychosocial characteristics should be researched. The objective of the APRN's marketing approach should be to focus on the potential employer and work with the employer to identify the needed and desired services (Dayhoff & Moore, 2004).

Identifying the APRN's product to the potential employer should include presenting one's education, certification, experience, and achievement. Highlighting unique attributes or skills that may distinguish the individual APRN from other APRNs or other disciplines may help the employer see the added value of the APRN. For example, identifying a special niche such as diabetes education, or a skill such as motivational interviewing, or expertise in treating mood disorders helps to define the added and unique benefit the APRN may have for the organization.

The APRN then needs to highlight what the product is worth to the organization. This may include additional services the employer can offer to patients, improved patient outcomes for the institution such as earlier discharge or prevention of readmissions, or development of other staff or providers by the APRN. The worth of the APRN must include salary and benefits that are based on the geographic and work setting standards or norms. Analyzing the competition (including other APRNs) and the current market through reviewing published salary surveys, websites of APRN professional associations, job ads, and personal, informal contacts are important. Direct questioning of the potential employer about the market and competition is an acceptable method for gathering additional information.

Researching the potential employer's work environment will help identify both what the APRN has to offer as a product and the worth or contribution the APRN can make to the organization. The environment includes both the relationships with professional peers and support staff and the physical space.

Is it important that APRNs are currently practicing in this environment? What are the characteristics of an environment that would make it conducive to APRN practice or present barriers to practice? Are the relationships collaborative? Are there productivity measures? Is there an assumed work ethic, which might suggest longer hours than stated or unpaid on-call work? Is physical workspace sufficient to promote the productivity and worth of the APRN in the organization?

Key APRN Marketing Tasks

Self-Inventory—Personal and Professional

Self-inventory and reflection are foundational components of professional career development and are part of an ongoing process throughout one's career. As Bolles (2014) states, "This [self-inventory] is a job-hunting method, and the most effective one, at that" (p. 111). Knowing oneself helps the APRN identify the product and worth she or he has to offer a potential employer. The self-inventory is an essential step and a guide for the job search and interview process. Exhibit 16.3 provides a list of questions for self-inventory.

Bolles (2014) provides multiple tools and exercises that may be useful for this self-inventory. Rath's (2012) popular book, *StrengthsFinders 2.0*, provides another tool for self-inventory that focuses on identifying one's strengths.

Exhibit 16.3 PERSONAL SELF-INVENTORY

Critical, reflective questions to ask may include:
What are my skills and abilities?
What do I enjoy doing?
What are my beliefs and values about work, my practice as an APRN, and my role in organizations where I work?
What are my needs?
Identify:
Abilities and skills: clinical, caregiving, communication, teaching, consultation, research, leadership, organization, computer proficiency, mentoring, writing, political action, achievements (and failures)
Interests: desirable professional activities, acquiring new skills, entrepreneurial activities
Values (principles or qualities that guide life and work): career, family, friends, work–life balance, spiritual, physical, emotional, social justice, organizational transparency, veracity (listing and prioritizing values can be helpful)
Needs: desired levels of control, power, salary, independence, security, recognition, creativity, achievement (consider satisfiers and dissatisfiers in prior work situations)
Characteristics: physical, emotional, intellectual (relevant to career and job performance) physical limitations, endurance, stress tolerance, enthusiasm, creativity, sensitivity, learning ability/style

---

Professional factors that will help the APRN be successful or prevent creation of barriers are important to identify. Exhibit 16.4 may provide some helpful questions to reflect on.

Ideal Job Description

Developing an ideal job description can be a helpful step in self-inventory. It is important to be specific about desired job functions and job benefits. Salary and benefit requirements including vacation and leave time should be included. The amount of time expected to be spent in various job functions should be considered, including time spent directly with patients (length of appointment time slots), communicating with other staff, returning phone calls, following up on laboratory results, providing case management services, and being on call for the practice.

Knowledge of Clinical and Professional Issues

Demonstration of clinical knowledge and competency is the cornerstone of the APRN's *product*. In addition to clinical knowledge and competency, APRNs must also possess knowledge about professional issues and the health care needs of the community. To successfully market the APRN role, APRNs must develop a working knowledge of the topics listed in Exhibit 16.5.

Exhibit 16.4 PROFESSIONAL SELF-INVENTORY

- What are my strengths as an APRN? What is special about me as an APRN?
- What are my weaknesses, and how am I working to improve them? What skills or knowledge do I need to develop further?
- What type of APRN job am I looking for?
- What do I enjoy most about working as an APRN? Least?
- Where do I want to live? What things are important about the place I live? How much am I willing to travel for work?
- What kinds of people do I like to work with? What kinds of people are difficult for me to work with?
- What things are stressful to me in my work? What do I need to manage stress?
- Am I comfortable working with a lot of autonomy? Would I prefer working closely with others? How much supervision is best for me?
- How many hours a day am I willing to work? How much call? How much weekend, evening, and night service? How many holidays?
- What is my ideal salary? What is an acceptable salary? Would I be willing to work for an hourly wage? Am I looking for productivity incentives in my pay?
- How important are the following benefits? How much of each do I prefer?
  - Paid vacation days
  - Paid sick days
  - Paid holidays
  - Retirement benefits (type, employer contribution, vesting)
  - Health insurance (individual and family coverage, portability, pre-existing condition coverage, pregnancy coverage, prescription coverage, optical and dental coverage, long-term care options)
  - Life insurance, short- and long-term disability insurance
  - Malpractice insurance (occurrence or claims made, gap or tail coverage requirements)
  - Licensing and certification fee reimbursement
  - Orientation period (duration and content)
  - Continuing education (travel, fees, meals, lodging)
  - Tuition reimbursement or waivers
  - Professional membership dues
  - Subscriptions to texts/journals
  - Office and supplies: private office, computer, e-mail/Internet access, medical supplies/equipment, personal digital assistant (PDA), cell phone, pager, parking
  - Mileage reimbursement
  - Interview and relocation expense reimbursement
  - Profit sharing
  - Academic freedom/intellectual property rights if I publish or patent my work
  - Employment contract

Exhibit 16.5 CLINICAL AND PROFESSIONAL ISSUES

- Standards for practice in clinical or specialty area
- Regulations affecting advanced practice, including licensure, certification, prescriptive privileges, institutional credentialing, and collaborative practice
- Reimbursement patterns and regulations
- Health care services provided and needed in the setting or community
- The presence of and services offered by competitors, either other APRNs or disciplines such as physicians, physician assistants, social workers
- Communication skills, including professional networking and negotiation skills
- The employer's perception and utilization of APRNs

The APRN may not have extensive knowledge about all these topics but should consider these as potential topics for an interview. Sources of information include professional APRN associations, publications, and government websites. A visit to state board of nursing website early in the employment process is a must because regulations affecting the scope and parameters of APRN practice vary widely from state to state. The Pearson Report, published annually, provides an up-to-date, state-by-state review of legislative issues and regulations affecting APRNs (Pearson, 2014). Professional organizations such as the American Association of Nurse Practitioners provides regular updates on regulatory changes in each state. (This information may be found at www.aanp.org/legislation-regulation/state-legislation-regulation.) Excellent information on issues, job opportunities, clinical guidelines, and regulations affecting the different APRN specialties is available online from the organizations listed in Exhibit 16.6.

Potential employers may not anticipate or believe all the benefits that the APRNs can offer. This may be a result of misinformation, personal bias, or previous experience with an APRN. Be aware, sensitive, and respectful of these perceptions. Often these perceptions will not be discussed with you or in some cases not be recognized by the potential employer. For example, APRNs with clinical doctorates may feel that they deserve higher compensation for services; however, the employer may not appreciate the additional skills associated with the higher academic degree. The APRN needs to be able to clearly articulate the value added and provide specific examples of how the additional knowledge and skill can benefit the organization.

Exhibit 16.6 APN PROFESSIONAL ORGANIZATIONS

National Association of Clinical Nurse Specialists	www.nacns.org
American College of Nurse Midwives	www.midwife.org
American Association of Nurse Anesthetists	www.aana.com
American Association of Nurse Practitioners	www.aanp.org

The APRN should be aware of the outcomes associated with advanced practice nursing care compared with other providers as reported in the literature. APRNs may be asked if they can function independently without supervision. They need to be clear about their comfort practicing independently, based on current experience and training. The systematic review of APRN outcomes (1990–2008) by Newhouse, Stanik-Hutt, White, and Johantgen (2011) can provide current research data. If the APRN role is not well defined, it is important to define this role and discuss the collaboration that may be required in this setting for the APRN to provide benefit to the organization (Shapiro & Rosenberg, 2002).

APRN Market Inventory

An inventory of the APRN target market is the next step. At this point, APRNs seek to determine what opportunities are available that may fit their "ideal" position. Analysis and inventory of the market ideally begins 6 to 12 months in advance of actual employment. The analysis continues throughout the interview process as the APRN evaluates the pros and cons of each potential employment setting. Many seasoned APRNs will continually inventory the employment market to identify career opportunities and trends. Exhibit 16.7 provides a sample APRN market inventory.

Exhibit 16.7 APRN MARKET INVENTORY

- What national standards will affect my practice?
  - Specialty certification requirements
  - Specialty certification process and time frame
- What state board of nursing regulations affect me?
  - Registered nurse licensure
  - APRN recognition/licensure
  - APRN scope of practice
  - Prescriptive authority regulations
  - Collaborative practice regulations
- What characteristics of this region are important to me?
  - Urban, small town, or rural nature
  - Population size, age distribution, ethnicity, and socioeconomic status
  - Educational system for me, my family, others
  - Cost of living
  - Health care organizations: type, size, focus
  - Transportation availability and accessibility
  - APRN practice in the area: roles/numbers of APRNs, practice settings, networks, typical salaries/benefits
- What characteristics of this organization will affect my practice?
  - Type of practice: acute/long-term/clinic, rural/urban, size, location, referral networks, satellite facilities, reimbursement mix
  - Organizational philosophy: indigent care, community outreach, educational partnerships, health promotion, research

---

(continued)

Exhibit 16.7 APRN MARKET INVENTORY *(continued)*

- Stability of the organization: age, financial, reputation
- Types of patients: age, gender, education, socioeconomic status, ethnicity, chronic/acute illness mix, diagnoses/conditions
- Medical providers (numbers/types/roles): physicians, registered and licensed practical nurses, physician assistants, therapists, medical assistants, social workers, psychologists, substance abuse counselors, specialists
- Support staff (numbers/types/roles): assistants, administrators, billing, medical records
  - Electronic medical record system
- Organizational policies/procedures: documentation, billing, quality improvement, performance appraisal
- Other APNs in the organization (numbers/types/roles)? Previous experience with APRNs? Good or bad? Seen as physician extenders or as collaborative colleagues?
- My role and responsibilities in the organization
  - Scope of clinical practice: typical patients, procedures, skill requirements
  - Level of autonomy, access to supervision, position in organizational structure
  - Collaborative practice policies, agreements, protocols
  - Employment contracts and stipulations to noncompete clauses
  - Credentialing requirements and procedures
  - Clinical productivity expectations: patient visits, call, weekend coverage, evening/night coverage, holiday coverage
  - Nonclinical responsibilities: administrative duties, committee work, education/precepting, research
  - Access to support services: billing, medical records, secretarial
  - Salary/benefit structure
  - Resource availability: office, computer, Internet/e-mail access, pager, cell phone, medical equipment, online clinical tools, journals/texts, parking
  - Performance appraisal frequency, criteria, evaluators
- Opportunities for growth: orientation, in-service training, continuing education

PRESENTING TO PROSPECTIVE EMPLOYER

Professional Portfolio

Once the self-inventory and a description of the ideal job are complete, the APRN is ready to develop a portfolio. The professional portfolio should contain evidence of professional knowledge, development, and achievement (Smith & McDonald, 2013a). Files such as a résumé or curriculum vitae (CV), published articles, presentations, and awards provide the APRN with a useful marketing tool (Billings & Kowalski, 2008; Hawks, 2012). Often the development of a portfolio (such doctorate of nursing program [DNP] capstone or final project) begins during the graduate educational program.

Electronic portfolios are the most efficient method for creating a record of the APRN's career. Typhon Group Health Solutions (www.typhongroup.com) and Digication (www.digication.com/highered) are two e-portfolios that APRNs may have had experience with as students. If the APRN's program did not require one to be developed, this period of job hunting is the perfect time to create a portfolio.

The APRN's e-portfolio should serve as the master file documenting career achievement. Generally, unless requested ahead of the meeting, the APRN should not bring a portfolio to the first interview. Several hard copies of the résumé and a copy of the cover letter should be brought, but follow-up interviews or contact are appropriate times to consider bringing examples of previous work. Developing the electronic portfolio is an important investment of time that provides a permanent record of the APRN's evolving career (Smith & McDonald, 2013b). Exhibit 16.8 lists items that APRNs may want to include in a professional portfolio.

One important element of the portfolio is the list of references. References should be individuals who can attest to the APRN's professional abilities, competence, and achievements. The APRN must contact each individual reference to determine the reference's willingness to provide a recommendation. Most employers will ask for three recommenders, so it is useful to have a pool of five to six so that the APRN can avoid overusing one, or be able to tailor the list to the organization. The list of references should include name, professional title, and complete contact information (address, phone, and e-mail).

Exhibit 16.8 APRN PROFESSIONAL PORTFOLIO

- Current résumé and/or curriculum vitae
- Official transcripts of all academic programs after high school
- Copies of nursing licenses and certifications
- Current list of references with addresses, phone numbers, and e-mail addresses
- Malpractice insurance policies
- Records of continuing education attendance
- Reprints of publications
- Abstracts or brochures documenting conference presentations
- Newspaper or media recognition
- Evidence of honors or awards
- Prior references, recommendations, and performance evaluations
- A sample job description listing desirable job functions and benefits
- Examples of clinical and leadership achievements such as patient education programs/tools, history and physical examinations, quality improvement projects, and research utilization projects
- Professional organization memberships
- Health records pertinent to APN employment (PPD, hepatitis B vaccine, tetanus, diphtheria and pertussis [Tdap], influenza)
- Volunteer and community activities

Advise the references that recommendations written specifically about the APRN to the hiring person in the organization are the best, rather than a generic letter. The APRN can "coach" the individual who is providing the reference by providing information about the potential employer and reasons for seeking employment with the organization.

Some potential employers may not be fully aware of the skills of an APRN; therefore, it is helpful to maintain a file documenting research, policy, and other documents describing and validating the APRN role. This information may also be useful when approaching legislators, insurance organizations, or other stakeholders.

Résumés, Curricula Vitae, and Cover Letters

Résumés and CVs are powerful tools for marketing the APRN. CVs are used to communicate professional credentials to prospective employers, current employers, and colleagues. CVs are more lengthy descriptions of professional career and qualifications. They are often called academic résumés because of their use in academic settings.

Résumés are one- or two-page overviews of an individual's professional career. They should be employer-focused, rather than reflecting the APRN's goals and hopes (Welton, 2013). An employer-focused résumé is directed to the employer needs. The résumé can be written in a format that focuses on function or on chronology or a combination of both. Functional résumés highlight areas of skill and expertise. Chronological résumés present the job history in chronological order. Exhibit 16.9 shows a typical chronological résumé for an APRN. Welton (2013) provides additional excellent ideas for preparing a résumé.

Critical information for any résumé or CV includes name, address, phone and fax numbers, e-mail addresses, education and degrees earned, professional employment, licensure, and certification. Additional information about specific clinical and electronic skills, languages spoken, publications, honors and awards, research and grants, presentations, teaching experience, consulting experience, membership in professional organizations, community service, or military service may be included. Some things should not appear on the résumé or CV, including social security numbers, names of references, salary expectations, and personal information such as age, gender, ethnic background, height, weight, marital status, or health status and disabilities.

Most academic institutions have career services and websites available to assist with résumé and CV composition and development. These documents should be kept up to date in an electronic and/or paper format. The physical appearance of these documents is extremely important. They are often the first impression a potential employer has of an APRN. Résumés should be free of spelling and punctuation errors, concise, well organized, and visually appealing. High-quality paper should be used in printing. White or off-white paper with black print is most commonly used to give a traditional, professional appearance to the résumé or CV. Finally, having colleagues review and proofread these documents is helpful.

Exhibit 16.9 APRN RÉSUMÉ—CHRONOLOGICAL

Marissa R. Butcher, MSN, CRNP, 4412 West Lake St., St. Paul, MN 55105, (615) 222-2222, butcher1234@online.com

Objective	Adult–Gerontologic Nurse Practitioner in a primary care practice
Education	2014 Master of Science in Nursing, University of Minnesota, Minneapolis, MN 2003 Bachelor of Science in Nursing, University of Michigan, Ann Arbor, MI 1998 Bachelor of Arts, English, University of Wisconsin, Madison, WI
Experience	2012–2014 Precepted clinical rotations: University of Michigan Family Practice: 180 clinical hours, acute and chronic primary care CVS Minute Clinic, Minneapolis, MN: 165 clinical hours, episodic care Westbrook Community Health Center, Minneapolis, MN: 220 clinical hours, acute and chronic primary care, including gynecologic care 2012–present, Clinical Coordinator, Eastbrook Long-Term Care Center, Roseville, MN 2008–2012 Nurse Manager—Coronary Care Unit Midwest Regional Medical Center, Ann Arbor, MI 2003–2007 Staff Nurse—Coronary Care Unit Midwest Regional Medical Center, Ann Arbor, MI
Licensure certification	Registered Nurse: Minnesota—active; Michigan—inactive Advanced Practice Nurse/AGNP: Minnesota—active Certification: AGNP–ANCC—expires 2020
Honors/Awards	2013 Gerontology Scholarship, University of Minnesota, Minneapolis, MN 2003 Sigma Theta Tau
Publications	Butcher, M. (2011). Assessing cardiac function in older adults. *Long-Term Care Nursing, 12*, 221–223.
Professional organizations	American Nurses Association, Minnesota Gerontology Association
Languages	Fluent in Spanish and French
References	Available on request

A cover letter should always accompany a résumé or CV. The cover letter introduces the APRN to the prospective employer and should be individualized to the position of interest. The cover letter is direct, brief (one-half to one page) and written in standard business format. Whenever possible, address the cover letter to a specific person. Be sure that the spelling and title of this person is correct. The letter should include the reason for writing and briefly explain why the APRN is a good fit for this organization. Exhibit 16.10 is a sample cover letter to accompany an APRN résumé or CV. It is important to follow up by telephone or mail on all résumés and CVs that have been sent. Follow-up indicates enthusiasm and persistence,

---

Exhibit 16.10 SAMPLE APRN COVER LETTER

Marissa R. Butcher, MSN, CRNP
4412 West Lake St.
St. Paul, MN 55105

September 1, 2015

Jillian D. Rodriguez, PhD, RN
Director, Clinical Services
Gerontology Nurse Associates
3640 Simpson Street
Minneapolis, MN 55455

Dear Dr. Rodriguez:
We spoke briefly at the Minnesota Long-Term Care Conference about a position for a nurse practitioner at Gerontology Nurse Associates. I am interested in applying for this position.

I understand that Gerontology Nurse Associates is one of the leading providers of primary care to older adults in Minneapolis and has been using many nurse practitioners. I have recently completed my master's degree and received certification as an adult–gerontologic nurse practitioner and feel well prepared to provide primary care to your patients. My prior clinical and leadership experiences in long-term care and cardiovascular nursing provide me with excellent skills and knowledge, which I believe will be beneficial in my role as a nurse practitioner. In addition, my fluency in Spanish could be an asset to the patients you serve at Gerontology Nurse Associates.

I have enclosed a copy of my résumé for your review. I can be reached at (615) 222-2222 or at butcher1234@online.com. Thank you for your consideration. I look forward to speaking with you.

Sincerely,
Marissa R. Butcher, MSN, CRNP
Enclosure

---

two attractive qualities in potential employees. This communication should occur within 2 weeks of sending the cover letter and résumé.

Cover letters and résumés or CVs have always been recommended to be sent by postal mail, but recently employers are requesting and receiving them by e-mail or online applications. Rather than assuming that a hard copy sent by postal mail is the best, call the potential employer and ask for their preference. Many organizations will accept only electronic versions and may not review hard copies efficiently. The electronic version allows the employer to quickly circulate the APRN's letter to many people in the organization who have an interest in employing the right person.

Locating Job Opportunities

For most APRNs, career opportunities result from networking. Finding opportunities requires persistence, openness, and assertiveness. Most positions are found through personal contacts or networks. Networks are built on relationships between colleagues, friends, and alumni. Every person the APRN knows or knows of should be considered a potential source of a contact that can lead to an opportunity. Professional organizations, other APRNs already working in the same role, nurse managers, and faculty are excellent sources of contacts. Telephone calls and personal meetings are both effective means of making contact. Making contacts solely electronically or mass mailings of résumés are generally not advisable and have a low yield (Bolles, 2014).

Traditional job search strategies should not be ignored. Weekly review of professional organization websites, newspapers, professional journals, and other website employment listings is important. For APRNs planning to use a professional job search firm, it is advisable to thoroughly research the track record of the firm and its experience and success in placing APRNs and whether any additional costs are involved.

Interviewing

Many books have been written about job interviewing; however, successful interviewing is not difficult. Essentially, the interview is an opportunity for the applicant and the prospective employer to meet, exchange information, and evaluate whether there is a "fit" between the organization and the candidate. Both parties are trying to determine whether they have something to offer each other by exchanging very subjective information and cues.

In a competitive environment, APRNs should expect to complete several interviews before locating an acceptable position. Typically, employers will conduct a series of interviews. Applicants are screened in initial interviews; then follow-up interviews are scheduled for applicants who progress beyond the screening. Patience is important. The interview process may take many weeks to complete.

Interviewing requires homework. As previously discussed, APRNs should be informed about characteristics of organizations they are interested in. Create a list of questions that you need to have answered or will discuss with a potential employer during an interview. Buppert (2014) has created a list of 20 questions that cover the crucial topics. Consider reviewing these before the interview as a way to be sure you are aware of important questions that should be asked, and to prepare responses and counter questions that may arise. Anticipating questions and responses is a way of reducing the anxiety of interviewing. Questions for APRNs to ask during an interview are easily generated from the ideal job description. Exhibit 16.11 is a list of questions typically asked of APRNs during the interview process.

Federal law prohibits asking certain questions during the interview. It is unlawful for an interviewer to ask about age, date of birth, children, age of children, race or ethnicity, religious affiliation, marital status, military discharge status, arrest records, home ownership, spousal employment, and organization and club memberships. When such questions are asked, it is usually not out of malicious intent. However, it is best to prepare a gracious way of not answering these questions.

Physical preparation for the interview is also important; first impressions count. Dress neatly and conservatively, arrive for the interview on time, and bring a folder that can be left with the interviewers that includes a hard copy of the cover letter and résumé that were sent before the interview. Psychological preparation is essential. Although nervousness during an interview is typical, the ability to project self-confidence is important. For APRNs unfamiliar with interviewing, Bolles (2014) offers detailed strategies for coping with interview anxiety.

During the interview process, maintain a positive attitude, interest, and enthusiasm. Be friendly, smile, and make eye contact. Listen as well as speak. Be professional in all interactions, focusing on the position, qualifications, and experience. Thank the interviewer for the opportunity and ask when the hiring decision will be made. Finally, follow up with a written letter expressing thanks and continued interest in the position.

Negotiation

During the interviewing process, it is expected that the APRN and the potential employer may have different perspectives about the job, roles

---

Exhibit 16.11 INTERVIEW QUESTIONS

- What type of position are you interested in?
- Could you tell me about yourself?
- What are your strengths? Your weaknesses?
- What do you know about our company?
- What would you do in this situation (typical situation described)?
- Why are you leaving your present job?
- What are your professional or career goals?
- What do you enjoy most about work? Least? Why?
- Why should we hire you for this position?
- What salary do you expect?
- What questions do you have about this position? This company?

and responsibilities, salary, and benefits. Negotiation is the process by which these differences are resolved. The lack of negotiation suggests that someone is losing out. Either the APRN is not fully communicating his or her needs or goals, or the employer has limited flexibility. Once negotiations have occurred and there has been give and take, both parties should be able to agree comfortably on an arrangement. It is acceptable to negotiate on several occasions, and generally is better to agree to a final arrangement after some period of review and consideration, which could be a few hours or a few days. Negotiation should be part of the process once there is acknowledgment that the APRN is interested in the position and the employer is interested in hiring the APRN (Berlin & Lexa, 2007).

In today's health care marketplace, the APRN should negotiate the employment agreement. Buppert's *Negotiating Employment* (2008) is an extremely helpful tool. It provides several scenarios of negotiation that the APRN may encounter and provides specific tables for estimating the APRN's worth to a practice or employer, which can guide the APRN's expectation for a salary offer. Specifically, it provides a list of sources of income and expenses associated with the addition of an APRN to the practice. By completing this process, an estimate of the worth of APRN services can be identified. Buppert's book also discusses employment contracts, including appropriate language that should be included and clauses that should be avoided.

The APRN needs to be clear in negotiations with a prospective employer about several key points. APRNs should know whether the position will classify them as an independent contractor or employee, whether their services will be billed under their name or "incident-to" a physician provider, whether they will be marketed, and how productivity will be evaluated.

Employment Contracts

Employment contracts have become the standard. In the past, APRNs were often hired based on an informal verbal contract and handshake. Employment agreements are legally binding contracts between employers and employees, which state the terms of a working relationship. The employment contract provides for job security in that it limits and specifies the reasons for termination. In addition, the contract provides a vehicle to describe salary, benefits, liability insurance coverage, productivity expectations, job functions, and hours of work. It helps to solidify the negotiation and verbal agreements made by each party. Before signing an employment contract, the APRN should carefully review the contract, negotiate areas of confusion, and consider having an attorney review the agreement (Blustein, Ancona, & Cohen, 2014; Buppert, 2008).

Employees hired without a contract are termed "at will." These agreements are not recommended because at-will employees may be terminated at any time without cause (Buppert, 2008). Most state laws provide some protection for employees who face termination without contract protection, but accessing this protection may be a lengthy process requiring legal action.

Noncompete and Termination Clauses

When negotiating an employment contract, APRNs should look for restrictive covenants or noncompete and termination clauses in the contract. A covenant not to compete is a clause in the contract that restricts an employee from practicing within a certain number of miles from an employer's business for a certain period of time after the employee leaves the position. Covenants not to compete are legal and enforceable. They protect the employer from competition in the event the APRN leaves the employer. The covenants not to compete restrict the ability of APRNs to continue to practice in a geographical area and prevent practitioners from taking their patients or clients with them when they leave a practice. APRNs should avoid a contract that includes a covenant not to compete (Buppert, 2008; McMullen, 2010; Roberts, 2010). Exhibit 16.12 contains an example of noncompete covenant.

Most employment contracts contain a termination clause that describes events that are the basis for termination of the employee "with cause." These events may include loss of license or certification, gross negligence, death, or conviction of a felony. Some employers will attempt to include a termination "without cause" clause. This states that the employee may be terminated at any time, for any reason, with 30 days' notice, for example. (This is not the same as a probationary 60- or 90-day period.) A without cause termination clause changes the contract significantly because it negates the intent of the agreement designed to assure both the employee

---

Exhibit 16.12 CONTRACT AGREEMENTS AND CLAUSES

Covenants Not to Compete
Restrictive: "Upon termination of employment for any reason, the CRNA agrees not to practice within 50 miles of any present or future office of this practice for a period of 5 years."
Less restrictive: "Upon termination of employment for any reason, the CRNA agrees not to practice within 25 miles of the current office of this practice for a period of 1 year."
Termination Clauses
Termination for cause: "The employer may terminate this agreement at any time by written notice to the CRNA for any of the following reasons:
a. The CRNA dies or becomes permanently disabled.
b. The CRNA loses his or her professional license.
c. The CRNA is restricted by any governmental authority from rendering the required professional services.
d. The CRNA loses his or her staff privileges.
e. The CRNA conducts himself or herself in a "grossly negligent way."
Termination without cause: "The employer may terminate this agreement at any time, for any reason, after giving the CRNA 30 days' written notice."

and employer of a continuous relationship for a specific period of time, usually a year. Generally, APRNs should not sign a contract containing a without cause termination clause because it effectively removes the employee job security that the contract provides (Buppert, 2008; Roberts, 2010). Exhibit 16.12 contains examples of with cause and without cause termination clauses.

Other types of clauses may be included. An evergreen clause is one that results in automatic annual renewal of the contract unless a request is made to change it. Another type of clause allows the employer to change the contract without notice or without consent of the APRN. An assignment clause allows an employer to sell the practice and reassign the APRN's contract to a new owner without agreement (Roberts, 2010). Asking for removal or amending one or several portions of a contract is acceptable and expected during negotiations. Accepting a boilerplate contract that the employer states is required by their attorney or administrators and cannot be amended or changed should signal to the APRN that genuine negotiation has not occurred.

Most employment contracts include discussion about liability insurance coverage. This is a critical contract issue for all APRNs. Contracts often specify the amount and type of liability insurance coverage. There are two types of liability insurance coverage: *occurrence* and *claims-made*. Occurrence insurance covers an incident that occurred during the period of coverage, regardless of when the claim is made. The claim could be made several years after the APRN left the organization; however, the APRN would be covered under this type of policy because the APRN was covered at the time of the incident. Claims-made insurance covers only claims made during the year of coverage, unrelated to when the incident occurred (Blaustein et al., 2014). Liability gap insurance may be needed when the APRN leaves an organization that provided claims-made coverage. Coverage limits (amounts) are usually specified by amount per claim and annual aggregate amount. Typical contract language would be "$1,000,000 occurrence/$3,000,000 aggregate." This means the insurance would cover $1,000,000 per claim and up to three claims a year of $1,000,000. Coverage amounts vary, but per-claim coverage should be at least $1,000,000. Although some APRNs will purchase their own coverage in addition to that provided by an employer, it may be useful to seek legal advice about the need for individual liability insurance.

Collaborative Practice Agreements

Some states require the APN to maintain a written practice agreement with a medical doctor (Pearson, 2014). Many states have removed this requirement from their state nurse practice act, but employers may not be fully aware of this change. In addition, some employers want to maintain this practice and require that the APRN have a formal written agreement with a physician. This can be a point of negotiation, but it is important for the APRN who is not legally bound by state regulations to be aware that this is a request of the potential employer, not a legal requirement. The APRN may find that this is acceptable or too restrictive. Other terms used for this agreement include *collaborative practice agreements, protocols,* and *standing orders.* The purpose of the practice agreement is to specify guidelines for provision of APRN care, including prescriptive authority. The agreement should be a positive mechanism to enhance interdisciplinary collaboration and integrate the delivery of health care.

Before establishing any practice agreement, APRNs must first review the state board of nursing requirements. These can be found online in most states. Some states allow APRNs to practice independently without physician collaboration. Others require on-site physician supervision for APRN practice. Most states encourage some degree of collaboration and/ or supervision. The APRN should enter the interviewing process aware of the state requirements.

Practice agreements can be controversial. Too much specificity in the agreement will limit the APRN's ability to individualize care and will also leave the APRN open to legal claims if the specifics are not followed precisely. Developing extensive protocols to address the details of every clinical situation is not desirable. Minimal and flexible guidelines that recognize APRN competence are preferred to those with extreme detail. The practice agreement should not prevent APRNs from delivering care that is within their scope of practice, education, and competence. In addition, the practice agreement should not require a level of supervision that limits effective clinical practice or reimbursement. Not having a practice agreement should also not negate or discourage collaboration with physicians and other health care team colleagues. If there is a written agreement, it should be reviewed and signed by the APRN and collaborating physician(s). States that require a written agreement generally provide a template, which the APRN uses to apply.

SUMMARY

Changes in the health care marketplace are generating new and increased opportunities for APRNs who demonstrate competence, enthusiasm, and commitment to the role. Marketing strategies enable APRNs to take full and timely advantage of these opportunities. Self-inventory, market inventory, and negotiation can be used to secure an APRN position and build a successful and rewarding career.

Acknowledgment

The author acknowledges the contributions of Jennifer Peters to this chapter in the previous edition.

REFERENCES

Auerbach, D. I. (2012). Will the NP workforce grow in the future? New forecasts and implications for healthcare delivery. *Medical Care, 50*(7), 606–610.

Berlin, J. W., & Lexa, F. L. (2007). Negotiation techniques for health care professionals. *Journal of the American College Radiology, 4,* 487–491.

Billings, D. M., & Kowalski, K. (2008). Developing your career as a nurse educator: The professional portfolio. *Journal of Continuing Education in Nursing, 39*(12), 532–533.

Blaustein, A. E., Ancona, L. J., & Cohen, Z. (2014). Understanding your physician contract. *Journal of the American College of Radiology, 11*(2), 112–113.

Bolles, R. N. (2014). *What color is your parachute? 2014: A practical guide for job hunters and career changes.* Berkeley, CA: Ten Speed Press.

Buppert, C. (2008). *Negotiating employment* (2nd ed.). Annapolis, MD: Law Office of Carolyn Buppert.

Buppert, C. (2014). 20 questions to ask a prospective employer. *Journal for Nurse Practitioners, 10*(1), 62–63.

Dayhoff, N. E., &, Moore, P. S. (2004). CNS entrepreneurship: Marketing 101. *Clinical Nurse Specialist: The Journal for Advanced Nursing Practice, 18,* 123–125.

Hawks, S. J. (2012). The use of electronic portfolios in nurse anesthesia education and practice. *American Association of Nurse Anesthetists Journal, 80*(2), 89–93.

Hethcock, B. (2014, July 10). Nurse practitioner, physician assistant demand soars. *Dallas Business Journal.* Retrieved from http://www.bizjournals. com/dallas/blog/2014/07/nurse-practitioner-physician-assistant-demand. html?page=all

Institute of Medicine (IOM). (2010). *The future of nursing: Leading change, advancing health.* Retrieved from http://books.nap.edu/openbook.php? record_id=12956&page=R1

McMullen, P. C. (2010). Non-compete covenants in NP employment agreements. *Journal for Nurse Practitioners, 6*(9): 685–690. doi:10.1016/j.nurpra.2010.07.021

Newhouse, R. P., Stanik-Hutt, J., White, K. M., & Johantgen, M. (2011). Advanced practice nurse outcomes 1990–2008: A systematic review. *Nursing Economics, 29*(5), 230–250. Retrieved from http://search.proquest.com/docview/89841 9565?accountid=11752

Pearson, L. (2014). *2014 Pearson report.* Burlington, MA: Jones & Bartlett Learning.

Rath, T. (2007). *StrengthsFinders 2.0.* New York, NY: Gallup Press.

Roberts, M. J. (2010). Plain talk about employment contracts. *The Nurse Practitioner: The American Journal of Primary Health Care, 35*(10), 12–13.

Shapiro, D., & Rosenberg, N. (2002). Acute care nurse practitioner: Collaborative practice negotiation. *AACN Clinical Issues. Advanced Practice in Acute Critical Care, 13,* 470–478.

Smith, C. M., & McDonald, K. (2013a). Transition to an electronic professional nurse portfolio: Part I. *Journal of Continuing Education in Nursing, 44*(7), 291–292.

Smith, C. M., & McDonald, K. (2013b). Transition to an electronic professional nurse portfolio: Part II. *Journal of Continuing Education in Nursing, 44*(8), 340–341.

U.S. Department of Health and Human Services. (2010). *The Affordable Care Act, section by section: Title V. Heath care workforce.* Retrieved from http://www. hhs.gov/healthcare/rights/law/index.html

Welton, R. H. (2013). Writing an employer-focused résumé for advanced practice nurses. *AACN Advanced Critical Care, 24*(2), 203–217.

Carole G. Traylor **17**

INAUGURATING YOUR ADVANCED PRACTICE CAREER

Where your talents and needs of the world cross, there lies your vocation.

—Aristotle

There is much to be done to launch a new advanced practice career. This is not just changing jobs; it is accepting the charge to change nursing practice in a new and exciting way. It is a chance to influence the lives of patients, families, and communities by rendering exceptional care while treating, teaching, and instilling health ideals in very tangible ways. This chapter is designed to give the reader the opportunity to envision the future and embark on a path that leads to this new future. No transition is easy. Understanding the stages and emotional adjustment that comes with each step of the process provides insight into what to expect along the journey of role transition.

The process of becoming an advanced practice registered nurse (APRN) begins during the educational experience and continues as one begins one's first job as an APRN. As the student moves through the educational requirements and clinical experiences, a sense of the new role begins to emerge. Certain components of transition must be experienced in order to successfully make the transition. In William Bridges's book on managing transitions (1991), he reiterates, "a transition is not a trip from one side of the street to the other but rather a journey" (p. 37). There are three distinct components that are fundamentally necessary to make the journey a success. To begin anew, one must let go of the old. As one leaves the role of the registered nurse to become an APRN, letting go often evokes feelings similar to those experienced during grieving. Leaving previous professional colleagues and a familiar work environment often produces feelings of sadness. The fear of the unknown in a new role may instill a sense of anxiety about the role. Feeling insecure in the role may be reflected in a wide variety of feelings including anger. The disorientation of transition may evoke a sense of loss. Having a supportive mentor can help the new APRN validate these feelings as normal and encourage him or her to move forward in the transition process.

After letting go of the old, one moves into a neutral zone, which is an emotional space with nothing to hold onto (Bridges, 1991). It is a time to see oneself with new eyes and begin to experience the new role and how the new role fits within the organization. As one achieves the transition, establishing learning opportunities to increase knowledge and skill will help the new APRN become successful in this new role. The neutral zone challenges the APRN to take time away from the chaos of change in the health care environment to reflect on the transition in order to gain strength in the new role and develop competency in it.

Brown and Olshansky (1997) discussed a similar process in going from "limbo to legitimacy" (p.46). Their work establishes four categories of transition. The first is a state of laying the foundation. This is the time when the APRN has finished school and has not yet completed the necessary steps to secure employment. This stage includes recovering from school and pursuing certification and licensing. The new graduate needs an opportunity to review the results of a self-inventory, as discussed in Chapter 16, and to develop a clearer vision of where his or her interests lie and what employment parameters meet his or her needs. Only then should the APRN begin a job search. Brown and Olshansky's work described launching as stage 2, which is at the beginning of the first position and continues for a minimum of 3 months (Brown & Olshansky, 1998). The underpinning of this stage is the early transition from expert RN to the novice APRN in a clinical setting. It is hard work.

Over time the transition process moves into stage 3, meeting the challenge (Brown & Olshansky, 1998), which is a time when the APRN's expectations become more realistic and helps the individual gain more skill and confidence. Internal support systems help the new APRN deal with the daily challenges of the current health care system. Stage 4, the final stage, is the broadening of the perspective of the APRN (Brown & Olshansky, 1998). It is in this stage that greater self-esteem is realized and a secure feeling of legitimacy begins.

In addition to the emotional transition, the APRN also experiences a concern about the lack of knowledge and skill. Although prepared academically, the myriad of patient presentations and required proficiency can be daunting for the new graduate. Becoming an expert occurs only over time as greater skill, knowledge, and experience are gained. Patricia Benner, in her book *Novice to Expert* (1984), describes the attributes of levels of proficiency in nursing. She uses the Dreyfus model to explore the levels of proficiency (Benner, 1984, 2004). These levels are novice, advanced beginner, competent, proficient, and expert. A novice with limited experience requires rules and guidelines to govern practice. A feeling of mastery does not occur until the competent level, which is still without speed and flexibility in practice (Benner, 2004). At the proficient level, the individual perceives the situation as a whole instead of separate equal parts, which is the viewpoint seen in previous levels. The expert demonstrates a deep understanding of the whole situation that is now intuitive (Brenner, 2004). Gaining skills and perspective allows the new APRN to move through the levels of proficiency. Transition in gaining proficiency begins with the movement from abstract principles to the use of concrete experiences in critical thinking. In addition, a change in perception now occurs when experiencing new clinical situations. This creates an action of becoming the involved performer from a previous position as the observer (Benner, 1984).

Based on the APRNs' previous nursing experiences and clinical learning situations during advanced education, graduates move through these stages at different rates. Although the progression is incremental, it may not necessarily be linear or step wise, nor may all individuals attain an expert level of skill (Porponsky, 2013).

In a qualitative study of role transition, the authors identified an overarching theme of the essence of nursing as a critical foundation for achieving this transition (Spoelstra & Robbins, 2010). Their work further addressed subthemes that reflected the importance of building a framework for nursing practice. Their findings suggested that the role of the APRN was to provide patient care based on empirical evidence through collaboration and consultation with both nursing colleagues and other health care professionals. The importance of direct patient care was another theme emerging from their study. Attributes that demonstrate this theme in practice included seeing the patient from a holistic view while demonstrating expert clinical thinking and skillful performance. Developing patient partnerships allowed the APRN to provide creative approaches for health and illness management. The final subtheme identified was the importance of exemplifying professional practice responsibilities. The manifestation of this theme was reflected in improved patient outcomes by the use of evidence-based practice, role modeling, effective communication, and collaboration in multidisciplinary teams. The findings in this qualitative study exemplify the core competencies and expectations of the APRN as set forth by national professional nursing organizations and accrediting bodies for advance practice education programs.

To successfully transition into this new nursing role, one must spend time in self-reflection to determine what current attributes support this new role. APRNs report that patient relationships are embedded in their overall job satisfaction (Szanton, Mihaly, Alhusen, & Becker, 2010). This is a time to reflect on previous nursing experiences and gain insight into what types of patient relationships have been the most meaningful. It is also a time to imagine a new role. Having a grasp of one's strengths and weaknesses is part of this, but self-reflection is more important. In her book *Reinventing You* (2013), Dorrie Clark recommends discerning what type of image one projects as a key component in carving out a new role and direction. There are many different ways to go about investigating your image. One quick way to see "what is out there" is to Google yourself. Search additional links such as Bing, LinkedIn, and so on, which may also have information about you. Meeting with colleagues to get honest feedback about your image is also helpful. Clark also suggests having colleagues and friends describe you in three words. Becoming more cognizant of who you are and the image you project allows you to identify areas that need attention to achieve the professional APRN image you wish to attain.

Just as competence, confidence, and judgment were frequent questions at the onset of the nurse practitioner movement, they remain critical elements to the successful implementation of the APRN role for the present and future (Houser & Player, 2004). Remaining active in professional nursing organizations keeps new graduates informed of changes in the nursing arena as they begin to develop their new role. Opportunities for participation and leadership roles within organizations can help the APRN carve out a unique place in nursing practice. National meetings and workshops provide wide ranges of networking with APRNs with immeasurable experience and who are committed to the goals of advance practice nursing. Staying connected with nursing colleagues gives the new graduate an opportunity to investigate solutions for identified problems in this new role. APRNs can become integral members of the health care team by participating in the the development of quality tools, as well as monitoring and analyzing patient outcomes (Stanley, 2011).

The advanced practice movement has been paved by revolutionaries and reactionaries demonstrating the values and goals of professional nursing (Joel, 2009). Colleagues before you and those who will follow strengthen the APRN role and nursing's critical position in today's health care arena. It is now time to actualize your vision and contribute to the knowledge and action as an advanced practice nurse.

The people who get on in this world are the people who get up and look for circumstances they want, and if they can't find them, make them!

—George Bernard Shaw

Acknowledgment

The author acknowledges the contributions of Michaelene Jansen and Mary Zwygart-Staffaucher to this chapter in the previous edition.

REFERENCES

Benner, P. (1984). *From novice to expert*. Reading, MA: Addison-Wesley.

Benner, P. (2004). Using the Dreyfus model of skill acquisition to describe and interpret skill acquisition and clinical judgment in nursing practice and education. *Bulletin of Science, Technology and Society, 24*, 188–199, doi:10.1177/0270467604265061

Bridges, W. (1991). *Managing transitions: Making the most of change*. Reading MA: Addison-Wesley.

Brown, M., & Olshansky, E. (1998). Becoming a primary care nurse practitioner: Challenges of the initial year of practice. *Nurse Practitioner, 23*(7), 46.

Clark, D. (2013). *Reinventing you*. Boston, MA: Harvard Business Review Press.

Houser, B., & Player, K. (2004). *Pivotal moments in nursing*. Indianapolis, IN: Sigma Theta Tau.

Joel, L. (2009). *Advanced practice nursing: Essentials for role development.* Philadelphia, PA: F.A. Davis.

Porponsky, C. (2013). Exploring the transition from registered nurse to family nurse practitioner. *Journal of Professional Nursing, 29*(6), 350–358.

Spoelstra, S., & Robbins, L. (2010) A qualitative study of role transition from RN to APN. *International Journal of Nursing Education Scholarship, 7,* 1–14. Retrieved from http://www.bepress.com/ijnes/vol17/art20, doi: 10.2202/1548-923X.2020

Stanley, J. (2011). *Advance practice nursing: Emphasizing common roles.* Philadelphia, PA: F.A. Davis.

Szanton, S., Mihaly, L., Alhusen, J., & Becker, K. (2010). Taking charge of the challenge: Factors to consider in taking your first nurse practitioner job. *Journal of the American Academy of Nurse Practitioners, 22,* 356–360.

INDEX